Friendships and Community Connections between People with and without Developmental Disabilities

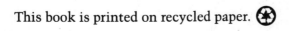

Friendships and Community Connections between People with and without Developmental Disabilities

edited by

Angela Novak Amado, Ph.D.
Human Services Research and Development Center
St. Paul, Minnesota

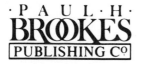

·P·A·U·L·H·
BROOKES
PUBLISHING CO.

Baltimore • London • Toronto • Sydney

Paul H. Brookes Publishing Co.
P.O. Box 10624
Baltimore, Maryland 21285-0624

Typeset by Brushwood Graphics, Inc., Baltimore, Maryland.
Manufactured in the United States of America by
The Maple Press Co., York, Pennsylvania.

Page 9: *The Poems of Emily Dickinson*, Thomas H. Johnson,
ed., Cambridge, MA: The Belknap Press of Harvard University Press, Copyright © 1951, 1955, 1979, 1983 by the President and Fellows of Harvard College, is reprinted by permission of the publishers and the Trustees of Amherst College.

Permission to reprint the following is gratefully acknowledged:

Page 17: "Dick and Jane" by Robert Williams (1989). *In a struggling voice:
The selected poems of Robert Williams*. Washington, DC: Author.
Page 36: "Gallant and Gaunt Their Beauty" by Robert Williams (1989). *In a
struggling voice: The selected poems of Robert Williams*. Washington,
DC: Author.
Page 343: "Little Gidding" by T.S. Eliot (1943). *Four Quartets*. Orlando, FL:
Harcourt Brace Jovanovich, Inc.
Page 349: "60" in *Complete poems, 1904–1962* by e. e. cum-
mings (1958). New York: Liveright Publishing Corporation.

Library of Congress Cataloging-in-Publication Data
Friendships and community connections between people
with and without developmental disabilities / edited by
Angela Novak Amado.
    p.   cm.
Includes bibliographical references and index.
ISBN 1-55766-121-9
    1. Mentally handicapped—United States.   2. Mentally
handicapped—Services for—United States.   3. Friendship
—United States.   4. Interpersonal relations.   I. Amado,
Angela R. Novak, 1951–
HV3006.A4F73   1993
362.3'3–dc20   92-47436
                                                    CIP

(British Library Cataloging-in-Publication data are available
from the British Library.)

Contents

Contributors

(612)- 698-5565 (handwritten)

Angela Novak Amado, Ph.D.
Executive Director
Human Services Research and
Development Center
357 Oneida Street
St. Paul, Minnesota 55102

225908 (handwritten)

Richard S. Amado, Ph.D.
InterBehavioral Technologies
1195 Juno Avenue
St. Paul, Minnesota 55116
and
Assistant Professor
Department of Psychiatry Clinical
Faculty
University Hospital and Clinic
University of Minnesota
Minneapolis, Minnesota 55455

Kathy Bartholomew-Lorimer
1929 W. Schiller Street
Chicago, Illinois 60622

Marian Cecelia Coverdale, M.S.
Director of Supported Employment
Services
Noble Centers, Inc.
2400 N. Tibbs Avenue
Indianapolis, Indiana 46222

Bill Gaventa, M.Div.
Executive Secretary
Religion Division
American Association on Mental
Retardation
and
Research Associate
The University-Affiliated Program
of New Jersey
Brookwood II
45 Knightsbridge Road
P.O. Box 6810
Piscataway, New Jersey 08855-6810

Elaine Jurkowski, M.S.W.
Research Associate
School of Public Health
The University of Illinois at
Chicago
2121 W. Taylor Street (M/C-922)
Chicago, Illinois 60612

Zana Marie Lutfiyya, Ph.D.
Department of Educational
Psychology
Faculty of Education
University of Manitoba
Winnipeg, Manitoba
CANADA R3T 2N2

Connie Lyle O'Brien
Responsive Systems Associates
58 Willowick Drive
Lithonia, Georgia 30038-1722

John O'Brien
Responsive Systems Associates
58 Willowick Drive
Lithonia, Georgia 30038-1722

Betty Pendler, M.S.
Member
New York State Developmental
Disabilities Planning Council
267 W. 70th Street #4C
New York, New York 10023

Robert Perske
Perske & Associates–Journalists
159 Hollow Tree Ridge Road
Darien, Connecticut 06820

Deborah Reidy, M.Ed.
Director of Training
Massachusetts Department of
Mental Retardation
160 N. Washington Street
Boston, Massachusetts 02121

Karin Melberg Schwier
Communications Coordinator
Saskatchewan Association for
    Community Living
3031 Louise Street
Saskatoon, Saskatchewan
CANADA S7J 3L1

Joseph P. Shapiro
Reporter
U.S. News & World Report
3701 Connecticut Ave. N.W.
#140
Washington, DC 20008

**Members of Speaking For Ourselves
    as told to Karl Williams**
Suite 625
One Plymouth Meeting
Plymouth Meeting, PA 19462

Cindy Strully, M.A.
Director of Service Coordination
Centennial Developmental
    Services, Inc.
3819 St. Vrain
Evans, Colorado 80620

Jeffrey L. Strully, Ed.D.
Executive Director
Jay Nolan Community Services
25006 Avenue Kearny
Valencia, California 91355

Rannveig Traustadottir, Ph.D.
Research Associate
Faculty of Social Sciences
University of Iceland
Odda v/Sudurgotu
101 Reykjavik
ICELAND

Bruce Uditsky, M.Ed.
Executive Director
Alberta Association for Community
    Living
11724 Kingsway Avenue
Edmonton, Alberta
CANADA T5G0X5

Jane Wells
Creative Community Options
4209 Oakmede Lane
White Bear Lake, Minnesota 55110

Sheila Conway Wilson, M.S.
Program Coordinator
Easter Seal of Del-Mar Program,
    Inc.
61 Corporate Circle
New Castle, Delaware 19720-2405

Foreword

To prepare for the decade of the 1990s, members of the Minnesota Governor's Planning Council on Developmental Disabilities took a new approach to make a difference in the lives of individuals with developmental disabilities and their families. Results from the Consumer Survey (conducted in preparation for the *1990 Report: The Heart of Community Is Inclusion*) reinforced the Council's observations—people with disabilities are lonely and isolated. The overwhelming concern was lack of friends and relationships, the essence of life.

The Council's focus had switched from federal priorities to making a positive impact upon individuals themselves. They addressed questions that focused on three issues: How do you fundamentally change a person's life? How can we create a cadre of citizen leaders in every geographic area? How can we fully realize the meaning of nonrestrictive environment found in the Americans with Disabilities Act?

Friendships aren't about new technologies, federal financial participation, special education methods, individualized service plans, accreditation, national data bases, or six-cycle logarithmic graph paper. Friendships are about:

- Interdependence
- Connectedness
- Equality
- Symmetry
- Give and take
- Support
- Unity

The direction was clear. As a future priority, attention must be directed toward helping people with developmental disabilities to achieve full integration and participation in the community—not merely to help them to be *in* the community, but to be *part of* the community as well.

The Council concluded that it must set a 10-year priority, not a 3-year cycle of compliance with federal law. The Council decided on the theme, "Leadership for Empowerment," and has committed its resources to projects and programs that will lead to greater self-determination, self-creation, and empowerment. There will be a growing number of educated people capable of exercising the highest levels of citizenship.

In more recent years, the Council has funded projects that have demonstrated self-determination: Vouchers, Parents as Case Managers, Personal Futures Planning, Friends, and Partners in Policymaking. The key is to empower people by providing them with timely information, by connecting them with resources and their communities, and by backing the choices and decisions they make about their own lives. It is through such empowered individuals that the system will get changed, beginning with each community and upward.

In August 1992, I listened to Lettitia Clay from Texas tell an audience of federal officials about her participation in the Texas Partners in Policymaking program. The effects on her family were tremendous. Her son Rodney was freed from the den of aversives. He had moved from behind a cyclone fence to full inclusion. Their family was able to thrive, not just survive.

Recently, Mrs. Clay called some families from her son's class. One father answered and said, yes, he knew all about Rodney. "My daughter talks about him all the time. They are friends." The father went on to say that he had fought in Vietnam, and as a result, he had trouble of his own. Because of Rodney, his daughter understands her father more and gives him hugs and kisses every day. This is only one of many stories about how people become empowered through friendships.

By pushing the boundaries, change occurs. We know we have succeeded in our efforts and the ripple effects are spreading.

Our Council invested in the development of friendships through the Friends Project. The authors of this book understand the magic of connections and relationships. Other projects, thinkers, and writers who are working toward the same goals in the United States and Canada have been brought together in this book to share what they have learned with all of us.

I hope you enjoy this book.

Colleen Wieck, Ph.D.
Executive Director
Minnesota Governor's Planning Council
on Developmental Disabilities

Preface

Fifteen years ago, in 1978, I started the doctoral program in Special Education at the University of Illinois in Champaign-Urbana. As part of learning about various ways of evaluating services, I attended a workshop in Milwaukee called PASS, the Program Analysis of Services Systems (Wolfensberger & Glenn, 1975). At that time, I already had 9 years of first-hand experience in services for people with mental retardation, had been taught by some of the "experts" in the country, and already had pretty strong ideas about what high quality in services meant. Yet, in that week in 1978, my eyes and heart opened to a whole new way of thinking about people with disabilities and their lives. The workshop took the perspective of the people themselves: who they were as human beings, what it was like to have other people's rules dominate every aspect of their lives, how it was to always live and work and travel in groups of other people with disabilities, how much they wanted simple things like everyone else wants from life.

In that first PASS workshop 15 years ago, the issue arose of relationships outside the services system with typical community members. The gulf, the grand canyon of isolation and separation that was everpresent in people's lives, was overwhelming. Throughout the next decade I participated in more PASS workshops, led teams in some, brought that perspective into other types of evaluations, used the ideas to conduct research, applied the principles as a state bureaucrat, and taught the values as a university lecturer. And every time since then that I have conducted an evaluation or workshop and met people receiving services, that gulf and grand canyon have been present.

Throughout the 1980s I followed many evolving ideas in school systems—mainstreaming, partial participation, full inclusion. I got excited hearing John O'Brien and John McKnight and reading and listening over and over to people speak of the importance of friendships and real community participation. I knew and even had some hand in helping many people move from institutions to apartments and foster homes. But even now, 15 years later, every time I walk into a program or meet people dependent on the services system, their isolation and separation from the rest of the community are still overwhelming.

In 1989, the Minnesota Governor's Planning Council on Developmental Disabilities funded projects reflecting the three federal priorities of participation, productivity, and independence. That first one hooked me—participation. I knew that the way "community participation" was practiced did not translate into friendships. But what did participation mean, really, except individuals with disabilities having friends and community members being friends with people in the services system? People could talk and talk about how important such relationships were, but what did it really take to make it happen? Although ideas were great, what was anybody doing about it? The jump from idea to reality led to our proposal to the Council to conduct the

"Friends Project," to actually find out what it took for staff to support real friendships in the community: Was it even possible, and what did it take to make such friendships happen?

Since the fall of 1989, when we started the Friends Project, I have learned about many other efforts focused on the encouragement of friendship and real community participation. Much more discussion and many strategies have emerged, even just in the last 3 years. I have tried to bring many of those ideas together here. Of course, so much is happening in this area that this book could probably have been three times as thick as it is. There are many others whom I could have asked to write a chapter. I have seen that what people consider to be friendship varies tremendously. I have also come to see that perhaps the best way to support and understand friendships is simply to *be* a friend oneself.

Most of the ideas presented here are about the services system, typically concerning assistance to adults; all of the many efforts in school programs regarding friendships between children are not addressed here. In addition, most of the authors here write about individuals with developmental disabilities. Other efforts are occurring for individuals with other disabilities, with some overlap in ideas and many unique concepts. I trust those readers interested in supporting individuals with other types of disabilities will also find many of the ideas here useful.

In fact, so many efforts and ideas abound that the cynics have once again charged that this issue of friendships and relationships is just another "hot topic" or "bandwagon." It may be, but what I do know is that I still visit group homes and apartments where people still tell me that they know hardly anyone except their staff and the other residents. When I first walk into a day program these days, people still approach me immediately, desperate to touch, to say hello, to tell me their names. I hope by bringing some of these many ideas together in this volume that we can make a difference in at least some of these individuals being less lonely.

When I meet people on an airplane or at a party and describe what kind of work I'm in, people will usually tell me they know someone who has a child with a disability or they know someone who teaches special education. More recently, they have also been telling me of people with disabilities who work at the same place they do. I have yet to meet a stranger who tells me about his or her own friend who has a developmental disability. I am committed that 15 years from now community relationships and friendships will be an outdated ideology in the history of human services—not because they passed out of professional fashion, but because community members without disabilities will have many friends who happen to have a disability, because communities will be nurturing in a rich diversity of very personal relationships, and because strangers I meet on airplanes and at parties will be proud to tell me of their own friendships.

REFERENCE

Wolfensberger, W., & Glenn, L. (1975). PASS 3: *Program Analysis of Service Systems handbook*. Toronto, Ontario, Canada: National Institute on Mental Retardation.

Acknowledgments

The production of a book, any book, takes effort and hard work from many people. This book is no different, but perhaps because of the topic at many times the effort has also seemed like a labor of love. It is in that spirit that I acknowledge many people.

First, Dr. Colleen Wieck, Ron Kaliszewski, and the grant review committee of the Minnesota Governor's Planning Council on Developmental Disabilities first supported the Friends Project grant to the Human Services Research and Development Center in 1989–1990. Fran Conklin was the extraordinary Project Director. From that project and the six Minnesota residential services agencies involved in it, my knowledge about many other efforts has followed and has resulted in this book. My profound appreciation and thanks go to all the persons who participated in that Project.

Second, the authors need to be thanked for their patience and diligence in working with me through the publication process. Cindy Olson and Patti Karlson significantly contributed to the word-processing, copying, and editing of this manuscript. The staff from Paul H. Brookes Publishing Co. have been extraordinarily patient and committed throughout the process. Vince Ercolano first accepted the proposal for this book and struggled with me through the early stages of labor. Sarah Cheney has done a remarkable job as overall editor, being able to balance the required obsessiveness with detail with deep appreciation for the issues as they affect people's lives. Sue Vaupel, Tania Bourdon, Roslyn Udris, Jennifer Lazaro, and Harriette Wimms-Cutchember have also made significant and much appreciated contributions in their particular roles as birthing assistants in the production.

My husband Rick has patiently not complained about the hours I huddle over the laptop in my office, and the hours I spend pouring over paper with red pen; the hours spent reading copy to each other; and the lively hours we spend sharing, arguing, and trying to understand the disjunction between friendships and human services. Such is one form of our mountain climbing and scuba diving together.

There are many people whose work over the years has significantly contributed to the ideas represented by the numerous authors in this book, including but not limited to John McKnight, Steve Taylor, Doug Biklen, John O'Brien, Connie Lyle O'Brien, Beth Mount, Marsha Forest, Judith Snow, Jack Pearpoint, Gail Jacob, and Wolf Wolfensberger. I have listened and learned from others all over the United States and Canada—Maggie Hanson and Kim Lyster, Kathy Bartholomew-Lorimer, Karin Schwier, Carolyn Carlson and Mary Romer, Sheila Wilson and Cecilia Coverdale, and many others who have been "learning through doing." All of us have learned from many people, many of whose names and stories are proudly used here in this text (unless they have requested that their names be changed). Many of the ideas have emerged and been clarified in long conversations driving all over Minnesota with Fran Conklin, Pat Lyon, Jane Wells, and Tom Fitzpatrick. Again, all these people need to be acknowledged.

Primarily, however, the ideas have come from the people we have met: Vicki, Muffy, Danielle, Mary Pieper, Patrick, Sandy, Art, Peg, Michelle, Bonnie, Jeff, and all the others who want friends, try to be friends, and try to support friendships. It is their spirit and their heart that are the real essence of this work, and in whose light these words on paper will always be only shadows.

To Bonnie and April, who challenge me and graciously allow me to learn how to be a friend. And to all the Bonnies and Aprils from whom we are all learning.

Friendships and Community Connections between People with and without Developmental Disabilities

1

Introduction

Robert Perske

Picture yourself as a community worker who places persons with developmental disabilities in neighborhood settings. You have a bachelor's and a master's degree, as well as 10 years of hands-on experience. You know a good locality when you see it. In addition, you have a sense for the best educational, vocational, and residential technologies in the area. So, with all this skill and your razor-sharp knowledge of the psychodynamics of personal relationships (backed up by 11 Qualified Mental Retardation Professional training seminar certificates), you place a young person named Robert in a good neighborhood. When you finish you have a sense of accomplishment. You note that Robert is the 582nd person you placed during your career.

Later, a reporter hearing about your work with Robert pays you a visit. He listens while you explain your agency's placement system and how it worked on Robert's behalf. You lead the reporter into believing that your agency is one of the best in the nation—even though there are numerous agencies across the country that deem themselves number one.

You and the reporter travel to Robert's home, and your success story continues. Suddenly, this reporter, who doesn't know a lot about such community placements, asks you a simple question: "Does Robert have any friends?"

The question catches you by surprise. You tell him, "I'm not sure. I can't think of any."

The reporter then asks, "Do you have any idea how he might make some friends?"

You stand for a moment in silence. Then you move around the house collecting documents for the journalist to view—Robert's individualized habilitation plan (IHP), the residence's latest accreditation report; and a sheet describing the home's guiding principles, called *The Four C's* (communication, consideration, cooperation, and contribution). Then you show him the posted meal schedule and the fire-escape plan.

Welcome to the 1990s, where a large number of visionaries and technologists have set off a wealth of ideas—all subsumed under the term *inclusion*. They say it is not enough merely to place persons with disabilities in a neighborhood—they must be connected to it socially. Their lives must interweave emotionally with the lives of others. According to these visionaries and technologists, good inclusion takes more than caring parents, committed professionals, and carefully matched volunteers. It also takes friendships—lots of friendships.

These promoters of inclusion talk about natural opportunities where one person becomes a scout, escort, bodyguard, or streetwise mentor for another. They talk about circles of friends in regular schools—even regular classrooms. They dream about building friendships in local diners and shops, religious congregations, recreation centers, as well as through common pursuits. According to these visionaries, all human beings possess unique gifts and energies that can enrich a neighborhood. If the interweavings of a truly inclusive neighborhood could be depicted by a colorful piece of fabric, one would find the vivid, colorful threads woven by people with disabilities in the fabric, too.

After writing about some of these promoters of inclusion (Perske, 1988), I began making a list of things I think friendships can and cannot do. This list continues to change and grow as it is pondered and challenged.

Friendship Is a Familiar but Elusive Term   Most people feel warmth when they call another person a friend. They profit from friendships in more ways than they can count. People consider friendships precious and believe their lives are enhanced by them. Yet, one only needs to consult a dictionary to find that the term *friend* can mean many different things and that researchers will have a hard time measuring it. Other hard-to-measure words are faith, hope, love, and jazz ("It's tough to define, but I know it when I hear it," said Miles Davis [1984]).

Families Provide Things that Friends Cannot   Friends may come and go, but a family provides birth-to-death ties that remain intact even if they are not honored. The birthing, family bonding, childhood nurturing, and family ceremonies and celebrations—even funerals—all give us a place in history. Therefore, people's familial relationships will last a lifetime, even if some relatives are not compatible.

For example, two friends may consider themselves "closer than sisters." One of them may have a sister she does not like. Yet, when that woman gets married, there is more than an average chance that the sister will be the maid of honor instead of the friend. In *Just Friends: The Role of Friendship in Our Lives,* social scientist Lillian Rubin draws on her study of 300 men and women, showing the marked distinction between blood relatives and friends. Interestingly, the whole study began after she struggled to understand why she was not chosen for an honorific place in a family ritual of her best friend. "My attention is caught by the stark clarity between family and friend. For the first time, I'm acutely aware of how undifferentiated I am from any of the other hundred or so friends and acquaintances in attendance" (1985, p. 2).

Families Can Be Limiting   I can recall returning to celebrations at home after several decades of adult life. At these happy times, relatives were quick to recall how "little Bobby" set the garage on fire at age four, and how he spit on an elderly woman who was trying to get him out of her cherry tree. Interestingly, these conversations made me feel like going back and being that kid again. After all, most parents watch with bewilderment at the type of people their sons and daughters become. Adult lives can be very different from what parents expect.

Friends Can Stretch Us Beyond Our Families   People do numerous things with friends that they would never want their parents, brothers, and sisters to know about. This does not mean that these activities were shameful, only that friendships are private affairs. Friendships stand outside the limiting judgments and protections of relatives. With friends, people can hope, dream, and dare afresh. With friends, people try new feats, fall flat, and try again; people make attempts with friends that they may never make with their parents watching.

Human Services Workers Do Things Friends Cannot Do   When persons with disabilities experience barriers or setbacks—medical, social, or others—a good team of workers may be able to rally around them. Each worker looks at the problem from the viewpoint of his or her own training and expertise. Together, the workers choreograph a healing or achievement that revitalizes the person with disabilities. Such outcomes are often beautiful to behold and they make life richer for the people being helped, even if a medical model or a specific educational technology has been used. (The intention is not to uplift one helping faction by suppressing another. For example, if a person suddenly suffers a heart attack, a medical team should be called in first—not a support circle.)

Friends Help People Move Beyond Human Services Goals   Friends provide a myriad of options that never could be programmed by a human services agency. The more friendships, the wider the range of options.

Friends Help People Rehearse Adult Roles   Sometimes people engage in courses of action that make certain relatives livid. Yet, the blood ties between them will remain intact. Misguided behavior with a friend, however, can dissolve a relationship immediately. Perhaps much of our adult development comes from losing certain friendships and subsequently pondering the consequences and adjusting the way we act with others.

Friends Serve as Fresh Role Models   Often, a person is attracted to someone who possesses mannerisms, attitudes, and skills he or she would like to have. This does not mean that the person will achieve what is admired, but that sometimes he or she is successful in copying certain desirable attributes of friends.

Professionals Cannot Program Friendships   Some service workers try to program friendships, but they often fail. However, others are remarkably skilled at helping people get to places where friendships can happen. These workers are also talented at reinforcing friendships when they see them happen.

The Quality of Friendship Differs in Males and Females   After interviewing 150 people for *Among Friends: Who We Like and What We Do With Them*, Letty Cotton Pogrebin (1987) found that young girls and adult women tend toward one-to-one relationships that may become intimate and emotionally intense (pp. 298–310). In them, some women share the deepest secrets of their lives. Males, however, do not consider opening themselves up like that to other men. Instead, they feel more comfortable being with a "gang of guys" who possess common interests and mutual enjoyments (pp. 257–275). For many males, loyalty to the group seems more important. These are only tendencies, however, and there are many exceptions to the rule.

Many Aspects of Friendships Are Mysterious   There is no explanation for why some people are compatible. There are no social contracts and no role requirements for getting people together. There certainly are not any rituals or institutional supports for holding them together. They can spark, thrive for a reasonable period of time, and then fade away without so much as a celebration, certificate, plaque, funeral, or divorce decree.

A Healthy Ebb and Flow of Friends May Be More Important than "Best Friends" and Lifetime Commitments   Damon and Pythias, the Lone Ranger and Tonto, and Don Quixote and Pancho Sanza provide friendship models well worth pursuing. Most people, however, will never be blessed with a single best friendship such as theirs. Furthermore, most people will be lucky if, at the time of their death, they can count one lifetime friend. As people move in different directions, they can grow away from certain friends. Growing apart is not bad, however, as long as people can look forward to other close friendships in the future.

Friendships Are Reciprocal   Both people must profit from a friendship. The nature of the personal invigoration and enrichment may, of course, differ for each person. Yet, each person must leave a friendship with something. Otherwise, all efforts in the relationship will lead to an agonizing or boring trip down a poorly paved, one-way street called "Benevolence," a street that will ultimately intersect with another called "Obligation."

Good Friendships Generate Their Own Energy   Two people may appear ordinary and mundane when they are apart, yet, when they get together, they generate much more energy than the sum of two people. They give off a supercharged effect. Their alertness, warmth, humor, and ease of interaction is heightened.

A Good Friendship Is Noticeable   People do not need a book of standards and an accreditation surveyor to indicate when a friendship is good. It is apparent from being around the friends for a while. Watch. Listen. It becomes clear.

A Good Friendship Can Be Attractive   People often take a second look at certain friendships in action. People are affected by what they see. They wonder if they could ever have as good a friendship. They wonder if these friends have some secret technique that others do not know about.

Each Friendship Is Unique and Unrepeatable   Each friendship is as distinct and separate as fingerprints. Once a good friendship is over, it can never be duplicated. Other good friendships will be created, but they will all be different.

Friendships Become a Haven from Stress   When life becomes stressful, it helps to know that there are some people who care about what happens. It is good to have a selective array of friends—different people ready to help with different situations. It is reassuring to know that these people are available if they are ever needed.

Some People in Authority May Frown on Friendships   Young workers in the field of disabilities may be surprised to learn that even as late as the 1960s, staff members in some institutions for persons with mental retardation were rotated every month so that they would not "get emotionally involved with the patients." C.S. Lewis (1971) may have provided us with one reason for this policy. In his book, *The Four Loves*, he says, "Men who have real Friends are less easy to manage or 'get at'; harder for good Authorities to correct or for bad Authorities to corrupt" (p. 115). Interestingly, this frowning upon friendships continues in other settings.

During Johnny Paul Penry's retrial for his life at Huntsville, Texas, the prosecution worked to prove that Mr. Penry "faked mental retardation." They claimed that he was intelligent and conniving. The defense put on the witness stand three death row inmates who had formed a protective circle of friends around the man because of his retardation. "I've never known a man in my life that wanted friends more than Johnny did," James Vanderbilt told the court (Perske, 1991, pp. 67–68). He went on to describe the man's childlikeness and vulnerability. Harvey Earvin explained how Penry's hunger for acceptance had set him up for ruthless exploitation until the circle decided to protect him. James Beathard testified that the circle even tried to keep him away from reporters "who could lead Johnny and get him to say almost anything they wanted to hear" (Perske, 1991). Shortly after the three men testified on Penry's behalf, prison officials moved all three to different cellblocks, away from Penry.

Friends Are No Big Deal   While being interviewed and observed for *Circles of Friends* (Perske, 1988), many parties in really good relationships wondered why one would want to write about or photograph them. They had a point. Ordinary friendships are not newsworthy; yet, a spate of newspaper articles now focuses on friendships that include a person having a disability. Why the sudden interest? Is it possible that for many years helpers in the field were so focused on their "services" that they never thought much about friendships? If people with disabilities are helped to have friends, writing on the topic will be passé. That day cannot come too soon.

Some of the most noble activities in life include having friends and being a friend. Friendships should occupy a strong place in everyone's human development. They call up the best parts of people—sometimes the fun-loving side and sometimes the serious. The saddest thing a person can say about someone is, "He doesn't have any friends."

REFERENCES

Davis, M. (1984, December). *Down beat, 51*(12), 16–19, 48.

Lewis, C.S. (1971). *The four loves.* New York: Harcourt Brace Jovanovich.

Perske, R. (1988). *Circles of friends: People with disabilities and their friends enrich the lives of one another.* Nashville: Abingdon Press.

Perske, R. (1991). *Unequal justice? What can happen when persons with retardation or other developmental disabilities encounter the criminal justice system.* Nashville: Abingdon Press.

Pogrebin, L.C. (1987). *Among friends: Who we like and what we do with them.* New York: McGraw-Hill.

Rubin, L.B. (1985). *Just friends: The role of friendship in our lives.* New York: Harper & Row.

I

DIMENSIONS OF FRIENDSHIPS

Although all of society has throughout history been challenged concerning how to relate to and include persons with disabilities, the phenomenon of supporting friendship between individuals who receive services and other community members is fairly recent. The first section of this volume presents various issues in our thinking about friendship between persons with and without disabilities, including the issues that have arisen as various persons and groups have attempted to build those friendships.

The first four chapters of this section present broad analysis of the contexts in which to try to understand friendship, the current emphasis on its importance, and various efforts to work on both supporting relationships and building community. In Chapter 2, John and Connie O'Brien begin this discussion with a thought-provoking analysis of four dimensions or aspects which affect friendships: attraction, the mystery by which two people are brought together; embodiment, the particular ways or practices by which a friendship is enacted; power, or the amount of personal control over one's life and the imbalances in such power that affect friendships between persons with and without disabilities; and community, or the contribution of a particular friendship to the life of a larger social body of people. In Chapter 3, Bill Gaventa provides a solid historical review of spiritual and classical thought regarding the importance and purposes of friendship for all people, and how these inherited cultural foundations affect current thinking in friendships between persons with and without disabilities. Richard Amado analyzes the research on the physical, emotional, and behavioral effects of loneliness in Chapter 4, and presents evidence that support for friendship is both beneficial and imperative in addressing these effects. Bruce Uditsky then proposes, in Chapter 5, very challenging arguments against many formal approaches that have been used to try to "arrange" friendship, and encourages greater understanding and use of the natural pathways which all people follow in discovering friendship.

7

The last three chapters of this section discuss particular issues which have arisen as more energy has been applied to supporting friendship and relationships for persons with disabilities. It has been consistently repeated and emphasized that the social networks of many individuals with disabilities are dominated by paid staff persons, and that relationships with unpaid community members need to be encouraged. However, in Chapter 6, Zana Lutfiyya presents evidence of the genuine friendships which do occur between staff and persons they serve; she also reviews the complex issues which affect such relationships, when staff do become friends. One of those issues is the fact that most human services staff, community integration facilitators, and community members who are friends with persons with disabilities are women; in Chapter 7, Rannveig Traustadottir discusses the various reasons why relationships with persons with disabilities are bound within such a strongly gendered context and how that context affects friendship. Finally, Elaine Jurkowski and Angela Amado discuss the most intimate types of friendship, those which include love, physical affection, and sexual expression; they discuss how important such intimacy is in the lives of everyone, including individuals with disabilities. They also discuss the importance of sex education which includes intimacy and affection in relationships, and problematic issues such as abuse prevention which must be taken into account when supporting relationships.

The ideas in these chapters are attempts to understand the many challenging and complex issues affecting this element of the lives of individuals with disabilities. Friendships and relationships are affected, as are most dimensions in the lives of individuals with disabilities, by both the human services system and the evolution of many cultural ideas and values in the larger society. In this last decade of the twentieth century, these ideas represent reflections of the current status in this part of the evolution toward a more diverse, pluralistic, and inclusive society.

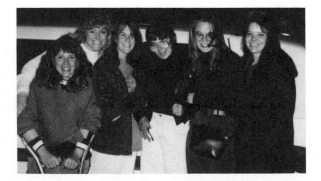

2

Unlikely Alliances

Friendships and People with Developmental Disabilities

John O'Brien and Connie Lyle O'Brien

> Nature assigns the Sun—
> That—is Astronomy—
> Nature cannot enact a
> Friend—
> That—is Astrology.
>
> Emily Dickinson

Friendships cannot be calculated by dispassionate observers, as the orbit of the sun can, but their meanings can be understood better by reflective participants, as other human mysteries can. Better understanding could make better friends and wiser assistants to people for

This chapter arises from continuing conversations with our friends Kathy Bartholomew-Lorimer, Barbara Buswell, Marsha Forest, Gail Jacob, Zana Lutfiyya, Beth Mount, Freeda Neumann, Jack Pearpoint, Jack Pealer, Beth Schaffner, Judith Snow, Jeff and Cindy Strully, Steve Taylor, and Alan Tyne.

Preparation of this chapter was supported through a subcontract from The Center on Human Policy, Syracuse University for the Research & Training Center on Community Living. The Research & Training Center on Community Living is supported through a cooperative agreement (Number H133B80048) between the National Institute on Disability and Rehabilitation Research (NIDRR) and the University of Minnesota Institute on Community Integration. Members of the Center are encouraged to express their opinions; these do not necessarily represent the official position of NIDRR.

Examples that are not otherwise referenced are drawn from notes and recordings we made during five, one-day—long focus group meetings on the topic of friendship and people with developmental disabilities. Three of these meetings involved parents and friends of people with developmental disabilities and were convened by the Association for Community Living in Colorado in January and June 1992 and by the Wisconsin Coalition for Advocacy in March 1990. One meeting involved people who use services for adults with developmental disabilities. This meeting was convened by INFO, a self-advocacy group active in the northwest of England, in November 1990. This meeting is also reported in Flynn (1991). The fifth meeting, which involved adult service providers and some of the people they support, was convened by the Ohio Society for Autistic Citizens in May 1985. This meeting is also reported in Pealer and O'Brien (1985).

whom friendships are unlikely alliances because they are separated and isolated by prejudice against disability.

English language dictionaries mirror the ambiguity of friendship. In common usage, someone attached by feelings of affection is a friend, someone who acts as a patron or benefactor is a friend, and someone who is simply not hostile is a friend. This ambiguity helps to illuminate a dispute between a special education teacher and a mother who has successfully advocated for her son's inclusion in high school. The young man's teacher points with pride to his many friends. The teacher notes that almost everybody in school knows the young man's name and says "hi" to him, and that some of the young women in his class have befriended him, as evidenced by their willingness to look after him on a class trip. The young man's mother says that, although he is well known in school, other students do not treat him as an equal or spontaneously involve him in their lives outside of school. She believes that people are friendly, but that he has no real friends to count on. She wants the people who assist her son to think more deeply about friendship and to work in a more focused way to support others to become his friends. She says that it worries and angers her that the teacher cannot understand her concern.

This disagreement over the meaning of friendship contains the questions that concern us in this chapter. What can people with developmental disabilities expect from their social relationships, particularly their relationships with people without disabilities? Is the meaning of "friend" exhausted by lack of hostility or by benevolent patronage? Or, are some deeper meanings possible, and, if they are, how can people understand them, call them forth, and support them? What challenges come with friendship?

These are difficult questions for three reasons, each of which offers a guide to the kind of discussion appropriate to the topic. First, modern patterns of practice and belief segregate and isolate people with developmental disabilities as a matter of course. Outside of families and human services settings, sustained relationships of any sort involving people with developmental disabilities are unlikely alliances. Instead of being able to consider many and varied experiences that extend over generations, people can only draw on a few experiences, most of which are measured in much less time than a decade. Therefore, this discussion must be tentative, a way to find the next steps in a new long journey.

Second, the stakes are high. People with developmental disabilities have suffered terrible consequences from being seen as less than human (Wolfensberger, 1975). However fuzzy or implicit the common understanding of friendship may be, most people would say that someone incapable of friendship is diminished in a basic quality of humanity. Aware of this, and moved by their own love, a growing number of parents of people with developmental disabilities hope powerfully for true, sustaining, and lasting friendships for their sons' and daughters' pleasure and protection. Jeff and Cindy Strully spoke for many other parents when they said, "It is friendship that will ultimately mean life or death for our daughter. It is her and our only hope for a desirable future and protection from victimization" (see Strully & Strully, chap. 13, this volume). Therefore, this discussion must be careful never to compromise the human dignity of people with developmental disabilities and cautious not to betray hope with inflated stories of easy success or perfect relationships.

Third, friendship is problematic. On one hand, friendship has stimulated beautiful, wise, and whimsical thoughts about some of the highest and best human possibilities (see Welty & Sharp, 1991). On the other hand, contemporary criticism exposes the elitist, individualistic, and patriarchal biases in the ways many thinkers have understood and shaped our society's written understanding of friendship (Heilbrun, 1988; McFague, 1987; Raymond, 1986). For instance, in some classical views, women could not be true friends, foreigners could not be true friends, and people of low status could not be true friends. All of these groups were thought to lack the qualities of intellect and spirit and the social position assumed necessary for friendship (Benveniste, 1973; Easterling, 1989). In some modern views, friendship is aside and apart from the real, fundamentally competitive business of life. It matters mostly to women and children and only to men as a brief respite from the daily fight for a living (Lasch, 1978; Traustadottir, chap. 7, this volume). Therefore, this discussion needs to be critical of assumptions about friendship.

FOUR DIMENSIONS OF FRIENDSHIP

Mary Hunt's (1991) consideration of friendship provides a good starting place because she calls attention to important aspects of friendship that are easily ignored in a culture given to individualism. Instead of focusing solely on its advantages to isolated individuals, Hunt sets friendship in the context of building a just community. Friendship, she believes, forms the goal of human community and the defining image of ethical relationships. "Justice involves making friends, lots of friends, many kinds of friends . . . [who] empower one another to keep making change [in the structures and conditions that make friendship difficult or impossible]" (p. 21). As shown in Figure 1, Hunt's reflections draw attention to four aspects of friendship; they have been adapted here in order to explore friendships that involve people with developmental disabilities.

Attraction points to the mystery that brings friends together and recognizes that friends feel some kind of unity that they can preserve, deepen, and express by being together. Friends may say they feel attracted by their similarities or by their differences. However it is explained, whether it is ever stated explicitly or not, attraction refers to the "something," noticed or discovered, that draws friends to one another and keeps relationships alive.

Embodiment identifies the particular ways people physically enact friendship, which differ from person to person and from relationship to relationship. People may embody a friendship by watch-

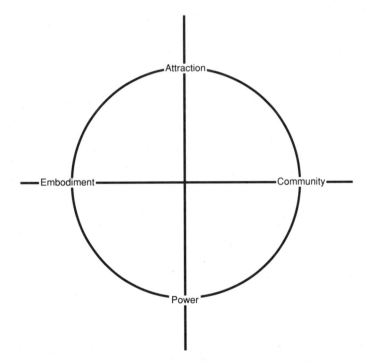

Figure 1.   Hunt's four aspects of friendships. (Adapted from Hunt [1991]. Hunt invites her readers to use her approach to stimulate conversation about friendships that will lead to new models [p. 100]. These authors have accepted her invitation, maintained the overall structure of her model, and modified its terms to better fit their reflections on friendships involving people with severe disabilities. Moving counter-clockwise around the diagram, Hunt identifies the four poles of the diagram as "love," "embodiment," "power," and "spirituality" [p. 99]. The words the authors have chosen retain the sense of Hunt's discussion.)

ing movies together, making music together, running a business together, exchanging the news of daily life, writing letters back and forth, meeting once a year to fish, or raising children together.

Power distinguishes the extent and the ways in which friends can make choices about their relationship, as well as the accommodations friends make to the personal and structural constraints that affect their friendship.

Community recognizes that friendships are situated within, and contribute to, the life of a civic and social body. The choices that friends make either build up or break down a community that can offer its diverse members justice and belonging.

These four dimensions do not exhaustively define friendship; they simply identify important elements of its meaning. These dimensions of friendship matter particularly for people with developmental disabilities because the social construction of disability can make friendship particularly difficult for them. The community aspect is important because people with developmental disabilities risk social devaluation—being seen as "not like the rest of us," even to the extent of being socially defined and treated as inhuman (Wolfensberger, 1991). Without the strength to resist, which is provided by a developing community, friendships cannot thrive. The power aspect matters because people with disabilities typically have less power than the amount people without disabilities take for granted. Without action to deal with imposed inequality, friendships cannot thrive. The embodiment aspect is important because people with developmental disabilities risk losing friends simply because they need assistance to undertake the activities that lead to and express friendship. Without effective assistance, friendships cannot thrive. Finally, the aspect of attraction matters because people with developmental disabilities have just as much capacity for friendship as any other people do. Because of the power of attraction, friendships can thrive.

THE QUESTION OF ATTRACTION

The question of attraction haunts many discussions about friendships for people with developmental disabilities. According to parents, there are at least three ways that others dismiss their concern for their children's friendships. Some people say that friendship is not a problem—people with developmental disabilities already have all the friends they need or want, especially among their "peers," the other clients of congregate services. Some people say that friendship, as people without disabilities understand it, does not matter to people with developmental disabilities because they lack the capacity to understand it. Some people say that friendships, particularly friendships including people without disabilities, are an unrealistic dream —people with and without disabilities have too little in common to make friends. These three dismissals have a similar element: each assumes that people with and without disabilities will not discover and pursue mutual attractions because of the way they perceive people with disabilities to be.

Are People with Developmental Disabilities Able To Attract People without Disabilities?

Summarizing his discussion of human development, Robert Kegan (1982) observed:

> Who comes into a person's life may be the single greatest factor of influence to what that life becomes. Who comes into a person's life is in part a matter of luck, in part a matter of one's power to recruit others, but in large part a matter of other people's ability to be recruited. People have as varying capacities to be recruited as they do to recruit others. (p. 19)

Does disability necessarily lead to low capacity to recruit and be recruited? Can people with developmental disabilities recruit people without disabilities into their lives? Are people without disabilities recruitable by people with disabilities?

The experience of many families clearly answers, yes! People with developmental disabilities can powerfully recruit others into their lives and activate good relationships through which people work for social justice. Based on his study of six families, three of whom adopted their children with disabilities, Biklen (1992) concludes that the kinds of positive relationships that these families work to achieve within themselves should guide public policy and educational practice. Schools should support all children, unconditionally, to be full participants in everyday life, as these six families strive to do. Professionals should recognize and assist people's natural desire to be fully involved in life, as these six families strive to do. Other people should make the chance to discover and enjoy people's individual gifts, as these six families strive to do. These families fully include and work to expand opportunities for their member with disabilities, not from a sense of pity or duty, but because their appreciation of his or her identity flows into a clear sense of what is right.

Dorothy Atkinson (1986) studied the relationship networks of the 28 women and 27 men discharged between 1971 and 1981 from the institutions serving one English county. She found that all but seven people had involved at least one neighbor in social and helpful relationships. Almost three fourths of the people had nondisabled acquaintances they saw regularly, and about half of the people had at least one supportive friend without a disability. She noted that these people without disabilities make a real and sustained contribution to the lives of people with developmental disabilities, offering information, advice, assistance, support, conversation, and company.

One reason that these positive images of relationships have not yet been influential in shaping policy and practice is that attention has focused elsewhere. During the past 25 years of service reform, concern for the rights of people with developmental disabilities overshadowed attention to their relationships.

As Steven Taylor and Robert Bogdan (1989) point out, many workers took up the sociology of deviance as an effective tool to explain, guide, and justify their reforms. This understanding of the negative effects of stigmatizing labels and practices fueled the fight for equal rights for people with developmental disabilities and led to much positive change, but "it has too often been interpreted in terms of the inevitability of rejection of people with obvious differences . . . labeling and exclusion of people with disabilities have become so taken-for-granted that instances of acceptance have been glossed over or ignored" (p. 25).

To complement the understanding offered by a sociology of deviance, Bogdan and Taylor have begun to outline a sociology of acceptance, based on the recognition that some people with and without disabilities have formed long-standing, close, and affectionate relationships that neither deny disability nor stigmatize a person on the basis of disability. In such relationships, people without disabilities see, enjoy, celebrate, and protect the positive qualities, abilities, and individuality of people whose disabilities loom very large to most people outside the relationship (see Bogdan & Taylor, 1987; Taylor & Bogdan, 1989).

Why Do So Many People with Developmental Disabilities Lack Friends?

If people with disabilities can recruit others into their lives, and if accepting relationships are possible, a reasonable person might mistakenly think that friendships will take care of themselves. Maybe people with disabilities will have few friends among nondisabled people, but certainly they will have many good friends among people with developmental disabilities.

A survey of U.S. residential programs asked knowledgeable staff about contacts between older clients of residential services and their friends (Anderson, Lakin, Hill, & Chen, 1992). The survey broadly defined a friend as a person other than a family member with whom the resident looks forward to spending time, either at the facility or somewhere else. Under this definition friends were found to be other residents (approximately 30% of the time), nondisabled persons (approximately 14% of the time), or other persons with disabilities. The survey estimated that about half of the people with mental retardation who were more than 63 years of age either had no friends at all or never saw their friends. Only 25% of those people staff identified as having friends actually saw a friend once a month or more. Compounding this group's isolation, about half of these people had no contact at all with their families.

Unfortunately, this level of isolation does not appear to result just from the age of the people involved. In a larger survey, representative of the whole U.S. population in residential programs for people with mental retardation, staff in close contact told interviewers that about 42% of people in community programs and about 63% of people in institutions had no friends, even among other residents or staff (Hill, Rotegard, & Bruininks, 1984). This study defined a friend as anyone the resident liked and did things with on the resident's own time. (Additional studies documenting the isolation of persons in residential programs are summarized in Amado, chap. 16, this volume.)

These findings call for action, and the researchers who report them have sensible recommendations to offer: use smaller residential settings rather than larger settings because the surveys show that smaller settings offer people more social contacts; increase people's involvement with neighbors (about two thirds of whom were described by staff informants in the study of older residents as either "warm and accepting" or "friendly"); increase people's use of ordinary community places such as shops, churches, libraries, and parks; increase attention to people's leisure time opportunities; and concentrate staff attention on building up people's social contacts. But these findings also deserve thoughtful, even meditative, consideration— why do so many people have no friends?

Do People Have Friendships that Are Invisible to Outsiders?

Perhaps these survey findings say more about the difference between life as people with developmental disabilities live it and those lives as seen by staff or other outsiders. Maybe there are many more friendships among people with developmental disabilities than are apparent to observers. Anne McDonald, who survived 15 years in an institution for "profoundly mentally retarded children," describes friendships among residents that were invisible not just to ordinary staff, but to her teacher, ally, and friend Rosemary Crossley as well. Some people that the staff assumed incapable of communication were, as it turns out, not babbling and shrieking, but conversing. Once Anne could communicate with staff, however, she kept these relationships secret for two reasons: she feared that even Rosemary, her closest ally, would not believe that her friendships were real; and she thought that if staff suspected that these friendships existed, they would break them up in order to retain control of the ward (Crossley & McDonald, 1984). Poet Robert Williams (1989) expresses this disjunction of perception in "Dick and Jane," who are institutionalized lovers who have "shared the same mat since they were children" and who find pleasure in one another's touch:

> They move an inch or two closer to each other
> hoping that the staff doesn't pick up on the subtleties
> of the moment;
> they don't of course. (p. 13)

Knowledge of the possibility of invisible friendships instills caution on two counts: people with the authority to move people with developmental disabilities around will consider their relationships when they make decisions about such movements (Berkson & Romer, 1981); and outsiders will be careful to remember the limitations of their point of view, keep open the possibility that much more is happening than they know, and inquire actively for different perspectives, especially the perspectives of the involved people with disabilities. However, the possibility of invisible friendships does not imply that all people in congregate residences and day programs have friends, and it does not engage the question of friendships between people with developmental disabilities and people without disabilities.

Indeed, if staff cannot even recognize some friendships among people with developmental disabilities, there could be such a gulf between the experiences of people with and without disabilities that friendship between them is unattainable. There is, however, a simpler explanation for this lack of staff awareness. The norms and beliefs that organize most service settings into distinct, unequal subcultures of keepers and inmates explain staff's blindness better than the argument that people with developmental disabilities are a distinct subspecies (Barnes, 1990; Glouberman, 1990). Concern for friendship means hard work to minimize the status and power differences between people with disabilities and the people who assist them. Only then will concerned people be able to better appreciate individual differences and more accurately describe the social worlds of people with disabilities.

Do Friendships Matter to People with Developmental Disabilities?

Even within the closed environments of congregate services, staff do see friendships. Staff surveyed in the studies summarized above said that about half of the people do have friendships—mostly with other residents. However, they may not think they are seeing friendships similar to their own. Many adults may remember that any possibility of friendship, even friendships among people with developmental disabilities, has been in question within their lifetime. MacAndrew and Edgerton (1966) summarized a thorough and sensitive description of a 10-year relationship with these words:

> We have outlined what we take to be the principal characteristics of a highly improbable, strikingly pervasive and intense friendship between two severely retarded young men. Hopefully, we have provided sufficient detail to convince the reader that this long enduring and highly elaborated relationship is indeed a *friendship* of a highly human order. The existence of such a relationship between two persons of such enfeebled intellect must be counted as compelling testimony to the essentially human character of even the most retarded among us. (p. 620)

A special education teacher in a segregated community program provided this explanation of why her students with moderate mental retardation had few social contacts: "They don't have friends because they don't have much in the way of a self concept. So they don't value the esteem of others" (Evans, 1983, p. 122).

Even when they are recognized, friendships among people with developmental disabilities may be trivialized. Patrick Worth (1990), a leader in the People First movement, shared his experience in a group home and a sheltered workshop:

> Staff put down our friendships when they didn't try and break them up. They acted like our friends were less than their friends. It's like they were saying, "Isn't it nice that you have your little friends to play with." When a friend got sick and you asked to go to the hospital and see him, they acted like you were being foolish. When a friend got in trouble and had to go to a discipline meeting, they acted like you were from Mars when you said you wanted to go to the meeting with him. "It's none of your business," they said. "We have to protect confidentiality," they said. Like we didn't talk to our friends about the trouble they were in. Like we didn't

owe our friends any help. And sometimes a friend got moved away without even having a chance for us to say good-bye.

Seeing friendship through the lens of quantitative research can also
have the effect of trivializing friendships. Defining a friend as a person "other than family or staff with whom the resident looks forward
to spending time" (Anderson et al., 1992, p. 493) powerfully documents people's isolation because only about one in five people had
weekly contact with such friends. However, that definition does not
begin to touch common understandings of friendship. Lining up a
corps of volunteers to provide individual recreation in facilities might
give residents an activity to look forward to, but it would only provide
them with friends in the most diluted sense of the term.

In a study that coded the behavior of 208 people living in 18 group
homes, based on observations at 15-minute intervals over a 2-day
period, Landesman-Dwyer, Berkson, and Romer (1979) operationally
defined friendship as "those pairs [of residents] who spent more than
10% of the observed time periods together" (p. 576). By this method,
they discovered 16 peer friendships. They concluded that "group
home characteristics are better predictors of social behavior . . . than
are individual variables. . . . For instance . . . in homes where the
average intelligence is higher, residents are likely to spend more time
in peer relationships" (578). This way of understanding friendship
sets people who live in group homes apart by both the peculiar, diminished image of friendship it projects and prescribes for them, and
by its loud silence about the possibility of friendships between residents and people without disabilities. The definition even rules out
residential staff as potential friends. The implications of the research
for practice are also of questionable utility. Manipulating the variables of group home design to increase the number of pairs of people
who spend 10% of their time together might not increase the number
of people with developmental disabilities who have others to share
with and count on.

As others listen better to people with developmental disabilities,
the gap between the worlds of people with and without disabilities
diminishes, and a common sense of friendship emerges. Consider the
powerful ordinariness of this woman's description of friendship,
taken from an anthology of writings and artwork by British people
with developmental disabilities:

As I've got older, I've got few friends and lots of acquaintances. A
friend is one who knows all about you and loves you just the same;
A friend to me is someone really special. Even if we don't see each

other for years we can pick up where we've left off. I've got one friend I've known for 34 years. (Atkinson & Williams, 1990, p. 78)

Can Relationships between People with and without Disabilities Be Friendships?

People with developmental disabilities share activities with people without disabilities, and people without disabilities establish accepting relationships with people with developmental disabilities, but some observers wonder about considering these relationships friendships. Assigned to identify the practical implications of Robert Perske's *Circles of Friends* (1988), some of the participants in a staff training course expressed skepticism about whether the relationships Perske described were really friendships. They asked: What do the people involved really have in common? Can these be equal relationships? What do the people with developmental disabilities contribute? Do people with limited language understand the relationship?

These questions reflect some sensible criteria for defining friendship: common interests, equality, mutuality, and understanding. In her careful study of four friendships involving people with and without disabilities, Zana Marie Lutfiyya (1989, 1990) makes two important points about these criteria. First, the meaning of any friendship is created by the ways in which its participants enact and talk about it. Commonality, equality, mutuality, and comprehension are best understood from the perspective of the friends themselves, rather than according to the measurements of a detached observer. Second, according to the people involved in the friendships, these criteria were satisfied in the relationships she studied:

> Despite the differences in opportunities and experiences, at least some people with disabilities have successfully formed friendships with nondisabled people. Through studying established friendships, we learn that both parties possess a respect for the other. The friends also experienced a mutuality in their interactions that may not be apparent to the outside observer. These feelings stem from a sense of identification between the two individuals. They come to see the "sameness" or commonalities between themselves and these serve as the basis of the relationship . . . (Lutfiyya, 1990, p. 74)

Jeff and Cindy Strully have grappled with the meaning of friendship for people with limited verbal communication as they have worked hard to support friendships for their daughter, Shawntell. They report (Strully & Strully, 1985, 1989; chap. 13, this volume) on her changing relationships from their perspective and from the perspective of the young women who are Shawntell's friends. Biklen (1992) provided a helpful metaphor for the construction of meaning in these relationships. He suggested that when someone's verbal communication is very limited, concerned others can read the person's behavior and expressions and give voice to them as if they were a text. Like the members of the families Biklen studied, Shawntell's friends read their shared activities and their reactions to one another as signifying friendship. Through time, Shawntell's responses to her activities with them—going out for dinner; taking holiday trips; going to concerts, sports events, and parties; listening to music; hanging out at school and around the house; and driving around town—all mean that they are friends. Her friends speak of sharing confidences with Shawntell. They can identify her preferences and interests, overlapping but distinct from their own. They speak of trusting her and of learning from her. They talk about keeping up with one another as their paths in life diverge. They identify themselves to others as friends.

It is worth considering the messages in these questions about whether people with and without disabilities can enjoy common interests, equality, mutuality, and understanding. The questions themselves suggest a sense of disability and of friendship narrowed and flattened by limited experience. Shawntell and Joyce are two young women of similar age and socioeconomic status who attended the same high school and choose to spend considerable time together. To wonder what they have in common, one would need to place very great weight indeed on the effect of developmental disability on a person's interests or on the way a person is perceived. To wonder about their equality, one would need to assume that disability necessarily means inferiority. To wonder about what they exchange, or whether Shawntell comprehends the friendship, one would have to estimate that expressed verbal intelligence plays the defining role in the friendship.

Notice the potential for self-fulfilling prophecy. Those who decide that disability overshadows anything that people might discover in common (i.e., disability equals inferiority) and that friendships are conducted primarily in spoken sentences, will neither seek nor support relationships between people with and without disabilities. Those who decide to share some of their life with someone apparently different, as Shawntell's friends have done, can create a relationship that seems significant but unremarkable to them. When outsiders ask about the "special" nature of their friendship, they will say, as Shawntell's friends do, that they are "just friends, no big deal."

Estimating a low potential for friendship because of apparent differences between people reflects a narrow and flat appreciation of friendship and how it grows. As the dominant modern way of understanding relationships, individualism assumes that each party acts as a separated, closed entity exchanging units of advantage or enjoyment with the other. The balance is like that on a bank statement. From this point of view, as long as the score balances out, the two parties can be said to have a friendship; if either scorekeeper predicts a low rate of return, no friendship can happen.

An understanding of friendship as dialogue offers a much richer medium for its growth. In this view, people reveal themselves as individuals when relating to a variety of different people. People learn who they are by developing new modes of expressing themselves with others. A relationship with somebody different can induct a person into new possibilities for self-expression (Booth, 1988; Taylor, 1991). Socrates communicates this in the form as well as the content of the *Lysis* (Plato, 1979). He demonstrates a way to make a friend through a discussion about friendship in which he enlarges his understanding of both himself and his circle of friends. Creating a friendship between a person with and a person without a developmental disability opens new kinds of self-expression and new definitions of self for both people. Balance in relationships understood as dialogue is more like the balance between dancers than the balance on a bank statement.

Clearly, friendship should not be ignored or trivialized because of developmental disability, and friendship need not be limited by disability. Among many others, Anne McDonald and her friends (Crossley & McDonald, 1984) show that people with disabilities can make friends, even in the most restrictive settings; that people with and without disabilities can make friends, even in those same restricted circumstances; and that these friendships can last and grow even stronger as the people involved come out of segregation. Along with Shawntell Strully and her friends, Anne McDonald and her friends demonstrate that these diverse relationships can thrive despite obvious differences in personal history, embodied experiences, abilities, and status. However, even when concerned people are inspired by its possibilities, friendships between people with and without developmental disabilities remain uncommon. Why?

THE CHALLENGES OF EMBODIMENT

Friends enact their relationship; they live their friendship in ways distinctive of the interests they share. As one man with a developmental disability said:

> I have two fishing friends and we fish. I have four football friends and we watch games and bet. I have three talking friends and we have a drink and talk—sometimes we go out and sometimes we come over to somebody's house. One of my friends is all three: fishing, and football, and talking. I also have a gardening friend and we ask about our gardens and talk about how to grow things and give each other cuttings. I also have a friend that was my teacher a long time ago and I go visit her and remember about bygone days.

Each embodiment of this man's friendships takes time and other resources specific to the activity. He needs to get to where the fish are and have the tackle to catch them, he needs the plot to garden in and the seeds to plant, and he needs the money to buy a round of drinks when his turn comes.

The social consequences of disability challenge the embodiment of relationships. Some challenges arise in the external world and some are part of people's personal experiences.

External Challenges

Difficulty in getting places easily and safely challenges friendships. Most people with developmental disabilities are pedestrians in a society that requires automobiles. Fewer and fewer neighborhoods offer a rich and accessible social life within walking or rolling distance, and many residential facilities are physically isolated. Convenient affordable public transportation remains uncommon. Always asking for rides, or being one of a group of passengers in the facility's van are typical experiences.

Most people with developmental disabilities are poor, and many activities cost money. One woman noted that she watches television most nights "because the TV's paid for." In addition, many places that people want to go together, including many people's homes, are either physically inaccessible or very inconvenient to use.

People's time may not be their own. For people who are full-time clients of developmental disability services, getting together with friends raises issues of control. Requirements for active treatment and restrictions on movement and outside contact, driven by service provider concern for regulatory compliance and liability, often leave people without free time, literally. Many people with developmental disabilities who live with their families report that their parents do not allow them to go out, or prefer that they not go out, except with the family or to supervised disability activities.

Staff concern for the isolation of people with developmental disabilities can result in direct, practical assistance in trying new experiences, making acquaintances, and making friends (see Firth &

Rapley, 1990; Richardson & Ritchie, 1989). This concern takes a different turn if friendship becomes the intended outcome of a rehabilitation process. In these cases, staff can decide that the road to friendship leads through correct performance on a professionally prescribed curriculum of social skills. A brochure describing one such program identifies 21 skills "selected to address the most common behavior problems exhibited by people with developmental disabilities," including "having a calm body and voice, interrupting the right way, [and] accepting no as an answer. . . ." Such approaches set up artificial prerequisites to friendship, based on an abstract analysis of assumed social deficiencies in people with developmental disabilities. This extension of staff control leaves many people waiting in vain for performance in role plays to result in real friends.

Lack of adequate help with mobility and communication inhibits the enactment of people's friendships. For example, facilitated communication is a method for assisting written communication by some people with autism and other physical problems in producing speech (Biklen, 1990). Facilitated communication has given some people whom others believed were asocial and incompetent the opportunity to communicate their interests and desires. With the physical assistance of a facilitator, Kim types,

---

my friends and me
at rye high school i have friends
they like me for me
it feels like some magic
how come i can't be like all the girls.

Delachesnaye, as cited in Bevilacqua, 1992

People with developmental disabilities are often socially disembodied. Friendships emerge among a variety of social relationships, including being part of a family, having a life partner, being a neighbor, being part of a workplace, and being a member of community associations (Ordinary Life Group, 1988). The more of these ties and connections a person misses, the fewer opportunities and supports the person has to meet and make friends.

Current policies and program designs seldom offer people with developmental disabilities flexible personal assistance to pursue activities with acquaintances and friends. Even staff from an exemplary supported living program reported, with remorse, that they are unable to consistently find time to help people become better connected to their community.

Pervasive unfamiliarity with people with developmental disabilities can make many people without disabilities uneasy about initial contacts. Uncertainty about whether one will understand a person, and when and how to offer help can keep people at a distance (Williams, 1977). Men are often uncomfortable offering help, especially with eating or using the toilet. This gendered reluctance can restrict people's friendships to women (see Traustadottir, chap. 7, this volume). People without disabilities, perhaps especially young men, may fear that their own status will suffer by close association with people with developmental disabilities.

Some thoughtful people with physical disabilities believe that friendships among people with different disabilities are easier, and in some political and cultural ways more desirable, than efforts to make friends with people without disabilities. They point to the continuing experience of being seen and treated by nondisabled people as somehow unfamiliar, unwelcome, and inferior, as a strong reason for putting priority on friendships with other people with disabilities. Judith Heumann (1993) writes:

> Disabled people's desire to be accepted by nondisabled people has been a cause of internal discrimination. I believe that we must first accept ourselves and then if nondisabled people don't accept us, so be it. (p. 235)

She goes on to provide welcome criticism of the assumption that

> The most important thing for us would be to be with nondisabled people. . . . I am very concerned about the continued discussion of the percentages of disabled people and the appropriate statistical balance of disabled and nondisabled people as opposed to a balance based on interests, social aspirations, and professional aspirations. (p. 245–246)

To the extent that people with and without disabilities come to feel that friendships among them are somehow incorrect, they will narrow their search for friends instead of widening it.

Accepting relationships are possible, but widespread, unthinking prejudice against people with developmental disabilities remains a fact of life. Some people act as though people with developmental disabilities are repulsive or dangerous and scorn or shun them. Some people act as though people with developmental disabilities are passive, pitiable creatures and intrusively try to be their helpers or saviors. Some people act as though people with developmental disabilities have no sense or will of their own and look for a trained staff person or a parent figure to talk to instead of relating directly to the person with disabilities. As one man with a developmental disability explained:

I think the hardest part is you gotta defend yourself. . . . You gotta fight a, a reputation. People decide they know everything they need to know about me before they meet me even. They never get close enough to see if there is something inside they might like after all. (Melberg-Schwier, 1990, pp. 161–162)

Personal Challenges

Making and keeping friends takes energy and willingness to extend oneself. People with developmental disabilities participating in a conference on friendship identified three negative, self-reinforcing patterns of personal effects of the external challenges to friendship. In the first pattern, a person lacks experience with other people, or has had bad experiences with reaching out to others, and therefore lacks confidence. Lack of confidence keeps the person from going out, engaging only in passive pursuits, such as watching television. This keeps the person from gaining experience, and, over time, further decreases confidence. This pattern gets worse when the person eats and drinks too much to deal with loneliness, and therefore decreases the amount of energy available for reaching out. Conference participants believed that repeated invitations and encouragement from others would help a person break out of this pattern.

In the second pattern, a person feels hurt inside because he or she has been hurt, rejected, or abandoned by someone important. For protection, the person makes a shell to keep others away. It may be a prickly shell that hurts a person trying to become close and therefore drives him or her away. It may be a hard shell that makes someone who tries to come close feel like the person does not care about him or her. A woman who responded strongly to the image of a shell said:

I know my parents love me and only did what they thought was best. But they put me in the institution when I was only a very little girl. For a long, long time I cried and cried because I missed them so much. Then I stopped crying. I think about this, but I still have my prickly shell. Knowing about it doesn't make it go away.

This pattern gets worse when people receive psychoactive drugs to control behavior that is unacceptable because staff and physicians have a poor understanding of the drugs' functions. As one man said, "The right pills might help, I guess. But if you get the wrong pills, they take all the interest out of you." Conference participants believed that others would need to be ready to take time and forgive a person caught up in this pattern of trying to hurt them, and that they would need to be unafraid and keep trying to make friends with the person anyway. They also thought it was important for others to tell the person when he or she was hurting them and for them to realize that the person may not want to be too close.

Maureen Oswin (1992) echoes this pattern when she describes the all too common practice of denying people with developmental disabilities the opportunity and support to grieve important losses. She explains this deprivation by identifying a mistaken notion that people with developmental disabilities lack the resources to comprehend, cope with, and grow through their losses. She associates failure to support people in bereavement with chronic depression, physical complaints, and "unexplained" anger.

In the third pattern, a person feels safe and comfortable because of the familiarity of the relationships he or she already has and because of fear of the uncertainty of change. As one man said:

> My mother and dad and me are very close. Sometimes I'd like to go out more on my own, but they really need me at home for company. My home could be a safe base to go out from, but it's a nice safe place to stay in. And I'm not sure other people would be as nice.

Conference participants felt that a person caught in this pattern should not be forgotten, but invited to share activities repeatedly, so that they know they have a choice.

This third pattern seems to be related to the decisions described by Robert Edgerton (1988, 1991) as he summed up his learning from more than 20 years of research with people with developmental disabilities who live in the community:

> Each person . . . realizes that it is sometimes, even often, necessary to seek help from others, and although these people may provide badly needed assistance, with that assistance may come unwanted advice, restrictions, or interference. When this happens, the person with mental retardation must decide, like the rest of us must, whether we need someone's help badly enough to surrender some of our autonomy. What is central in the lives of these older people is the search for well-being, and that search involves an ever-shifting calculus that attempts to balance freedom of choice against the need for the help of others. (Edgerton, 1991, p. 273)

Aware of these personal barriers to enacting friendship, some people advocate individually focused counseling or training as the way to friendships. Aware of the negative effects of socially devaluing attitudes, others call for large scale public education as a prerequisite to integration. Neither of these approaches seems preferable to vigorous effort alongside people with developmental disabilities to tear down those external barriers that are within reach. Many challenges to making friends result, directly or indirectly, from the negative effects of common practices by the staff and programs that people with developmental disabilities rely on for assistance. Work to reverse these practices makes the best investment in improving the chances for good relationships.

Some people with disabilities, and some people without disabilities, want and could benefit from counseling to sort out personal difficulties in making and keeping relationships. However, greater autonomy, more money, better transportation, more flexible and available personal assistance, and more respect from those who provide assistance seem prerequisite to the effectiveness of counseling or skill teaching.

Widely held prejudices will only change slowly with increasing personal contact between people with and without disabilities, and it is unlikely that prejudice will ever be eradicated. It makes more sense to offer people practical help to realize that prejudice co-exists with the potential for acceptance than it does to wait for implementation of grand plans to educate the public. People who act on this realization will encourage people with developmental disabilities to find and build the many accepting relationships that are already potentially available.

ISSUES OF POWER

Power enters into friendships between people with and without developmental disabilities in two connected ways. First, friends have to deal with constraints imposed on their relationships by outsiders who control the lives and circumstances of people with developmental disabilities. Second, friends have to negotiate power differences between themselves. Failure to respond effectively to either of these issues of power threatens the strength and endurance of the friendship.

Pushing Back Constraints

Many people with developmental disabilities live and spend the day in situations where others have power over them. Even when staff in direct contact treat people with respect, impersonal others—service administrators and policymakers —retain power over them. This imbalance of power, and the responses friends make to it, shapes their friendships.

Most residential settings manage friends' access to one another. This control is sometimes explicit, as when friends must have their contacts approved by an interdisciplinary team, when friends without disabilities are required to undergo some form of training as a condition of spending time with their friend, or when staff members are forbidden to invite a friend home for a meal because it would violate wage and hour regulations. Other times, control of access is less direct: people have no privacy, visits with friends are interrupted by program routines, messages get lost, or activities that require some cooperation from program staff break down because someone did not pass along the right permission slip or the van was re-routed.

One of the greatest powers service settings exercise is the power of definition. Staff define whom the person with a developmental disability is and what is good for him or her. They assert the right to say how it really is for a client. Often this process of definition reflects a preoccupation with finding fault in the person. A staff member describes a person with a developmental disability to the person's friend as manipulative, and cautions the friend against being "sucked into" or "feeding" the person's dependency. A staff member nods knowingly when a friend makes a positive comment about a person with a developmental disability and says sagely, "I thought that, too, when I first met her." A staff member discounts ideas about a positive future as "unrealistic" or "inappropriate for someone who functions at that level." A staff member passes along comments about syndromes and symptoms.

Even when service workers enthusiastically endorse a plan for change, the systems they work in often respond ineptly and painfully slowly. Months can pass between a victory in a planning meeting and the first hint of real change.

Friends have to decide how to respond to these expressions of power over the person with a disability. The person's continuing need for assistance makes this issue of power a complex problem. Some people with developmental disabilities fear offending the people they rely on. Some people without disabilities doubt their own perceptions when they run counter to professional judgments.

Friends may decide to push back. Nicola is a 21-year-old woman who attends a day program for people with developmental disabilities. A group of six of her friends, with whom she regularly shares a variety of social activities, reviewed her individualized program plan (IPP) together and wrote a letter to her IPP team that begins:

> It's Tuesday night and we're all together with Nic. In the pub. We have just read your report . . . with disbelief, we're not so sure that we are discussing the same person . . . We don't see Nic in the same light as you do, and we feel you need to see the Nic that we know, because otherwise we don't think Nic's best interests will be served.

Nicola's friends go on to make several concrete suggestions for assistance that they believe would be more relevant and better focus her strengths. The service system made no effective response to their comments.

The response from a threatened system can be much less benign. Working as a staff trainer in an institution, Rosemary Crossley discovered that several residents were able to communicate, given assistance by someone who cares about what they have to say. Rosemary's discovery created close, increasingly personal relationships between her and several of the young people involved, including Anne McDonald, who ultimately came to live with Rosemary and her partner (Crossley & McDonald, 1984). Her personal engagement led her to challenge the constraints of the institution in a number of ways, including: spending her free time with Anne and other residents; taking Anne home for weekends and holidays; creating techniques and materials to support further communication; feeding Anne and other residents; working the bureaucratic system for a variety of resources; and, ultimately, helping Anne get a lawyer to free her from the institution. From very early in their relationship, these activities threatened the institutional system, which reacted by invoking medical authority to publicly discredit Rosemary and her assertion that Anne and several other young people were able to think and communicate, demoting her, forbidding her to visit outside work hours, transferring her, and separating the group of young people involved. Elks (1990) helpfully analyzes the situation, as shown in Table 1, by contrasting the approach of Rosemary, a personally involved ally, with the institution's professional approach.

Negotiating Differences in Power

Power issues arise within any relationship. Questions between friends about how to make decisions, how to share resources and tasks, and how to deal with conflicts, which are common to all relationships, are sharper in a friendship between a person with a disability and a person without a developmental disability. This is because there is typically a power difference between the friends: one friend can come and go relatively freely and the other friend's time and movement may be under staff control, one friend may have more disposable income than the other, one friend may have transportation while the other does not, one friend may be seen by others as capable while the other is not, and one friend may feel confident about changing jobs or living places while the other is unable to do so. The person with less power usually sees and feels this difference more clearly than the more powerful person does. People without disabilities take for granted many small everyday powers that are privileges in the world of the person with a disability.

Table 1.   Contrast of the approaches of an ally and an institution

Dimension of difference	Personally involved ally	Institution professionals
Overriding concern	Quality of life	Efficiency of operation
Involvement	Personal, daily, all hours, hands on, informal	Professional consultation, formal, day appointments only
Assessment issues and standards of proof	Open to all, informal, commonsense, anecdotal, subjective	Professionals only, formal, scientific, controlled, objective
Sources of support and power	Friends, media, courts, independent professionals	Bureaucratic and professional authority, legislation
Preferred way to make change	Personal and direct response to needs	"Normal (official) channels"
Gender	Female	Male
Status	Low	High
Conceptualization of controversy	Civil rights versus institutional denial and obstruction	Professional judgment versus irrational and emotional lay opinion

From Flks, M (1990) Lessons from Annie's coming out. *National Council on Intellectual Disability: Interaction*, 4(1), 7–17; reprinted by permission.

When a person with a developmental disability needs regular physical or cognitive assistance from a friend, the friendship can be strained. One woman with a developmental disability said, "I liked my friend a lot, but I stopped calling her because she can't come to the group home because it's so noisy and so I was always having to ask her for rides." This kind of resource sharing is easier to resolve, once people bring it up, than the issues that arise when a person with a developmental disability has limited experience with relationships or a limited repertoire of expression, and treats his or her friend as if he or she were a staff person, a parent, or a servant.

Sometimes the friend with a developmental disability has very few ties and connections to anyone other than the friend without a disability. This isolation can leave the person who has a wider social network feeling like the person with a developmental disability wants more from the relationship than he or she can give. This problem is exaggerated when the friends embody their relationship in a narrow range of activities. As one man with a developmental disability put it, "We love the same football team. So some parts of the year we see each other all the time. Other parts of the year, I miss him a lot."

People with disabilities may strongly and repeatedly test their friends because their personal history makes trust crucial to them.

Anne McDonald risked her freedom and jeopardized Rosemary Crossley's credibility by refusing to cooperate with examinations that would prove her ability to communicate to outsiders. As she explained in a conversation with Rosemary after refusing to respond compliantly to an investigating magistrate's questions, "Stubbornness is both my salvation and my besetting sin. . . . If surviving depended on any characteristic it was stubbornness: not letting the bastards grind you down" (Crossley & McDonald, 1984, p. 239). Someone whose life experiences have not included living in an institution or living with continual discrimination may have difficulty comprehending these tests of trust for what they are—opportunities to deepen and strengthen the friendship.

Finally, friends can fail in their efforts to deal with injustice or achieve the cooperation necessary from others to move toward a better future. Failure can bring hurt, uncertainty, and even resentment. Friends without a disability may wonder if they have done enough. Friends with a disability may even feel that somehow they have let their friends down.

Signals of real differences in power between friends can make dealing with these hurts and conflicts harder. Anthropologist Mary Catherine Bateson (1988) observed the American people's discomfort with relationships that do not seem to be symmetrical:

> The ethical impulse in American culture is toward symmetry. . . . Nothing in our tradition gives interdependency a value comparable to symmetry. It is difference that makes interdependency possible, but we have difficulty valuing it because of the speed at which we turn it into inequality. This means that all of the relationships in which two people complement each other—complete each other, as their differences move them toward a shared wholeness—man and woman, artist and physician, builder and dreamer—are suspected of unfairness unless they can be reshaped into symmetrical collegiality. But symmetrical relationships and exchanges alone are limiting . . . . (pp. 104–105)

Real differences in power create the possibility that people with and without disabilities can transcend ordinary social patterns and develop a friendship that allows interdependence.

THE CONTEXT OF COMMUNITY

Within the larger context of community, there are at least two dimensions in which friendships between people with and without developmental disabilities can be viewed. Rather than an individualistic phenomenon between two people, classical and medieval thinkers saw friendship as an avenue both for the maturity of human beings and as a contribution to the whole community. The survival of any friendship between people with and without developmental disabilities may be more likely if that friendship is situated inside a larger community, such as a community of resistance.

Friendship as a Way to Human and Community Development

To sustain friendship through struggles with external constraints and internal contradictions, friends need a deeper way to understand friendship than many contemporary accounts offer. Friendship, especially friendship across a structural imbalance in power, requires endurance, discipline, and courage. American society tends to understand friendship individualistically and therapeutically, as something done primarily for the improvement of individuals (Bellah, Madsen, Sullivan, Swidler, & Tipton, 1985). In this view, friendships are not supposed to be a source of problems, but a means to achieve pleasure, relief, and personal betterment. Friendships are a private, individual matter, arising from the spontaneous feelings of the people involved. If the feelings turn bad, many people think the friendship is over. This may make one or both people sad, but nothing important is lost to anyone besides the friends. This way of understanding friendship offers little support for people who need to struggle with power issues in order to maintain their friendship.

In contrast, classical and medieval thinkers saw in friendship a way to mature as a community member. Friendship imposes disciplines worth mastering, both for one's own sake and the sake of one's community. In his lectures on friendship, Aristotle (1976) identifies friendship as the basis for effective government; as a foundation for practical knowledge of human affairs; and as a realization, a kind of harvest, of individual virtue—people become good in order to be worthy friends. He recognizes that "the wish for friendship develops rapidly, but friendship does not" (p. 264) and says that people must spend time together, over time, to develop knowledge and trust. He measures friendship in terms of the number of meals people eat together, allowing that friends will not know each other well until they have eaten a "bushel-and-a-half of salt" together.

Ailred (1942), Abbot of Rievaulx in the mid-12th century, saw friendship as a way to strengthen a whole community and to deepen spirituality by directly experiencing, through moments in the friendship, an image of the divine. Thus, he saw friendship as worthy of working at and teaching about once a person has the experience of friendship to draw on. He distinguishes childish friendship, which is based on calculation of mutual advantage or a fantasy of the friend's perfection, from mature friendship. Mature friendship begins when the friends live through disillusionment with one another. Ailred teaches that an extended period of what he calls "probation" is an essential stage of mature friendship. In this stage, friends test one another to try the other's trust. One result of this testing is that a friend can perform one of the central duties of friendship: giving criticism that upholds the ideals that the friends share in the context of mutual respect and affection. Ailred counsels that friendship should not be dissolved lightly, only because of betrayal of the friendship itself.

These ideas seem a bit odd to people accustomed to thinking about friendship in individualistic terms, but they provide a corrective for some of the negative effects of individualism on friendships. Ailred's idea is that older people in a community have a duty to instruct younger people in friendship, first by example, as well as by providing advice, encouragement, and teaching, and by insisting that the whole community work to achieve the civility necessary to support friends as they struggle. Aristotle's idea is that friendship is not just a private matter between individuals, but that the positive effects of friends working to stay together for the long haul are a key resource to the whole community. Most people do not live in a world as physically small as the Athenian *polis* or the Cistercian monastery, and most people would not want to; however, the men who formed these places have some important lessons for people trying to make friends today. If people think about what these philosophers had to say, they will remember: friendship is not just spontaneous; it is intentional, involving duties and virtues that are worth working to develop. In addition, friendship is not just for the self-improvement of individuals, it contributes to the good of a community.

Communities of Resistance

Friendships between people with and without disabilities are unlikely alliances, not because people are unable to attract and enjoy one another, but because of difficulties imposed on making and keeping relationships by the social construction of developmental disability. Dealing with the consequences of beliefs that justify the social exclusion and therapeutic control of people with developmental disabilities is far more than a two-person job. To survive effectively in a fragmented society with little room for people with developmental disabilities, friends may need to make a conscious choice to situate their friendship within a community of resistance.

A community of resistance is simply a group of people who, among other shared interests, recognize the negative effects of common beliefs and practices on their friendships and their friends and support one another to get on with their lives. They contradict the notion that friendships must be purely private, exclusive, and only one to one (Hunt, 1991).

For instance, Judith Snow, Jack Pearpoint, and Marsha Forest sustain their 14-year friendship by reaching out to include people in their friendship (see Pearpoint, 1990). They purposely seek people who join them in celebrating diversity and, therefore, counter the notion that there is something odd or saintly about them. They purposely seek individuals who will join them to fight the injustice of systems that divide and violate people. They purposely seek people with whom they can have a good time. Their friendships are not compartmentalized and separated from the rest of their lives, but complex and mixed-up with their whole lives. Each is friends with the other and each has other friends, but their constellation of friendships is more than permutations of one-to-one relationships. The power of such a complex web of friendships can be considerable. It has sustained Judith's system of personal assistance against repeated bureaucratic attempts to standardize her out of existence, it has energized a large network of people committed to inclusive education, it has supported Jack and Marsha in their transition from ordinary job roles to the uncertainties of working freelance for social change, and it has given them all a good deal of pleasure.

A community of resistance creates and gives life to a story that counters the dominant social beliefs that devalue the community's members and their relationships (Welch, 1990). This story relieves its members of the debilitating fear that there is something crazy or foolish about their friendship. As the lore grows about how its members have responded to challenges, the community's story guides and sustains action.

A community of resistance contains the hurts of its members, hurts that are too big for two individuals to hold between themselves alone. If it is to sustain real people, such a community cannot promise to fix its members or magically remove their pains with some technique. Indeed, Jean Vanier (1992) points out that community develops out of people's willingness to walk with one another in their shared weakness as well as their strength. "Community is the place where are revealed all the darkness and anger, jealousies and rivalry hidden in our hearts" (p. 29). People do not need to be perfect to hold one another's hurts, they simply need to be willing to listen, to look for ways to act together when action makes sense, and to find ways to bear with each other when action does not help.

In the context of a community of resistance, people will be able to deepen the attraction that draws them together, regardless of disability; they will be able to work against the barriers to embodying their friendships; and they will be able to struggle creatively with the power issues that arise around and between them. By so doing, they will contribute to a modest revolution built of the daily activities of people who are unlikely allies against the beliefs and practices that make friendships difficult. As the community of resistance to the separation of people with developmental disabilities grows, more people will be able to realize the promise of meeting the challenge posed by Robert Williams (1989) as he speaks on behalf of the people he has come to know in his work as an advocate with people in institutions.

Look deep,
deep into the hearts of
my people:

Witness their horror,
Witness their pain.

Horror and pain
your spoken words alone
will never soothe.

Do not try to explain it away,
they will never believe you . . .

Gallant and gaunt, their beauty.

Beauty,
your spoken words can never
capture. (p. 19)

REFERENCES

Ailred of Rievaulx. (1942). *Christian friendship*. (H. Talbot, Trans.). London: The Catholic Book Club.

Anderson, J., Lakin, K.C., Hill, B.K., & Chen, T. (1992). Social integration of older persons with mental retardation in residential facilities. *American Journal on Mental Retardation, 96*(5), 488–501.

Aristotle. (1976). *The ethics of Aristotle: The Nicomachean ethics, Books 8–9*. (J. Thomson & H. Tredennick., Trans.) London: Penguin Press.

Atkinson, D. (1986). Engaging competent others: A study of the support networks of people with mental handicap. *British Journal of Social Work, 16*, Supplement, 83–101.

Atkinson, D., & Williams, F. (Eds.). (1990). *Know me as I am: An anthology of prose, poetry and art by people with learning difficulties*. London: Hodder & Stoughton.

Barnes, C. (1990). *'Cabbage syndrome': The social construction of dependence*. London: Falmer.

Bateson, M.C. (1988). *Composing a life.* New York: Atlantic Monthly Press.

Bellah, R., Madsen, R., Sullivan, W., Swidler, A., & Tipton, S. (1985). *Habits of the heart: Individualism and commitment in American life.* Berkeley, CA: University of California Press.

Berkson, G., & Romer, D. (1981). A letter to a developmental disabilities administrator. In R. Bruininks, C.E. Meyers, B. Sigford, & K.C. Lakin (Eds.), *Deinstitutionalization and community adjustment of mentally retarded people.* AAMR Monograph, No. 4. Washington, DC: AAMR.

Benviniste, E. (1973). *Indo-European language and society.* Coral Gables, FL: University of Florida Press.

Bevilacqua, C. (1992, May). Poetry by students using facilitated communication. *TASH Newsletter, 16*(5), 6.

Biklen, D. (1990). Communication unbound: Autism and praxis. *Harvard Educational Review, 60*(3), 291–314.

Biklen, D. (1992). *Schooling without labels: Parents, educators, and inclusive education.* Philadelphia: Temple University Press.

Bogdan, R., & Taylor, S. (1987). Toward a sociology of acceptance: The other side of the study of deviance. *Social Policy, 18,* 34–39.

Bogdan, R., & Taylor, S. (1989). Relationships with severely disabled people: The social construction of humanness. *Social Problems, 36*(2), 135–148.

Booth, W. (1988). *The company we keep: An ethics of fiction.* Berkeley, CA: University of California Press.

Crossley, R., & McDonald, A. (1984). *Annie's coming out* (rev. ed.). Ringwood, Victoria: Penguin Books Australia.

Dickinson, E. (1951). "#1336." In The complete poems of Emily Dickinson. Boston: Little Brown.

Easterling, P. (1989). Friendship and the Greeks. In R. Porter & S. Tomaselli (Eds.), *The dialectics of friendship.* New York: Routledge.

Edgerton, R. (1988). Aging in the community: A matter of choice. *American Journal on Mental Retardation, 92*(4), 331–335.

Edgerton, R. (1991). Conclusion. In R.B. Edgerton & M.A. Gaston (Eds.), *"I've seen it all!": Lives of older persons with mental retardation in the community* (pp. 268–273). Baltimore: Paul H. Brookes Publishing Co.

Elks, M. (1990). Lessons from Annie's Coming Out. *National Council on Intellectual Disability: Interaction, 4*(1), 7–17.

Evans, D. (1983). *The lives of mentally retarded people.* Boulder, CO: Westview.

Firth, H., & Rapley, M. (1990). *From acquaintance to friendship: Issues for people with learning disabilities.* Kidderminster, Worcester: British Institute of Mental Handicap Publications.

Flynn, M. (1991). *Moving On 2: Report from a conference of service users exploring friendship.* London: National Development Team for People with Learning Difficulties.

Glouberman, S. (1990). *Keepers: Inside stories from total institutions.* London: King Edward's Hospital Fund for London.

Heilbrun, C. (1988). *Writing a woman's life.* New York: Norton.

Heumann, J. (1993). A disabled woman's reflections: Myths and realities of integration. In J.A. Racino, P. Walker, S. O'Connor, & S.J. Taylor (Eds.), *Housing, support, and community: Choices and strategies for adults with disabilities* (pp. 233–249). Baltimore: Paul H. Brookes Publishing Co.

Hill, B., Rotegard, L., & Bruininks, R. (1984). Quality of life of mentally retarded people in residential care. *Social Work, 29,* 275–281.

Hunt, M.E. (1991). *Fierce tenderness: A feminist theology of friendship.* New York: Crossroad.

Kegan, R. (1982). *The evolving self: Problem and process in human development.* Cambridge, MA: Harvard University Press.

Landesman-Dwyer, S., Berkson, G., & Romer, D. (1979). Affiliation and friendship of mentally retarded residents in group homes. *American Journal of Mental Deficiency, 83*(6), 571–580.

Lasch, C. (1978). *The culture of narcissism.* New York: Norton.

Lutfiyya, Z. (1989). *The phenomenology of relationships between typical and disabled people.* Doctoral dissertation, Syracuse University, Syracuse, NY.

Lutfiyya, Z. (1990). *Affectionate bonds: What we can learn by listening to friends.* Syracuse, NY: Center on Human Policy, Syracuse University.

MacAndrew, C., & Edgerton, R. (1966). On the possibility of friendship. *American Journal of Mental Deficiency, 70,* 612–621.

McFague, S. (1987). *Models of God: Theology for an ecological, nuclear age.* Philadelphia: Fortress Press.

Ordinary Life Group. (1988). *Ties and connections: An ordinary community life for people with learning difficulties.* London: King's Fund Centre.

Oswin, M. (1992). *Am I allowed to cry? A study of bereavement amongst people who have learning difficulties.* London: Souvenir Press (Educational & Academic).

Pealer, J., & O'Brien, J. (1985). *Personal relationships for people with developmental disabilities.* Proceedings of a Conference on Informal Support. Columbus, OH: Ohio Society for Autistic Citizens.

Pearpoint, J. (1990). *From behind the piano: The building of Judith Snow's unique circle of friends.* Toronto: Inclusion Press.

Perske, R. (1988). *Circles of friends: People with disabilities and their friends enrich the lives of one another.* Nashville, TN: Abingdon Press.

Plato (1979). The *Lysis.* In D. Bolotin (Ed.), *Plato's dialogue on friendship: An interpretation of the* Lysis *with a new translation.* Ithaca, NY: Cornell University Press.

Raymond, J. (1986). *A passion for friends: Toward a philosophy of female affection.* Boston: Beacon Press.

Richardson, A., & Ritchie, J. (1989). *Developing friendships: Enabling people with learning difficulties to make and maintain friends.* London: Policy Studies Institute.

Schwier, K.M. (1990). *Speakeasy: People with mental handicaps talk about their lives in institutions and in the community.* Austin, TX: PRO-ED.

Strully, J., & Strully, C. (1985). Friendship and our children. *Journal of The Association for Persons with Severe Handicaps, 10*(4), 224–227.

Strully, J., & Strully, C. (1989). Friendships as an educational goal. In S. Stainback, W. Stainback, & M. Forest (Eds.), *Educating all students in the mainstream of regular education* (pp. 59–68). Baltimore: Paul H. Brookes Publishing Co.

Taylor, C. (1991). *The malaise of modernity.* (CBC Massey lecture series, 1991). Concord, Ontario: Anansi Press.

Taylor, S., & Bogdan, R. (1989). On accepting relationships between people with mental retardation and non-disabled people: Towards an understanding of acceptance. *Disability, Handicap & Society, 4*(1), 21–36.

Vanier, J. (1992). *From brokenness to community.* The Wit Lectures, Harvard Divinity School. New York: Paulist Press.

Welch, S. (1990). *A feminist ethic of risk*. Minneapolis: Augsberg Fortress Press.

Welty, E., & Sharp, R. (1991). *The Norton book of friendship*. New York: Norton.

Williams, P. (1977). *Our mutual handicap*. London: Campaign for the Mentally Handicapped.

Williams, R. (1989). *In a struggling voice. The selected poems of Robert Williams*. Washington, DC: Author. (Available from The Association for Persons with Severe Handicaps (TASH), 7010 Roosevelt Way, N.E., Seattle, WA 96115 (206) 523-8446.)

Wolfensberger, W. (1975). *The origin and nature of our institutional models*. Syracuse, NY: Human Policy Press.

Wolfensberger, W. (1991). *A brief introduction to social role valorization as a high-order concept for structuring human services*. Syracuse, NY: Training Institute for Human Service Planning, Syracuse University.

Worth, P. (1990, July). Presentation to The Summer Institute on Inclusive Education, McGill University Faculty of Education, Montreal, Quebec.

3

Gift and Call

Recovering the
Spiritual Foundations of Friendships

Bill Gaventa

Theologian C.S. Lewis (1960), in his classic book, *The Four Loves*, notes that friendship was the most human of loves in the ancient world; yet, it is by and large ignored in the modern world. If, however, the ancients were right, he says, one "can hardly write a chapter on it except as rehabilitation" (p. 57).

The basic premise of this chapter is similar. Until recently, friendship has been ignored in both theory and practice within the world of developmental disabilities. Friends, even in the form of volunteers, have been seen as nice but not necessary, more unusual than usual. Individual growth and development has meant movement up a career ladder, one that depends on the acquisiton of skills rather than the acquisition of friends. As in a modern, mobile society, personal success in growth and development has been more important than ongoing relationships, ties, and bonds with friends and family. Yet, as the phenomenon of friendship has emerged as a key component in assisting people with developmental disabilities to become part of community life, caregivers and advocates cannot begin to explore the importance, meaning, and experience of friendship without a fundamental "rehabilitation" of the way they view their "clients," systems of care, and roles as professionals and caregivers in the context of community life.

Part of the professional struggle is caused by the fact that as the importance of friendship in community living is validated, professionals are pushed to look at ways that the power of friendship has been evident all along, either in its presence or absence. I expect that my experience is not much different from that of many other professionals. Many of us have had the experience of working in segregated caregiving facilities where the greatest tragedy has not been the disabilities of the persons served, but their separation from any opportunities for ongoing friendships with others. Limited numbers of staff, even with skills and commitment, could not fulfill the overwhelming needs for friendship. There are "clients" whose demeanor changes when they are lucky enough to receive a visit or a phone call from a friend. Lives change when a friendship develops where previously there had been none. Institutional "residents" continually request and enjoy songs and music that speak of friendship and love, such as "God is my friend," or "Jesus loves me." People who began as volunteers have become genuine friends, establishing bonds that are not easily explainable other than by saying the relationship is a gift to them, and that it answers a deep call within them to something very important in their own lives. I have personally struggled with a professional role in which I knew I was the only friend for many people, and in which I have seen other staff members and caregivers also form deep friendships with "clients"; yet, our work was in a system where the "program" rather than the "person" was paramount.

Only recently have we begun to talk about the gifts and positive attributes of people with developmental disabilities, partially in response to the research that has been done by the Turnbulls at the Beach Center on Disabilities in Kansas, which allows parents and friends to talk about the "positive contributions" made to their family, class, or community. We have just begun to be honest enough to talk about the gifts that persons with disabilities bring to "professionals." We have also just begun to talk about values and vision, and are taking steps toward describing the spirit that drives and motivates us in our work (i.e., our understanding of mission, vocation, and call).

This process of rehabilitation compels professionals to re-examine personal assumptions, beliefs, and experiences of friendship. It calls for a search for those voices in the present and past who can help to explain the transforming power of friendships that has been witnessed in the lives of people who are called "clients" and "consumers," but whom professionals seldom permit or allow themselves to call "friends." In short, it pushes us to examine what we believe about friendship, the reasons for its absence in professional literature and practice, and the challenge to change. No wonder the topic has been avoided; the concept and experience of friendship lay claim to understandings of person, policy, and practice in ways like no other.

The purpose of this chapter is to summarize some of the ways that "friendship" has been understood, both in spiritual and philosophical traditions. (This discussion is limited by the fact that most of my experience and research, and probably that of most readers, is around issues of friendship in the context of a western classical and Judeo-Christian tradition. The rich understandings of friendship and community in eastern, Native American, and African traditions awaits other research and interpreters.) On that foundation, how can this system of care be understood and critized? As "community" becomes a clearer vision and experience, how are caregivers called upon to reframe, or perhaps recover, their understanding of their vocation as "professionals" who are friends and enablers of friendships? Finally, some helpful strategies are discussed for working with the religious community, in the form of local congregations, to facilitate the development of friendships between people with developmental disabilities and congregational members. Throughout, my hope is that caregivers can recover the rich traditions of understanding friendship in the context of both gift and call.

HISTORICAL FOUNDATIONS

As the field of developmental disabilities has become more aware of the importance of friends and friendships, even if it is by first noting their absence, much of the focus has been on the importance of friendship as a relationship characterized by mutual enjoyment, reciprocity, and acceptance in contrast to relationships in which a person is continually a "client" or "consumer" and is constantly being treated, programmed, or fixed (Lutfiyya, 1988). There is, therefore, an understanding of two of the three basic elements of friendship in the classic philosophical and Judeo-Christian traditions:

1. Friends enjoy each other's company (an acceptance and appreciation of gifts).
2. Friends are useful to each other (reciprocity).

The third component in those traditions is the moral or spiritual dimension of friendship, the sharing of a common commitment to the good, that which forms the basis of a good life or a good society (Bellah, Madsen, Sullivan, Swidler, & Tipton, 1985). The current theoretical and practical work in the system of care with persons with disabilities to clarify what is "good," "valuable," and "quality," especially in the context of a caregiving, inclusive community, leads us directly into a renewed dialogue with these classic understandings of the moral and spiritual dimensions of friendship.

The Classical Tradition

In classic essays on friendship by Plato, Aristotle, Cicero, Augustine, Bacon, Montaigne, and others, friendship (*philos* in Greek) was viewed as the most important of all human forms of love (Lewis, 1960) and

the most "instinctual natural basis for all positive social relationships" (Graham, 1990). Friendship was associated not only with mutual love and usefulness, but also with the development of a virtuous
life. Friends were needed to help understand the purpose for which
life had been given (Waddell, 1989).

Friendship, or *philos*, differed from other forms of love, while at the
same time retaining some of their elements. Its mutuality made it
different from altruism or charity, which implies a giving to others
that is not necessarily reciprocated. Although friendship may have
had sexual dimensions, it was not primarily sexual, and therefore, it
was not sexual love (*eros*). It also was not the same as affection, such
as the care of a parent for a child. Because friendship is by definition a
relationship with particular others, indicating a preference, it was not
agape, an understanding of love that is universal, inclusive, and sacrificial. These distinctions are important differences that form part of
the historical uneasiness of professional caregiving with the concept
and experience of friendship.

C.S. Lewis notes that friendship in classical thought was the most
"human" of all loves because it was "the least natural of loves; the
least instinctive, organic, biological, gregarious, and necessary" (Lewis,
p. 56.). Sam Keen (1983) describes that same difference between
friendship and other forms of relationships in a way that brings this
philosophical discussion into a modern context:

> Friendship exists as a sanctuary that is situated between the private
> world of the family, the ambiguities of sexual love, and the public
> world . . . Friendship is a sanctuary precisely because within it we
> may be *more* than, and *different* from, the destiny we must wrestle
> with in the family, or roles we must assume to enter the contrac-
> tual order of civility . . . Friendship also sets us free, for a moment,
> from the sweet burden of sexuality. (p. 215)

In classic Greek philosophy, the dilemmas of friendship focused
not around sexuality, but around the relationship between teacher
and student. The question was whether or not "good men" needed
friends. The answer was that friendship was necessary to understand
and participate in the universal values (Hunter, 1990). Its characteristics of mutuality, acceptance, and reciprocity did not mean an unconditional acceptance that led to an abandonment of moral standards
(Bellah et al., 1985). Instead, particular friendships led one beyond
oneself to the nature of that which was universally good. Therefore,
Aristotle would say, "No one would choose to live without friends,
even if he had all other goods" (Meilander, 1981, p. 13).

In classic traditions, then, friendship was a great gift and treasure, but also an imperative. It was not simply a source of mutual pleasure that differed from other more "natural" pleasures. Whereas a key dimension was reciprocity, or mutual usefulness, Bellah and his associates (1985) point out that friendship was not solely a utilitarian tool for developing economic success and power (e.g., *How to Win Friends and Influence People*) or individual well-being and health (i.e., modern therapy) (pp. 118–135). It was instead, a pathway to the understanding of truth and knowledge about oneself, one's community, and the meaning and purpose of life. In C.S. Lewis's words, friendships are "about something," a seeing or caring about a common truth (p. 61).

The Biblical Tradition

At the risk of being too simplistic, one could summarize the classical philosophical view of friendship as important because it was necessary for an understanding of universal values and truth. In the biblical tradition, friendship reveals the grace, love, and call of a caring God. In the classical view, friendship was a human pathway to the universal or divine. In the biblical tradition, it is a pathway of the divine to humankind, a gift of grace that calls for human response.

This discussion will not pretend that there is a single biblical understanding of friendship. As opposed to a single understanding, there is rather a rich weaving of biblical stories, traditions, and themes that relate to friendship. Friendship is rarely used in the Bible as a description of the relationship between the human and the divine. God is not often called a "friend," but rather human friendships reveal many of the characteristics of God's love for humankind. Nor do the various expressions of the divine voice in the Bible describe human beings as God's friends, except for some significant exceptions that will be described. The more common metaphors used for the relationship of God and humans are those of creator, Lord, and parent (usually images of father, but sometimes of "mother"). Humans are not called to be God's friends, but rather to love and befriend others as a way of responding to the gift of God's creation and love. Thus, friendships are one of the expressions of God's grace, a grace that compels the reciprocal actions of both loving God and loving God through loving others.

Rather than a single understanding of friendship, there are a number of biblical themes that relate to friendship as ways of both describing God's love and grace for humankind and as a response to that gift in love and service. These themes include the following:

1. We are created in God's image for relationship.
2. In the acceptance of friendship, we see a vision of God's acceptance of us.
3. In the steadfastness of friendship, we see a vision of God's faithfulness to humankind and ongoing covenant with us.
4. We are called to love others in the same way God has loved us (i.e., through a sacrificial, universal, and inclusive love).
5. We are called to love and serve through the gift of hospitality, the grace of befriending a stranger in ways that see and/or find (as in number 1 of this list) the image of God in every person.

Each of these dimensions needs to be described in more detail to relate them to biblical understandings of friendship. There are significant differences with some of the classical understandings of friendship, especially in the biblical understanding of love as agape, a love that attempts to mirror God's love for humankind. However, there are also great similarities between the biblical and classical views because the spiritual views of friendships in the biblical tradition also describe the experience of friendship as treasure and moral imperative (i.e., as gift and call).

Created in God's Image for Relationship   The basic value of humankind comes from the very fact and gift of creation. Every person is created, in biblical understanding, in the image of God, and called into a relationship with God and others. The two great commandments in the biblical tradition are the call to love God and the call to love your neighbor as yourself (Deut. 6:5, Lev. 19:18, Luke 10:27, Matt. 22:37–40). Not only is the act of creation an act of God's love and grace, but, also in the biblical tradition, God over and over again reaches out and redeems humankind because of that relationship:

> But now thus says the Lord, he who created you, O Jacob, he who formed you, O Israel: Fear not, for I have redeemed you; I have called you by name and you are mine . . . Because you are precious in my eyes, and honored, and I will love you. (Isa. 43:1,4)

The first biblical answer to the "Why?" of friendship and love is that we have been given value by virtue of our creation, not because of our abilities or accomplishments, and are thus called to see that value in every person. John Landgraf (1989) describes this sense of love and friendship in this way:

> I love you. This means "I perceive you to be precious," infinitely worthful, priceless. No matter what kind of body you may have, no matter what kind of mind you may have, no matter what kind of talent you may have, no matter what kind of performance you put

on. None of these has anything to do with the fact—and it is a fact
—that you are precious. You are precious simply because you *are*,
whatever your equipment and however you may use it. You were
born that way—created in the image of God and given life by the
breath of God. To see that and be grasped by the reality of it is to
love. (p. 3)

Friendship as a Mirror of God's Love and Acceptance   Much of
the human importance of friendship simply comes from the gift of
acceptance, which comes from a friend. A friend is someone who
loves and accepts another unconditionally. In the face of a person feeling unworthy, unloved, and/or lonely (or, as more commonly expressed in the field of developmental disabilities, devalued, stig-
matized, labeled, or isolated), the gift of friendship provides first of all
acceptance of the other person; indeed, on the basis of being created
in God's image, it provides celebration of the other.

In biblical stories, we are simply called to love with that kind of
acceptance because God first loved us (1 John: 4:11). Acceptance of
another as friend, or by another who is our friend, is a gift not of our
control and doing, but an expression or evidence of God's acceptance
of us. Images of that acceptance include: God's choosing of a people;
the importance of the Lord's house as sanctuary; affirmations of
God's presence wherever one goes (Psalm 23); and what is known as
the Golden Rule, being called not only to give what we have been
given, but to "do unto others what we would have them do unto us."
We cannot say that we love God and then hate our neighbor (1 John
4:20). In both the Old and New Testaments, God's choosing, freeing,
and saving of the people are evidence of God's acceptance and commitment not because of human accomplishments or abilities, but
usually in spite of them. We are saved, not by works, but by grace.

Friendship as Covenant   "A faithful friend is a sure shelter, whoever finds one has found a rare treasure. A faithful friend is something
beyond price, and there is no measuring his worth. A faithful friend is
the elixir of life" (Eccles. 6:14–16). In the Bible, friends are both faithful and unfaithful. Job complains bitterly to friends that they have
vanished, scorned him, failed him, or, like God, pursued him. In
times of trouble, writes a Psalmist, "my friends and companions
stand aloof from my plague, and my kinsmen stand afar off" (Psalms
38:11). Friends can be too quickly tied to wealth (Prov. 19:6-7), and the
wrong friends (e.g., friendship with an "angry man") can lead a person astray (Prov. 22:24) and quickly deceive (Jer. 38:22). But, as the
writer of Proverbs says, "There are friends who pretend to be friends,
but there is a friend who sticks closer than a brother" (Prov. 18:24).

Therefore, a faithful friend is a sure shelter. "Your friend, and your father's friend, do not forsake, and do not go to your brother's house in the day of your calamity. Better is a neighbor who is near than a brother who is far away" (Prov. 27:10).

Throughout the Bible, it is God's faithfulness that is evidence of God's commitment to a relationship. The relationship is one of covenant, a promise of continual and ongoing presence if God's commandments are obeyed. In true friendship, as in covenant, there is a sense both of choosing and being chosen. The choosing and faithfulness imply and build the kind of bond that is at the heart of an everlasting friendship. The few times that an individual is called "God's friend" in the Bible are used to point to the eternal nature of God's covenant:

> Didst thou not, O God, drive the inhabitants out, and give it forever to the descendants of Abraham thy friend? (2 Chron. 20:6)

> Israel, Jacob, the offspring of Abraham my friend, you whom I took from the ends of the earth, saying "You are my servant, I have chosen you and will not cast you off. Fear not, for I am with you, be not dismayed, I am your God. I will strengthen you, I will uphold you." (Isa. 41:8–10)

> Abraham, called the friend of God. (James 2:23)

> Thus the Lord used to speak to Moses, face to face, as a man speaks to his friend. (Exod. 33:11)

Loving Others as God Loves Us: The Challenge of Universal Love
In the New Testament, there is only one place where Jesus calls his disciples friends, but it is a passage that is central to Christian understanding of friendship as a response to God's love and choosing of humankind, as well as a measure of the vulnerabilty and self-disclosure of the relationship:

> This is my commandment, that you love one another as I have loved you. Greater love has no man than this, that a man lay down his life for his friends. You are my friends if you do what I command you. No longer do I call you servants, for the servant does not know what his master is doing; but I have called you friends, for all that I have heard from my Father I have made known to you. You did not choose me, but I chose you and appointed you so that you should go and bear fruit and that your fruit should abide; so whatever you ask the Father in my name, he may give it to you. This I command you, to love one another. (John 15:12-17)

This passage and many others in the New Testament point to the sacrificial, risk-taking character of God's love for humankind, a tradition that continues the Old Testament themes of God's refusal to give up on the people of God in spite of the anguish they may have caused. The call to love others in ways that risk one's own well being (agape) is a call to love others in the same radical, impartial, universal, and inclusive way that God has loved. "When you give a feast, don't invite friends and neighbors, lest they invite you, and you be repaid. But when you give a feast, invite the poor, the maimed, the lame, the blind, and you will be blessed" (Luke 14:12). The call to love in this way is sometimes a call to paradox, that in giving one receives, and in losing one's life, it is found. It is a call beyond the usual boundaries to love one's neighbor; as in the parable of the Good Samaritan, it is a call to love wherever or whomever that turns out to be. It is the call to love in the way that one loves a friend willingly at a cost to himself or herself.

The Gift of Hospitality: The Challenge of Particular Love   "The task of all life is to make of every enemy a friend, and of every stranger a neighbor" (Menachem Begin, Camp David [reprinted in Ripple, 1980, p. 25]). At the heart of all three major western religions (i.e., Christianity, Judaism, and Islam) is an injunction to welcome the stranger in the act of hospitality (Palmer, 1986). It is through the act of hospitality that the host creates a space where a stranger feels welcome and accepted in a way that gives to others the same kind of sanctuary that the host has received. However, the paradox in the three traditions is that the gift is not just from the host to the stranger because in welcoming the stranger, the host is often the one who receives. The stranger turns out to be a messenger or a revelation from God. The angels appear to Abraham as the strangers. The disciples welcome the stranger on the road to Emmaeus. "As you did it to the least of these, so you did it unto me" (Matt. 25). "Do not neglect to show hospitality to strangers, for thereby some have entertained angels unaware" (Hebrews 13:3). The stranger can be the leper, the child, the blind man, the woman at the well—anyone unknown and/ or thought to be beyond the scope of God's people and love. The call to hospitality to the stranger turns out to be a gift for everyone involved.

As stated earlier, the call to hospitality in the scriptural tradition also brings one back full circle to being prepared and ready to see and welcome God's spirit or image that is in every person. Part of the importance of hospitality as one of the dimensions of friendship and love in the Bible is that it balances the challenge of universal love with the specificity of particular people. To love equally, fairly, justly, and universally, as God loves everyone, is a challenge that can overwhelm and lead, paradoxically, to a disengagement and distance from others.

In the next section, the way that the call to universal love has affected professional caregiving and friendship is discussed. The gift and call to hospitality remains one of the biblical traditions that pulls us back to the stories of a universal and just God who acts in specific, limited, and particular relationships. It is also a way of describing how, in the gift of friendship, the sum often feels much greater than the parts:

> The Friendship is not a reward for our discrimination and good taste in finding one another out. It is the instrument by which God reveals to each the beauties of all the others. They are no greater than the beauties of a thousand other men; by Friendship God opens our eyes to them. They are, like all beauties, derived from Him, and then, in a good Friendship, increased by Him through the Friendship itself—so that it is His instrument for creating as well as for revealing. At this feast it is He who has spread the board and it is He who has chosen the guests. It is He, we may dare to hope, who sometimes does, and always should, preside. Let us not reckon without our Host. (Lewis, 1960, p. 83)

The Classical and
Biblical Foundations—Dilemma or Paradox?

On one level, there are profound differences between classical understandings of friendship (*philos*) and biblical understandings of love and friendship (*agape*). In the classical philosophical traditions, particular friendships were formed by mutual attraction and reciprocal relationships. They were seen as necessary for development, growth, change, and for understanding the true values of the society and universe.

In biblical understandings, good friendships were an expression of God's grace and love, a way, as C.S. Lewis described earlier in this chapter, of creating and revealing. The major difference from the classical traditions was in the call to love your neighbor, the call to universal, sacrificial love, which was just as important, if not more so, than the gift of friendship. *Agape* was a way of expressing and showing God's universal, self-giving love for every person. Thus, to celebrate particular friendships seems, at first, to be preferential in ways that God is not. Meilander (1981) summarizes that historical debate succinctly by noting, "When streams of classical thought about friendship and the Christian teaching of *agape* flow together, the ideal of particular friendship becomes haunted by the requirements of universal love" (p. 7). Campbell (1985) captures the dilemma with this picture: "Outside the warm circle of personal friendship there is the needy neighbor who is also the Christ. *Agape*, Christian love, perpetually unsettles us in the name of a greater peace" (p. 15).

Therefore, understandings of *agape* historically form part of the understanding of what today constitutes good "professional care," in that caring and loving others must be done impartially, and, at best, demonstrate a sacrificial service to others (Campbell, 1985; Meilander, 1981). One who "professes to serve" is to love others equally as God loves all, and to give without thought of mutuality and reciprocity because that is a demonstration of the gift of grace in God's first and ongoing love of humankind.

In the call to *agape*, the seeds can be seen as a kind of caring that detaches from personal relationships that appear to be preferential. This theological theory matches the historical reality that the concept "profession" first meant to separate one's self from family and friends to serve God, and that the practical reality of loving everyone equally with the same kind of self-giving love demonstrated by God is a human impossibility. The historical seeds of understanding caregiving as charity can also be seen because people were to give to others without thought of reciprocity or mutuality. Hence, a person called to serve was called to benefit others. This sense of caregiving also makes it hard for the caregiver to see the person served as a friend, even when there is a profound awareness of mutuality and reciprocity in the relationship. Friends do benefit each other, but the role of "benefactor" in a friendship is awkward and, as C.S. Lewis (1960) says, "accidental, even a little alien, and embarrassing" (p. 66). The importance of listening to the historical discussions of these questions in light of current discussions of the beneficial and harmful effects of "charity" in the context of community and friendship is captured by a fascinating quote by Jeremy Taylor in an essay on friendship in 1847: "When friendship was the noblest thing on earth, charity was little" (Meilander, 1981, p. 2).

The two historical strands of understanding the spiritual foundations of friendship would, therefore, appear to lead in opposite directions—one that celebrates particular, preferential friendships and one in which the call to love is not preferential or even necessarily mutual. As seen in the earlier discussion of biblical dimensions of friendship, however, the dilemma is more paradoxical than contradictory. The call to universal love or friendship is to be acted out in the context of hospitality to particular neighbors or strangers, in which the sense of gift and of giving becomes profoundly reciprocal, and the bond that recognizes, accepts, and celebrates inherent value in one another as part of God's creation and covenant is profoundly mutual. Therefore, in the biblical tradition, particular friendships both demonstrate the valuing, choosing, accepting, and welcoming qualities of God's steadfast relationship with humankind and challenge or call us to share that gift with others.

More important than the dilemma or the paradox is the similarity between classical and biblical understandings of the spiritual qualities of friendship. Although each uses different words and concepts, both focus on the importance of friendship as gift and grace, a celebration of mutual enjoyment, acceptance, usefulness, reciprocity, and caring that is different from other human relationships. There is always, as Amado, Conklin, and Wells (1990) say in *Friends*, a sense of magic or a feeling that something in the friendship is greater than the sum of its parts. In addition to being felt as gift, grace, or magic, the second fundamental spiritual foundation of friendship in both the classical and biblical traditions is that it calls us beyond and out of ourselves to new understandings of ourselves, others, community, and God. The question then becomes how those rich traditions of philosophical and spiritual understandings of friendship inform our newfound awareness as professionals, advocates, and caregivers of the importance of friendship. Paradoxically, the question may just be the reverse: is our newfound awareness of the importance of friendship leading to a sometimes hesitant recovering of the spiritual foundaions of friendship that challenge the way we understand ourselves in caregiving relationships and communities?

LIVING OUT OF GIFT AND CALL: THE CHALLENGE OF FRIENDSHIP FOR PROFESSIONAL CAREGIVERS

Looking at the Present Through Ancient Eyes

Given the preceding summary of the historical understandings of the spiritual foundations of friendship, it is no wonder that friendship is both a concept and experience that challenges current systems of care and current understanding of the role of caregivers. First and foremost, if friendship is as fundamental and important a human need as proposed by both philosophical and scriptural traditions, it has been a need that has certainly been overlooked, unappreciated, and/or devalued in the field of human services. At one level, segregated facilities and services have too often made friendships improbable, impossible, and/or unacknowledged. However, as friendship has received growing attention because of its importance as a key to integration or inclusion in community life, affirmation of its importance is often reluctant in the field because it challenges the understanding of caregiving roles at so many levels.

If, for example, a person asks about friendship in current practices in light of classical understandings, the questions begin with "Where do people called "clients" have that experience?" Other questions quickly follow: Where is or are there places and relationships characterized by mutual appreciation and enjoyment? Where are there opportunities for a sense of reciprocity and usefulness to others? It is perhaps the third dimension of classic understandings of friendship as posed by Bellah et al. (1985) (i.e., friendship is necessary for growth and mutual understanding of the common good) that is the current back door by which the importance of friendship is being reaffirmed. The only difference is that we are coming at friendship in a reverse direction. Rather than affirming that friendships lead to an understanding of the universal good, the field, in its search for the universal good in community, has rediscovered the importance and power of having friends. The central question in the field is, "What constitutes community, or a "real" or "good" experience of community?" Research in response to this question leads to the answer that friendship means having friends.

In light of the biblical dimensions of friendship, the indictment of the current system perhaps is even stronger. As stated at the beginning of the chapter, we have just begun to talk about the inherent value and giftedness of each person, what the Bible symbolizes in the "image of God." But we continue to struggle with our ability to see and affirm the uniqueness and value of each person who has a birth name other than "client" or "consumer." Professionals struggle with the label or name to call people whom they serve. Can the name be "friend"?

We have also been part of a system of care in which there has been very little focus on the grace and gift of mutual acceptance at the heart of friendship, which is captured in the old gospel song, "Just as I am." Acceptance, celebration, and reward, in fact, too often come in a behavioral system after an accomplishment and achievement of a goal (i.e., in biblical terms, a system that operates based on being "saved," or "made whole," by "works," not by grace). The underlying message of caregiving systems is still too often, "You are not okay." Both the biblical and classical affirmations of friendship are that friendship frees one to grow, learn, and develop. Jean Vanier and L'Arche communities have led the way in reaffirming and demonstrating the power of acceptance and creating communities in which people are not first characterized by entrance and exit criteria, but rather by mutual acceptance and celebration.

The third biblical dimension discussed earlier is the way in which friendship illustrates a steadfast, eternal relationship or presence. In the services system, the symbol for long-term or abiding care has been the solidness of an institution, not a focus on the importance of continuity in relationships. How often have "clients" been moved with no thought of the importance of helping them to maintain long-term relationships with those whom they see as their friends, whether they be professionals, family members, peers, volunteers, or others? Perhaps caregivers have denied the importance of long-term relationships as friends because of their basic belief that individual (and client) success, and also, as Bellah et al. (1985) point out, professional success, has come to mean "moving up and away" from a community rather than "embedding in it."

In the biblical view, a long-term relationship is also one of covenant, in which each person has freedom of choice. Ethicist William May captures the importance of covenant by asserting that the system of professional caregiving is not based on a sense of responsibility that comes from an understanding of covenant, but rather one that comes from code and contract (Campbell, 1984, p. 103ff). If professionals meet the standards or code, that is "good." If they understand a person as a "client" or "consumer" with whom they have a contract, then "better." But, as others have said, "consumer" means that choices can be made and one can take them back if not satisfied. Most "clients" don't really have that right, and should more properly be called "receivers" (Nisbet, 1992). Building relationships among caregivers, families, and consumers must be characterized by choice and also is a central issue in quality improvement and empowerment.

Through the fourth and fifth biblical dimensions of spirituality (i.e., the call to universal love and the gift of hospitality), it is possible to frame two of the dilemmas facing professional caregivers. First, in spite of all of the obstacles to friendship in current systems of care and historical obstacles that have come from injunctions against friendship in professional care, many caregivers and staff have been, and are, the only friends for many people with developmental disabilities. This fact has rarely been acknowledged or accepted, much less celebrated as a gift. There are special relationships between staff and "clients" all over the country that go far beyond job expectations (see Lutfiyya, chap. 6, this volume). Jean Edwards's (1983) book, *My Friend David* provides one of the few examples of people who have been courageous enough to talk about what caregiving professionals have re-

ceived as well as given. Persons in the field are just beginning to find a
professional language and image that allow caregivers to talk about
enjoyment of "clients," feelings of mutuality and reciprocity in their
relationships, and the ways that both parties have been called beyond
themselves to a deeper understanding of what is good (Amado et al.,
1990; O'Brien & O'Brien, 1991; Perske, 1988).

Second, the call to hospitality spells out a fundamental challenge
for caregivers. It is first a reflection of the changing roles of professional caregivers as we seek to enable community for people we call
"clients" by tapping the hospitality that is potentially present in so
many parts of community life (McKnight, 1985; O'Connell, 1988;
Vanier, 1989). (The last section of this chapter explores some of the
ways that role can be acted out in relation to the religious community.)

As the boundaries change, however, the call to hospitality also
means that professional caregivers have to practice what we preach.
As people with developmental disabilities become part of community, it means "they" become part of "our" communities, part of
"our" congregations, clubs, organizations, and neighborhoods. Rather
than keeping traditional boundaries between "professional" and "client," the very direction of our work compels a recognition and celebration of the possibilities of friendship within the context of professional care. Prior to a discussion about enabling, facilitating, or building
friendships between people with developmental disabilities and others, it is necessary to take a hard look at what that support for friendship means in caregivers' relationships with the people they serve. To
widen the circle of friendship, people usually become friends through
shared activities and through introducing friends to other friends. The
first issue for "professionals" may be that we have to start this work
with ourselves.

Reframing "Professional" To Include "Friend"

Why has it been so difficult for professional caregivers to confess to
the reality and importance of friendship? There is no clear or easy
answer, nor is there space within this chapter to explore that question
in the depth that it has been approached by others (Bellah et al., 1985;
Campbell, 1985; Lewis, 1960; Meilander, 1981; Palmer, 1983a; Vanier,
1989; Waddell, 1989). Just as this book is evidence of the beginning of
a recovery for the importance of friendship and the movement to
community is a recovery of basic understandings of what it means to
be "in community," so are professionals called to recover what it
means to be "professional." That recovery, at its heart, is a spiritual
journey to reframe "profess-ional," which also leads back to reaffirming gift and call.

A fundamental question in this area has often been, "Can you be a professional and a friend?" Some families and consumers talk about the difficulty of finding (or when they do, appreciating) a "friendly professional." To be a "professional friend" feels like a contradiction in terms and a violation of a basic human feeling about friendship— a friend is not someone you pay (see also Lutfiyya, chap. 6, this volume).

The historical spiritual seeds of that dilemma are partially based in the dilemma discussed earlier between the particularity of friendship and the universal call to love. Does recognizing and affirming a friendship with a "client" mean preferential treatment and a violation of the injunction that equal care should be provided for all? If the question is not so much a dilemma of "either-or," but the challenge to live with the paradox of "both-and," then there are other reasons which make this such a difficult issue for people who call themselves "professionals."

One reason is that professional has come to mean "expert" and "detached problem solver." "To profess" meant originally to make a commitment and/or to take vows for a religious order. As the meaning of "profession" widened to include other kinds of service to the community or humankind, it became more attached to science, medicine, and other forms of knowledge connected with a university. To be a professional also meant knowing how to "fix" or "cure." As understandings of knowledge became more objective, rather than focused on faith and a vow of commitment, profession came to mean mastery of a body of knowledge, including facts, theories, and methodologies (Palmer, 1983a). The very core of the pursuit of new knowledge through scientific research implied a detachment between the "knower" and the "known," or, as caregiving professions became more scientific, between the "professional" and the "patient" or "client." When the impetus toward the detachment is combined with the understanding of the spiritual call to service as universal, impartial, and sacrificial love, it is not difficult see how religion and science combined forces to shape an understanding of a professional caregiver as an impartial, dedicated, knowledgeable dispenser of care and help in relationships that were neither mutual nor reciprocal.

These historical strands were accompanied by the understanding that reciprocity comes by being paid, only as subsistence at first, but as more income when the term *profession* became disconnected from vows of faith and poverty. "Profession" came to mean a career path that offered honor and advancement (Bellah et al., 1985). It also became a social class of distinction, with rights, privileges, and, not least of all, power and position (Campbell, 1984). To guard against overzealous or inappropriate expressions of religion or commitment in caregiving relationships, professionals were cautioned not to let their values or beliefs get in the way of their professional care. Friendships thus became suspect, because of their implications of exclusivity, preferential treatment, or challenge to objectivity in care. In any social order where there is concern for maintaining power and control, friendships have been and are suspect because of the very way they empower (a mutual recognition of gifts) and lead to (call for) a questioning of what exists in that social order in light of new understandings of the common good.

This discussion is not meant to dismiss the importance of recognizing and utilizing boundaries in human caregiving relationships. Appropriate boundaries are first and foremost an awareness of limits, something with which "professional experts" have not been very effective nor mastered. Neither is it a call for professionals to be friends with everyone whom they serve.

However, it is an affirmation that reframing professional roles in light of changing understandings of community and care means recovering what it means to be "profess-ional." To profess is to make a declaration of one's faith and values. Making that declaration requires examination: what motivates you? What are your intentions? One was to "profess" in response to both a sense of the gifts of God and the call. In addressing current roles, such "profession" may mean being more honest about what professionals receive from the people they serve. The question is not just what gifts do they have for families and communities. What gifts do "clients" bring to professionals? What do "they" do for "us"? Each caregiver can pointedly ask himself or herself: What does he or she do for me, in the course of my relationship with him or her? Honest answers may mean that perhaps the gift of one's self and one's friendship has been much more important to "clients" than the gift of professional skills or knowledge.

"To profess" is also "to follow," to recognize and respond to the call to use one's gifts in service to God and community. It was, at least in early religious and caregiving professions, also a sense that one was giving up something (agape's call to universal love) in order to serve. It was a commitment of permanence, a covenant of new bonds other than family or civic status, and a willingness to "stand with" others in a shared community.

Responding to the call and the challenge of friendship may still pose the question of what one is willing to give up in order to serve what is understood to be the common good. Professionals may be called to give up some of the detachment, status, or boundaries they have maintained between work and community in response to the call inherent in friendship. It pushes them to ask what kind of commitment they are making to people whom they serve "over the long haul. To facilitate the experience of belonging inherent in friendship and community means to share, and perhaps give up, ownership. Can caregivers learn how to give knowledge away to others in the community? Learning how to empower others means a reversal of the age-old stance of empowering special services by asking others for adequate funding. Responding to the call also certainly pushes caregivers to give up some of the temptation to over-manage or control.

To affirm the gift of friendship means that caregivers do not create or control the magic or grace inherent in that relationship. The call inherent in friendship continues to push them along the path of clarifying the values inherent in what they do. It means being willing to try new patterns of dialogue, relationship, and caregiving that enhance experiences of acceptance and mutual enjoyment (celebration). It means developing new understandings of reciprocity and covenant that honor both choice and long-term relationships. Can we admit that, in fact, we as professionals depend upon those we serve in ways other than paychecks? Can we let choice be a real option in the context of a long-term commitment to a covenant relationship? Can we recognize, as Lutfiyya (1988) says, the ways "people with disabilities often become slowly desperate for connections with others that are not governed by control"? (p. 4). Can we find intentional ways to nurture and maintain long-term relationships and friendships, just as we are beginning intentional ways to build circles of friends?

As we begin to live, work, play, and worship in a community together with the people we serve, professional caregivers are faced with the dual task of honoring the gift and call inherent in friendship and that of reframing our own concept of the gifts and call we bring to our role as caregivers. Part of our gifts include what we know about people with developmental disabilities, but part also includes what we have learned from and through the people we serve about ourselves and the meaning of life itself. Thus, part of our call is to believe that others may discover some of the same things we have learned without having to be, or needing to become, "experts." The call of friendship is that caregivers and persons with disabilities walk together into new understandings of life and spirit. The song of the Chaverim Group, a social and religious program with Jewish people with developmental disabilities in Rochester, New York, captures the challenge:

Don't walk in front of me, I may not follow.
Don't walk behind me, I may not lead.
Just walk beside me and be my friend
And together we will walk in the way of God.

BUILDING FRIENDSHIPS
THROUGH RELIGIOUS COMMUNITIES

The intention of the final section of this chapter is not to develop an extensive argument for the importance of tapping religious communities as a resource for friendships for people with developmental disabilities. Readers of this chapter and/or book probably already either know or believe in that resource. That knowledge and belief is perhaps based on one or more of the following reasons:

Simply their own personal experiences, an awareness of the huge number of congregations in communities, and/or common sense about the ways that "typical people" often utilize church or synagogue as a way of finding friends and becoming embedded in community

Personal experience with many people with developmental disabilities whose primary place of community involvement outside residence and work is a church or synagogue, such as the network of religious education programs around the country that intentionally call themselves "Friendship Ministries"

Awareness of the growing numbers of intentional congregational ministries, services, resources, and efforts to include people with disabilities and their families more effectively in congregational and community life (AAMR Religion Division, 1992; Gaventa, 1986; National Organization on Disability, 1992)

Rather than a plea to tap religious communities as resources for friendship, the final section of this chapter continues the central themes discussed above. This section is an appeal to hold on to the principles and symbols of "gift" and "call" when beginning and/or strengthening efforts to facilitate inclusion in congregational life and/or the development of friendships. To hold on to "gift" means to first view congregations as places and settings with rich opportunities for the development of friendships. It means "going to church" is not just duty, but, if facilitated with care, the possibility for contact and relationships with people in the community in many different kinds of activities.

Rather than a plea to tap religious communities as resources for friendship, the final section of this chapter continues the central themes discussed above. This section is an appeal to hold onto the principles and symbols of "gift" and "call" when beginning and/or strengthening efforts to facilitate inclusion in congregational life and/or the development of friendships. To hold onto "gift" means to first view congregations as places and settings with rich opportunities for the development of friendships. It means "going to church" is not just duty, but, if facilitated with care, the possibility for contact and relationships with people in the community in many different kinds of activities.

Holding onto "gift" means approaching congregations, or individuals and groups within congregations, with the belief that the gifts of friendship and inclusion are both present and possible for everyone concerned. To believe and perceive that "gifts" are present is to approach congregations with a perspective that does not tell them what they should be doing. It also does not imply that to include a person with developmental disabilities means that congregational members have to receive special training. Viewing people with developmental disabilities through their strengths rather than their deficits also translates into trusting the strengths of congregation members. It means helping individuals and congregations to see that the simple parts of congregational life, inclusion and relationships, are strengths and gifts they already have in abundance, and could make a significant difference in the lives of people who often have neither. It means helping congregational members to see that they have many gifts to give, as well as knowing how to articulate some of the gifts that people with disabilities can bring to them.

Holding onto "call" sharply focuses the need to approach the art of making introductions (O'Brien & O'Brien, 1991) or facilitating friendships (Lutfiyya, 1991) with a belief in both the gift and call of hospitality—a belief that people will respond most genuinely with love to others when they act in response to their own sense of call and commitment. Call means believing that others may in fact commit themselves to a relationship and friendship in ways that defy explanation. It means operating from the framework that friendship is a covenant relationship, not a relationship characterized by giver—receiver or by the service system's reliance on "compliance with code." A covenant means space for individual choice, an awareness that relationships and friendships often grow slowly and/or fluctuate in intensity. It is an awareness that friendships arc not controlled or fixed. Helping friendships begin and develop is more like planting seeds and nurturing, always being aware that the growth cannot be controlled (1 Corinthians 3:6–7). It means rediscovering that truth in relationships is different than truth in a science that operates on objective facts, and a recovering of truth as "troth." Through seeking truth in the context of relationships, people become "betrothed" (Palmer, 1983a). Perhaps the best injunction for professionals in service systems who are so easily tempted to use relationships as tools for growth, development, or inclusion, is to remember that the art of befriending is characterized much more by "courtship" than it is by "control" (Landgraf, 1989).

The skills of making introductions and facilitating friendships in and through congregational settings are not very different than in other settings. Just as one might take time to get to know potential employers or co-workers in a supported employment setting or do preparatory work in a community association or recreational setting, it is important to be intentional and careful when it comes to congregations. Professionals, advocates, or other friends who are seeking to facilitate friendships must first of all be sensitive to both parties. Just as in relationships between nondisabled people, there are no guarantees that friendships will develop in a congregational setting or that they will do so without time and work.

Other than being intentional and sensitive, it is important to be prepared. Preparation means knowledge of the kinds of resources that may be available for a congregation to use from either their own faith group or others (AAMR Religion Division, 1992). It means taking time to discover, within a particular congregation, the opportunities, rituals, and traditions for entry into that community. In each congregation, it is important to ask: What does it mean and how does one become a "member"? What are ways a congregation may already have for welcoming strangers? How can those ways be extended to a person with developmental disabilities? Preparation means trying to understand and use congregational language for friendships and relationships rather than relying on diagnostic or treatment language.

It may also mean being aware that many congregations initially welcome strangers through an intentional ministry or service "to" or "for" others, which can feel like and be more of a charity, one-way relationship. That type of relationship is sometimes avoidable by careful introductions and beginnings, but sometimes it is perfectly "typical" for a particular congregation. In these instances, it is important to remember that these types of "ministries" often change, and that ministries "to" or "for" can often become ministries "with" or "by," characterized by awareness of mutual gifts and call (Gaventa, 1986).

In the face of a bewildering number and variety of denominations, faith groups, religious practices, and religious traditions, a facilitator's search for and approach to congregations for the purpose of inclusion, relationships, and friendships should rely on the five spiritual dimensions of friendship discussed above. Holding onto gift and call in approaching congregations can thus mean the following:

1. Start with a theology of creation. People with developmental disabilities are people created, like others, in the image of God. They are, as are all of us, God's children and part of God's family. Therefore they belong, whether it has been practice or not. If their gifts have not been seen and used in the context of the people of God, it is the congregation's call to discover them, just as it is their call to do so with everyone.
2. Articulate the value that acceptance has in the lives of everyone, but particularly in the lives of people with developmental disabilities. Be able to talk about acceptance in biblical, psychological, social, and very personal terms.
3. See the importance of congregational involvement as a way of enhancing spiritual identity and journey over time, as well as developing relationships that can be friendships characterized by steadfastness, long-term commitment, and covenant. "Typical" people often talk of their faith or congregation being an "anchor" in seas of transition and change. Can both service providers and congregations see the importance of honoring and nurturing those long-term relationships with people who have often been given little choice or opportunity to do so?
4. Help interpret the risk and/or fear that others may have in relationships with people with disabilities as an expression of the call to love in ways that are inclusive; risk-taking (sacrificial); and part of the second great commandment, "to love they neighbor as thyself." The irony is that most "typical" people feel "disabled" in their capacity to relate to people with developmental disabilities. Holding onto gift and call means helping others to see that God has promised to be with them as they reach out in service to others in ways that feel risky, and being aware of the ways that such service lives out God's love for humankind and can lead to new discoveries of grace, gift, and presence in oneself and others. It also means being prepared to support others who make that commitment, and to learn from and celebrate both the difficulties and the joys.
5. Be able to balance the spiritual call to universal love with the specific gift of hospitality that welcomes particular individuals. Help congregations to envision inclusive ministries with people

with disabilities not as "special ministries" that require "special people with special gifts and call," but as part of the biblical injunction to welcome the stranger. Thus, the call is to the congregation's own tradition and strengths, rather than to becoming another form of a social service agency or human services program. Practicing the gift of hospitality may mean doing things differently, but it is an attitude of "doing what it takes" to welcome and include, with a vision that the stranger can become the giver and the friend.

However one approaches the art of inclusion and befriending in relation to congregations and people with developmental disabilities, it is crucial to remember that this call challenges individuals and congregations at many levels. It can push individuals and congregations to re-examine basic understandings of personhood, faith, congregation, and community (Gaventa, 1986). It can push congregations to look at how they reach out to anyone and everyone. Is "everybody welcome" as the signs so often say? Can people get here or get in? How do people intentionally care for each other in sensitive, individualized ways? What are everyone's limits and gifts? Where are they met and used? What does it mean for caregivers and congregation members to be friends with those whom they serve or to whom they minister? Friendships, in spiritual traditions, can be transforming; so can the call to welcome and befriend.

CALLED TO BE FRIENDS

As service providers, advocates, families, clergy, lay people, individuals with developmental disabilities, and others rediscover the power of the gift of friendship, the challenge for everyone is to reaffirm, in the best of both the classical and spiritual traditions, its inherent call to new forms of relationship, profession, and community. Friendship means being able to operate with a high tolerance for paradox because as a gift it is not a tool, but a resource. A particular and special friendship is celebrated for its mutual enjoyment and usefulness to each member, but also for the way it calls both parties beyond themselves to universal values and/or to God. People respond to the call and need for friendship through choice, and it cannot be controlled. People are challenged to love fairly and equally; yet, in each stranger and neighbor there is the possibility of a new friend. Developing friendships takes intentional work and commitment on the one hand and a celebration of gift and discovery on the other.

The ultimate paradox, of course, is the awareness that in relation to relearning the art of friendship, it is probably people with developmental disabilities who are the teachers and experts. If cultivating friendships means doing things such as giving priority to relationships; being open with feelings, thoughts, and affections; practicing acceptance; learning the gestures and touches of warmth; listening; and seeing in every stranger a potential friend, then "we" are the learners from "them" (Landgraf, 1989; McGinnis, 1979; Vanier, 1984, 1989; Wolfensberger, 1988).

Operating from a spirit of friendship as professionals, advocates, and caregivers means practicing new roles in addition to that of learner. To use a metaphor from music, the universal language of friendship and community, it means learning how to sing common songs with new voices. It means that caregivers must learn to talk about the basic values and symbols of those values in what they do, and to share the images that bring meaning to their work. It means, in the best of spiritual traditions, being a "witness" to the power of relationships with people who have been called "clients." If caregivers want others to become friends with people who receive services, they have to be willing to tell stories about, or give witness to, the ways their friendships with these individuals have brought value to them. Such stories would begin, "Let me tell you about my friend," rather than describing a client. Reframing a role as professional reaffirms the ancient spiritual role of guide and companion. It is not a "fix-it" guide or a "how-to" guide, but a guide that walks with others in their mutual response to gift and call, and helps introduce, facilitate, accommodate, and interpret. This role also means a willingness to see and celebrate the inherent gifts of all others, and the gifts discovered in response to call (Gaventa, 1991).

"I will no longer call you servants [consumers, clients, patients, or providers], but friends" (John 15:12–17). It is indeed difficult to write about friendship, except as an act of rehabilitation.

REFERENCES

AAMR Religion Division. (1992). *Dimensions of faith and congregational ministries with persons with developmental disabilities and their families: A bibliography and resource listing.* Princeton, NJ: AAMR Religion Division.

Amado, A.N. (1992, May). *Advice to churches on friendship and inclusion: Lessons learned from the Friends Project.* Paper presented at the 116th annual AAMR conference, New Orleans.

Amado, A.N., Conklin, F., & Wells, J. (1990). *Friends: A manual for connecting persons with disabilities and community members.* St. Paul, MN: Human Services and Research Development Center.

Bellah, R., Madsen, R., Sullivan, W., Swidler, A., & Tipton, S. (1985). *Habits of the heart: Individualism and commitment in American life.* New York: Harper & Row.

Bogdan, R., & Taylor, S.J. (1989). On accepting relationships between people with mental retardation and non-disabled people: Towards an understanding of acceptance. *Disability, Handicap, and Society* 4(1), 21–36.

Campbell, A. (1984). *Professional care: Its meaning and practice.* Philadelphia: Fortress Press.

Campbell, A. (1985). *Professionalism and pastoral care.* Philadelphia: Fortress Press.

Doherty, F. (1989, March/April). Friends. *Stauros Newsletter,* 28(1–4).

Eareckson-Tada, J. (1987). *Friendship unlimited.* Wheaton, IL: Harold Shaw Publishers.

Edwards, J. (1983). *My friend David: A sourcebook about Down's syndrome and a personal story about friendship.* Portland: Ednick Communications.

Gaventa, B. (1986). Religious ministries and services with adults with developmental disabilities. In J. Summers (Ed.), *The right to grow up: An introduction to adults with developmental disabilities* (pp. 191–226). Baltimore: Paul H. Brookes Publishing Co.

Gaventa, B. (1991). Think ecumenically, act parochially. (Available from Bill Gaventa, Religion Division, American Association on Mental Retardation, Washington, DC.)

Graham, L.K. (1990). Friendship. In R. Hunter (Ed.), *The dictionary of pastoral care and counseling* (pp. 446–447). Nashville: Abingdon Press.

Hunter, R. (1990). *Dictionary of pastoral care and counseling.* Nashville: Abingdon Press.

James, M., & Savory, L. (1979). *The heart of friendship.* New York: Harper & Row.

Keen, S. (1983). *The passionate life.* San Francisco: Harper & Row.

Landgraf, J. (1989, Fall). Love and friendship. *Minister's Magazine,* X(1), 3–9. Publication of American Baptist Churches in the USA.

Lewis, C.S. (1960). *The four loves.* London: Fontana Books.

Lutfiyya, Z. (1988). *Reflections on relationships between people with disabilities and typical people.* Syracuse, NY: Syracuse University, Center on Human Policy.

Lutfiyya, Z. (1991). *Toni Santi and the bakery: The roles of facilitation, accommodation, and interpretation.* Syracuse, NY: Syracuse University, Center on Human Policy.

McGinnis, L. (1979). *The friendship factor.* Minneapolis: Augsburg Publishing Co.

McKnight, J. (1985, November). *Regenerating community.* Address to the Canadian Mental Health Association Search Conference, Ottawa.

Meilander, G. (1981). *Friendship, a study in theological ethics.* Notre Dame, IN: University of Notre Dame Press.

National Organization on Disability. (1992). *That all may worship: An interfaith welcome to people with disabilities.* Washington, DC: National Organization on Disability.

Nisbet, J. (1992, May). *Natural supports.* Presentation at the multi-disciplinary session at the AAMR National Conference, New Orleans.

O'Brien, J., & O'Brien, C. (1991). *Members of each other: Perspectives on social supports for people with severe disabilities.* Lithonia, GA: Responsive System Associates.

O'Connell, M. (1988). *The gift of hospitality.* Evanston: Northwestern University, Center for Urban Affairs and Policy Research.

Palmer, P. (1983a). *To know as we are known: A spirituality of education.* San Francisco: Harper & Row.

Palmer, P. (1983b). *The company of strangers.* New York: Crossroad Publishing.

Palmer, P. (1986). *The company of strangers.* Keynote presentation at Merging Two Worlds Conference, Rochester, New York.

Perske, R. (1988). *Circle of friends.* Nashville: Abingdon Press.

Ripple, P. (1980). *Called to be friends.* Notre Dame, IN: Ave Maria Press.

Vanier, J. (1984). *Man and woman he made them.* Mahwah, NJ: Paulist Press.

Vanier, J. (1989). *Community and growth.* Mahwah, NJ: Paulist Press.

Waddell, P. (1989). *Friendship and the moral life.* Notre Dame, IN: University of Notre Dame Press.

Wolfensberger, W. (1988, April). Common assets of mentally retarded people that are commonly not acknowledged. *Mental Retardation, 26*(2), 63–70.

4

Loneliness

Effects and Implications

Richard S. Amado

There is much said in this volume in favor of friends and friendships and almost everyone would agree that it is enjoyable to have friends. However, staff and agencies supporting persons with developmental disabilities, advocates, and policymakers might question if friends are really all that important. Is it really worth the effort to support people having friendships, especially with community members? Because many individuals with disabilities are vulnerable and live without adequate or guaranteed services, perhaps efforts would be better spent ensuring adequate care, better quality of care, or better programs. Is friendship a luxury, knowing how many other pressing problems there are in people's lives?

INTRODUCTION

It is a fact that most people with developmental disabilities who are dependent upon the services system have very limited social networks and very few friends (Hill, Lakin, Bruininks, Amado, Anderson, & Copher, 1989). Although this fact is generally known and accepted, providing the basis for all of the community-connecting efforts described in this volume and elsewhere, very little examination has occurred regarding the effects of this social isolation. Whereas there is substantial research on the effects of loneliness in the general population, the effects of loneliness on persons with disabilities in the services system has not been thoroughly discussed.

Indeed, many services practices and difficulties in supporting people might be a result of this issue; the loneliness of people with disabilities might be contributing to their health problems, moods, and behavior. Program planners might be responding to those problems, moods, and behavior without recognizing the true cause. In this chapter, some of the current information regarding loneliness is summarized, including what loneliness is and how it affects human beings. Other issues that are examined include: how some of our current practices in human services are related to loneliness, the effects of displacing loneliness with friendships on the behavior of persons with disabilities, and implications for service delivery.

WHAT IS LONELINESS?

Identifying Loneliness

Dictionary definitions of "lonely" progress from "being without company" to "not frequented by human beings" to "sad from being alone" to "producing a feeling of bleakness or desolation" (Webster, 1979, p. 672). Loneliness and its effects have been studied extensively in the population at large and different researchers have contributed and developed different definitions of this phenomenon. For instance, Perlman and Peplau (1982) have defined loneliness as ". . . the unpleasant experience that occurs when a person's network of social relationships is significantly deficient in either quality or quantity" (p. 15). Weiss (1982) distinguishes between two types of loneliness. First is the absence of attachment to one figure and second is the absence of community. He further comments that the first is experienced as an "aching emptiness," and the second includes feelings of marginality and exclusion. Weiss clarifies that absence of community is not a geographical event—people can be living in an institution and be within close geographic proximity of their former homes, yet, still be functionally isolated. For those whose lives are bound by institutional regulation, restriction is not simply associated with a large fenced institutional campus; it can also be imposed through the policies and practices of service providers.

Hojat and Crandall (1989) reviewed several studies regarding loneliness and concluded that the experience of loneliness is independent of the amount of social contact a person has. That is, even if a person was surrounded by staff, had a weekly case manager visit, and spent several sessions with a volunteer each week, he or she might still experience a great degree of loneliness.

Three central conclusions regarding loneliness can be drawn from the work of Hojat and Crandall (1989), Perlman and Peplau (1982), and Weiss (1982):

1. Loneliness is a subjective event, a feeling that is individually defined. (Given the same set of circumstances, one person might experience loneliness and another person might not.)

2. The quality of social relationships, not just the quantity of social contacts, affects the feeling of loneliness and associated behaviors.
3. Loneliness is an unpleasant condition, an aversive context in which to live life.

These definitional conclusions have several implications for determining the degree of loneliness a person experiences and for evaluating the effects of loneliness in the lives of people with disabilities.

Assessing and Measuring Loneliness

It cannot be assumed that a person is not lonely simply because people are always around him or her (Luftig, 1988; Taylor, Asher, & Williams, 1987). For instance, many persons with disabilities in the services sytems are constantly surrounded by other people, 24 hours a day, and are never physically alone. This does not mean they do not feel lonely. Simply counting the frequency of social contacts will not provide an accurate measure of loneliness.

In addition, people might be physically present in social situations, but not actually be participating with others. At the first level, then, it is important to distinguish between physical presence and social participation. Second, it is important to distinguish between social participation and specific friendship interactions. Taking direction from a supervisor or correction from a teacher is very different from chatting about a topic of little consequence and mutual interest with a peer. Although persons with disabilities may now be experiencing more opportunities to be physically present and to participate with community members, they still may not have specific friendship interactions or be any less lonely.

Determining the existence of loneliness or measuring its degree may be problematic. Chadsey-Rusch, DeStefano, O'Reilly, Gonzalez, and Collet-Klingenberg (1992) have suggested measuring the degree of loneliness by asking the individuals themselves if they are lonely. However, the responses of people with mental retardation are often influenced by a lack of understanding and by their desire to please others (Sigelman et al., 1980); hence, responses to the question by the individuals themselves may not be accurate. Other researchers have used measures of the quality of lifestyle to clarify the degree or experience of loneliness. Lifestyle measures have included frequency of social contacts with people who are not paid to be there or with formal volunteers (Newton, 1989), opportunities to choose preferred people with whom to do things, and the size of a person's social network (Schalock, 1992).

As suggested by Hojat and Crandall (1989), it is also useful to look at the nature and quality of social interactions when assessing the degree of loneliness. Social interactions initiated by others can be characterized as predominantly corrective, supervisory, and coercive; acknowledging, supportive, and empowering; or they can fall anywhere in between. In addition, questions regarding the social interactions that do occur can include: Does the person choose to interact with the people who are available and willing? What are the person's reactions to interactions initiated by available people—avoidance, evasion, aggression, and self-injury; boredom and listlessness; or approach, joyful participation, and thoughtfulness to their appearance?

Many life factors influence the actual occurrence of the experience of loneliness. To determine the existence of the experience or the degree of it, the nature of social interactions, quantity of interactions with different people, and self-report can be taken together to provide a good indication of a person's experience. However, typical program and clinical assessment instruments used by services supporting persons with disabilities usually do not evaluate the size, scope, or quality of social networks or the individual's experience of that network.

Factors Associated with Loneliness

Woodward (1988) has summarized current research and identified seven factors that are associated with the occurrence of loneliness:

1. *Gender*   In the results of recent studies, either women tended to report more loneliness than men or there was no difference between the sexes. Woodward explains this difference as a function of gender-distinct priorities. (See also Traustadottir, chap. 7, this volume.)
2. *Transportation*   People with adequate transportation were generally less lonely than those without it. People without adequate public or private transportation were isolated and restricted in their social contacts.
3. *Self-esteem*   In the studies in which it was measured, individuals with low self-esteem were the loneliest of people.
4. *Ease in making friends*   Individuals who found it easy to make friends were the least lonely and also tended to have high self-esteem.
5. *Happiness*   The happier subjects reported they had been during the last year, the less lonely they reported they were. Happiness was also closely related to the respondent's closeness to family members.
6. *Money*   To the degree a person perceived his or her money as adequate, he or she was less likely to be lonely. When money was seen as inadequate, activities were often limited, contributing to feelings of inadequacy and loneliness.

7. *Days and seasons*   While no season stood out as being associated with loneliness, weekends were likely to be lonely times.
This finding was attributed to the lack of social contact people
have when they are away from work.

Woodward also discussed the interrelationship of these factors. For
instance, is a person more happy because he or she has more friends?
Does having fewer friends result in lower self-esteem, or are people
with low self-esteem generally unhappy and unlikely to attract
friends? Certainly there are interrelationships between these factors
of friendship, self-esteem, and happiness; however, further research
is needed to clarify the interconnected nature of these factors. Does
being happy result in having friends, does having friends result in
being happy, or does some yet-to-be identified factor produce both?
The causal relationships are likely to be reciprocal and multifactoral.

Given the life circumstances of many individuals dependent on the
human services sytem, it is probable that many of these interrelated
factors are at work influencing the quality of life and the experience
of loneliness. For instance, many of these people have little income
and no independent transportation. Given that many of them also
have few friends, self-esteem, happiness, and ease in making more
friends are all affected.

EFFECTS OF LONELINESS

Loneliness Affects Physical Well-Being

Weiss's (1982) reference to an "aching emptiness" suggests that certain physiological reactions may correlate with the experience of
loneliness. To the degree these physiological events are internal and
unobservable, they are difficult to include in routine assessment procedures. However, the presence of physiological involvement in loneliness raises questions about the effects of loneliness on physical
health.

The "aching emptiness" of loneliness is a physiological phenomenon, a biological reaction to certain external events. Weiss suggests
this physiological reaction is provoked by an absence of individual
and community relationships. The relationship between psychological factors and physical health has long been recognized by medical
and mental health professionals. Ulman and Krasner (1975) provide
an extensive review of the variety of known physical maladies that
are psychological in origin. Perlman and Peplau (1982) also review the
psychosomatic symptoms associated with loneliness, including
headaches, poor appetite, and tiredness. Lynch (1977) has extensively

reviewed the research on the effects of social-emotional factors on physical health and provides substantial data documenting that isolation affects longevity. In particular, heart-related illnesses and deaths are highly related to disruptions in interpersonal relationships and the lack of close family and community ties. Lynch advises medical practitioners to make people aware that their family and social life are every bit as important to health as dieting and exercising. He concludes, "We must either learn to live together or increase our chances of prematurely dying alone" (p. 14), and "simply put, reflected in our hearts there is a biological basis for our need to form loving human relationships. If we fail to fulfill that need, our health is in peril" (p. xiii).

In another review of 20 years' worth of research studies, House, Landis, and Umberson (1988) concluded that social isolation was a greater mortality risk than smoking. After controlling for the effects of physical health, socioeconomic status, smoking, alcohol, exercise, obesity, race, life satisfaction, and health care, they found that research documented that those with few or weak social ties were twice as likely to die at a given age than were those with strong ties. This evidence leaves little room for doubt that loneliness contributes significantly to poor physical health and increases the likelihood of illness and premature death.

Loneliness Affects Mental Health

The relationship between loneliness and mental health is also well documented. Perlman and Peplau (1982) report studies documenting increased anxiety, neuroses, general maladjustment, depression, and aggressive conduct associated with loneliness. Loneliness in males is also associated with a greater proclivity toward rape. Although both the psychological and physical symptoms referenced in the previous section are very real to the person experiencing them, all of these psychosomatic symptoms also reflect significant mental health issues. Polansky (1986) has identified relationships between loneliness and: 1) narcissism, 2) rejection of all relationships, 3) parental neglect and abuse of children, and 4) prolonging a relationship with an abusive partner.

The Effects of Loneliness on Behavior

Several of the results of loneliness discussed above also indicate that loneliness can have a profound effect on a person's behavior, with a potential to lead to rape, abuse of one's children, and staying with an abusive partner. Loneliness is also an unpleasant and aversive condition, whether it is due to a brief period of loss or it is a chronic condition. Any length of duration can be very punishing.

Specific behavioral reactions to aversive, punishing conditions were first clearly identified 40 years ago (Skinner, 1953) and since then have been further analyzed and explicated in numerous formulations and with various populations. In his classical formulation, Skinner defined an aversive event or condition as any event or condition the withdrawal of which strengthens behavior. In this paradigm, loneliness is by definition an aversive condition if, when the loneliness is terminated, the behavior that terminated it is strengthened or becomes more frequent when the person is lonely (i.e., any actions that successfully terminate the experience of loneliness are more likely to occur the next time the person experiences loneliness.)

However, in this complex world, there are very few behaviors that occur for only one reason. Despite this complexity, escape from loneliness probably contributes to a variety of activities in the general population, including: frequenting singles bars, cruising shopping malls, over-working, unnecessary visits to physicians and counselors, over-eating, joining clubs, and volunteering. Although most people seek solitude from time to time, loneliness is an aversive condition for most people. Although individuals adapt differently to the condition, with different habits and changes in their behavior, there are some general principles about reactions to aversive conditions that are shaping those individualistic actions. If it is assumed that loneliness may be the cause (perhaps previously unrecognized) for many behaviors, the principles of reactions to aversive conditions can be applied and people's behavior can be understood in a very different light. Several examples of the applications of these principles follow.

One effect of the onset of an aversive condition such as loneliness is the cessation of behavior in the immediate situation. However, the immediate result might not have an effect on the ceased behavior in the future. For example, when a loved one leaves during an argument, the experience of loss and loneliness will likely result in apologetic and conciliatory behavior (i.e., the cessation of arguing). Despite this change in behavior, as many divorced couples and estranged parents will testify, the momentary discomfort does not prevent subsequent arguments. Group home staff are familiar with many instances of residents who exhibit the same pattern of argument, concern over the withdrawal of a preferred staff member, apologies, and repetitions of this cycle.

A second effect of aversive conditions is the development of emotional responses. Some of this emotional response behavior includes reactions by the glands and smooth muscles; the "aching emptiness" discussed above might be just such a reaction. These emotional responses often serve to suppress behaviors that provoke them (i.e., if we feel bad enough we will stop the behavior that created the loneliness). They also often create a condition of physical discomfort. These emotional responses are one way we experience shame or guilt and they can be accompanied by self-deprecating or self-blaming statements. "I should have never said . . ." or "If only I had done . . ." are statements commonly expressed by people who were subjected to an aversive event. Furthermore, these reactions of the glands and smooth muscles can create conditions making disease and illness more likely. Headaches, butterflies in the stomach, diarrhea, "24-hour flu," heartburn, and ulcers can all be a function of aversive conditions.

A third effect of aversive conditions is the development of conditioned aversive events and situations. Any person, place, thing, or activity that becomes associated with loneliness intentionally or accidentally will develop aversive properties, serve to suppress behavior, and provoke emotional responses. This conditioning effect is particularly important because it can result in the proliferation of aversive events in a person's life. For example, a group home resident might be experiencing a great deal of loneliness. It is possible for staff, housemates, and co-workers to be accidentally associated with the loneliness and therefore become conditioned aversive stimuli for the individual with disabilities. The results of such a conditioning process could appear in a range of behavior varying from avoidance of the persons associated with loneliness, mild suppression in their presence, or violently reacting to their presence. All of the emotional effects of aversive events discussed above can also be produced by these conditioned aversive elements.

Skinner considered this result the most important effect of punishment because it strengthens conduct that avoids the array of conditioned aversive events. For instance, a person may have sought out social relationships but then been disappointed or hurt in their interactions with others. Then that person might find himself or herself "too busy" or "simply not interested" in significant relationships; the person is then exhibiting this extreme avoidance behavior to social relationships. Over time this effect diminishes because the behavior of being too busy or not interested allows the person to successfully avoid contact with the primary aversive event, causing a concomitant reduction in the power of the conditioned aversive events. At this point the person who was "too busy" finds opportunities to spend some time with people over. The person returns to socializing with certain social expectations. However, if the time spent with others results in sufficient disappointment again, it is likely that withdrawal will occur and the cycle will start over. When staff, housemates, or co-workers become conditioned aversive stimuli in this way, they will be cyclically avoided and their presence could result in the suppression of an array of behavior. Residents might avoid staff presence, move away from staff, not make requests, or speak very little.

There are a number of unfortunate by-products of aversive stimulation. The first is the conflict between the behavior that avoids the punishment and the behavior that produces it. These behaviors are often of similar strength and are always incompatible with each other. When people do not want to stay home alone but complain that it is too much trouble to go out, they are exhibiting this conflict. The person who at the last minute refuses to get in the car to go to the mall might also be exhibiting conflicted behavior; so might the person who gets excited about having guests, but hides or sulks when the guests arrive.

Another unfortunate by-product of exposure to aversive events is the intense emotional reaction that can result from the suppression of very strong behavior. This intense emotional behavior is commonly recognized as fear or anxiety; it can result in physical symptoms or otherwise interfere with normal daily activities. Temper tantrums for "no apparent reason," anxiety and fear over some event that may or may not happen, and depression or resentment can be the behavioral manifestations of this by-product. A person in a day training and habilitation program who vacillates between listless and angry is displaying behaviors that could be the by-product of punishing circumstances.

Finally, aversive conditions will often provoke aggression or other lashing out at any person, place, or thing that is available. In the absence of an outside target, this reaction can be self-directed, resulting in significant self-induced tissue damage. People (e.g., staff) who have become conditioned aversive stimuli through an association with loneliness can by their very presence provoke aggression or self-injurious behavior. It is worthwhile to note that although self-injury and aggression can be very intense and destructive, the behavior that occurs as a function of the mechanism described here is not *voluntarily* directed at anyone; staff do not have to "take it personally." At the same time, the role of loneliness in the occurrence of these behaviors is virtually never considered by those concerned with the person's behavior.

Loneliness as an aversive condition creates a context for life that can promote personal conflict, emotional distress, poor health, anti-social and potentially dangerous behavior, and premature death in the population at large. When viewed in this way, the wealth of research on the primary and secondary effects of punishing conditions can be applied to understand the powerful capacity of loneliness to interfere with the ability of people with disabilities to have a full, rich life.

HOW CURRENT HUMAN
SERVICES PRACTICES AFFECT LONELINESS

Human services agencies are regulated by a variety of federal, state, and local laws; rules; and regulations. Due to several factors in the historical evolution of social services that have contributed to the design and funding of services, including the fact that many services are funded in part with federal Medical Assistance funds (Title XIX of the Social Security Act), many of the overall governing rules still reflect a medical model of intervention. The underlying assumption of this medical model is that what an individual needs is treatment for an illness or disease that interferes with normal functioning and/or causes discomfort. It further assumes that specially trained persons must oversee or personally deliver certain diagnostic and treatment services and that the consumer is often too incompetent to understand the sophisticated technology behind the treatment services being delivered. Typically, the more severe the illness, the more dependent the patient is on others for care, supervision, and decision making, often including very personal decisions.

In recent years, this model has been and continues to be seriously challenged in the medical arena. Patients have successfully reclaimed their rights to in-home health care, the hiring and supervision of their own in-home care staff, having babies at home, and even choosing the time and place of their death. In human services, greater emphasis is also being placed on consumer-driven services, self-advocacy, and more "person-centered" services (Mount, Ducharme, & Beeman, 1991). However, no matter how consumer-driven an agency is, service providers still must account to regulatory agencies, licensers, and funding sources. Partly due to this historical medical model and for other reasons, the regulations that govern these funding sources have typically been slow to recognize consumers as total human beings rather than as the disabilities that make them eligible for services.

The focus on disability rather than the whole person has resulted in a variety of program practices and designs that interfere with the development of friendships and normal social relationships and that promulgate loneliness, including congregation of people in groups, segregated buildings, and special recreation programs. Programs have devoted years to trying to fix annoying or challenging behavior *before* allowing a consumer contact with the public and instead of designing situations to foster typical behavior in typical integrated settings. Rules requiring minimum training and medical and criminal background checks of people who would have routine, on-going contact with a consumer have been used to exclude friendships as an option. Personal data privacy rules often prevent even acknowledging that a consumer is known by an agency. This focus of the rules and regulations on fixing, protecting, and preventing additional damage has resulted in practices that interfere with the development of normal friendship relationships and thereby promote all the ills associated with loneliness. The services themselves have been designed around fixing the resulting ills, rather than addressing the causal loneliness or being redesigned to promote normal relationships and prevent loneliness in the first place. A multi-million dollar industry is literally engaged in an array of practices that, at a minimum, are inconsistent with what the industry says it is for, and, in the worst cases, are destructive to people.

The picture may, however, not be so glum. After all, there are many friendless people who have learned new skills and stopped engaging in culturally undesirable behavior within the current human services system. Many of the lonely people who have failed to learn the new skills and who have persisted in undesirable behavior have had their mental health and behavioral issues successfully managed through the application of psychiatric and behavior suppression methods. Heavy doses of tranquilizers and mood-altering drugs have stopped many friendless people from engaging in self-injurious behavior and aggression. When a sufficiently skilled practitioner has been available, the same behaviors have been addressed by the use of differential reinforcement and token economies; if competent practitioners have not been available, time-out, restraints, and skin shock have usually been effective for containing the problem. People who have adapted to their loneliness by displaying withdrawal and resignation have largely been accepted the way they are with little interference because they do not ostensibly create such a drain on the system's resources. And, of course, medical technology has comprehensively treated all of the physical ailments of lonely and friendless people (except when welfare reimbursement rates have been too far below scale fees). Whereas a variety of medical and psychological responses to the outcomes of loneliness have been developed, loneliness itself has not been even acknowledged as a potential cause of many of these problems. It has not been recognized that it is service practices and policies that promote isolation and loneliness, thereby creating a "vicious cycle" of additional ailments, mental health problems, and behavioral difficulties.

FRIENDS AS AN ALTERNATIVE

Several authors have documented the changes in behavior and health that result when social relationships with typical community citizens are supported (Baker & Salon, 1986; Berkman & Meyer, 1988; O'Brien & O'Brien, 1992; Tyne, 1988). Amado, Conklin, and Wells (1990) also reported changes in people's patterns of behavior as the result of establishing friendships and connections with typical community members. For many of the individuals in this study, similar to the other efforts referenced above, typical interventions had previously failed or proved insufficient. Efforts to support these individuals in acquiring new relationships were not initiated in order to change behavior; such behavioral changes were an unexpected and surprising by-product of efforts to support friendship and community connectedness. Three examples from this study follow and describe the changes in individuals when friendships were supported.

Michelle

Michelle is 17 and lives in a 13-bed group home with people who are mostly older than she is. She speaks very little, mainly one word statements like "mama," "no no," and "baby." It was often difficult to get her up in the morning and get her onto the school bus. She would often sit in front of her cereal bowl, and not initiate eating or asking or reaching for the milk. Staff worked on goals for a long time to try to have her be more "motivated," and to speak more. (Amado et al., 1990, p. vii)

Staff were already actively working on training Michelle and certainly behavioral programming could have been used to motivate her and to teach her to talk. An ideal program would likely have included a token economy that would allow Michelle to earn desired things by moving faster and meeting certain time-limited objectives in her program plan. She also could have been taught language through the use of an augmentative communication system and language training incorporated throughout day-to-day life experiences.

When her residential services agency began working on supporting individuals to have more friends with community members, her group home staff helped Michelle make friends with two girls from her school. Initially when the girls came to visit Michelle at the group home, they brought a crafts activity with them. The staff informed them that they would prefer it if the girls just "hung out" with Michelle, had fun, and did what they did with their other teenage friends. The girls proceeded to do regular "teen" things with Michelle.

With her programs already going on and with new anticipation of going to school, Michelle started getting up much more easily, reaching for her milk and finishing her cereal. One morning when it was time to get on the school bus, the staff were running around trying to find her—then they realized she was already out on the bus, waiting to go.

The three girls do teenage stuff together. They look at Michelle's pictures, listen to music, shoot baskets, play computer games, etc. They spent one afternoon putting on makeup and fixing their hair. A couple of days after this visit, a staff person walked by the bathroom and saw Michelle primping herself. She was saying emphatically to herself in the mirror, "you're cute!" They have never heard that much from her before. (Amado et al., 1990, p. vii)

Michelle apparently became more interested in life as a result of having new, meaningful social relationships. Her lack of motivation, which might have been a result of loneliness, started to be resolved when there were good reasons for participating in life. Although she needed and will continue to need assistance to acquire friends in the future, she proved capable of participating in and contributing to a friendship relationship. "When the girls were asked about what they were getting out of being Michelle's friend, Melissa said, 'Now I have something to look forward to on Friday afternoons'" (Amado et al., 1990, p. vii).

Arthur

Arthur is 40 years old and lives in his own home with two other men. He loves books and history, and has a fascination with cemeteries and death. He was described by the staff as hesitant to try new things. They said, "We have to go slow with Arthur." Arthur also tended to be a "yes-man," willing to comply with whatever staff asked or expected him to do. Staff had been working on the goal of Arthur being more "assertive" for quite some time. (Amado et al., 1990, p. 69)

An appropriate behavioral intervention for Arthur might include various social skills programs for assertiveness training and desensitization to novelty; in fact, various social skills programs had been tried to improve his assertiveness. A different approach was taken when his agency started to focus on people having more friends and being more a part of their community. Using his interest in books to hopefully lead to more social relationships, Arthur was assisted in beginning to volunteer at the community library. He had the job of dusting the book shelves; he reported on the importance of his visits to the library. After his first visit, the staff inquired as to how it went. Arthur replied, "The books were really dusty. They really needed me."

Arthur also almost immediately began to assert himself more. When the library staff gave him a name tag with his name misspelled, he immediately requested a new one. In addition, there was a marked transformation in his hesitancies.

> Staff were willing to go with Arthur for as long as necessary, but after just two visits Arthur told them that they didn't need to come along anymore—he could walk by himself and handle it himself. One staff said, "But Arthur, what about walking home? It will be dark out." Arthur told her firmly, "But Sandy, there are street lights!"
>
> Arthur also tried other things for the first time. He agreed to stay for the coffee hour between church services and went to the adult Bible class. One Sunday, he sat way up in the front so that he could attend communion. Art said he was "proud of himself for trying." (Amado et al., 1990, p. 69)

Arthur's sense of playing a valued role at the library catalyzed a whole new lifestyle for him. Whereas many of these changes could have been produced with enough programming time, when he had a role with community members that he found valuable, and when he had a chance to participate and contribute in a community setting totally separate from his agency programs, a qualitative shift happened that programming could not provide. Programs, no matter how good they are, and no matter how good their results are, perseverate the model of providing programs. Within the programming paradigm, the only thing programs lead to is the next program.

Vicki

Vicki lives in her own apartment and works at the sheltered workshop. She is pretty independent, but usually gets attention from people by doing negative things. For instance, she would call her landlord constantly to come and fix things in her apartment. When she scheduled a birthday party, she called her guests to tell them what to bring her as presents. At one point, a few days before the party, she was calling people every 15 minutes. Although she is one of the best workers at the sheltered workshop, she has a reputation for "inappropriate behavior" in her relationships with co-workers. That is one of the reasons the workshop considers her "not ready" for community employment. When the Friends group first started meeting, some members of her group despaired of finding people who would like her, because she had a reputation of being annoying. (Amado et al., 1990, p. 81)

One way of addressing Vicki's behavior would include social skills training and a reinforcement and response-cost program in which socially pleasant behavior would be reinforced and annoying behavior would be fined. A well-designed program implemented by properly trained staff would likely produce the desired results with enough time. In fact, the staff working with Vicki had used a variety of programs (addressing both physical and verbal aggression) over several years without success. When her agency began working on individuals having more community members as friends, Vicki's friends' focus group found someone her own age who shared her interests.

Vicki and Muffy live only a few blocks away from each other. They have become great friends. Vicki is thrilled to watch Muffy's children with her. The two of them talk on the phone, go for long walks and shopping together, and sew together. Muffy helped Vicki enter one of her pillows in the County Fair craft competition. Muffy really likes Vicki, and thinks she is "really funny." Vicki is not at all annoying with Muffy, and really is a delightful person to be with. (Amado et al., 1990, p. 81)

Once her relationship with Muffy was established, Vicki also joined Weight Watchers and lost 30 pounds, joined a women's group at her church of which Muffy is also a member, and became more proud of herself. Her behavior also improved significantly. Rather than seeing her as "the problem" that she used to be, her staff are also very proud of her. Her agency also assisted her to buy her own home.

As with Michelle and Arthur, Vicki's behavior changed substantially as a function of a major qualitative change in her life. Major shifts across broad spectrums of conduct are not typically achieved through contemporary habilitation practices. However, by addressing loneliness, a lifestyle factor that has broad behavioral influence, many supposedly unrelated behavioral changes can be effected.

IMPLICATIONS

The degree to which the aggressive, self-injurious, and nonconstructive behavior of human services recipients is a result of and artifact of the human services system is unknown, but it is probably fairly significant. Perhaps the human services system is simply continuing to generate more institutions and more variations of institutionalized behavior, even in small community-based settings. This discussion has reviewed the extreme toll on human well-being extracted by practices in human services that promote social isolation in human beings and the role those practices play in generating anti-social and dangerous behavior by forcing people to live in the aversive condition of loneliness.

Given the information reviewed in this discussion, there are at least four implications for practices and policies:

1. Human services rules and regulations that contribute to the isolation of people must be changed immediately and replaced with designs, practices, and policies that support the building of social networks.
2. It is no longer acceptable to address behaviors of concern with behavioral programs or behavior- and/or mood-modifying medications without ensuring the person's quality of life is at least as good as that of a typical member of society, especially in such areas as size of the social network. To do otherwise might result in forcing a person to tolerate personally unacceptable conditions in the guise of mental health services (e.g., counseling a prison inmate so that he will like prison, or using behavioral programs in prisoner-of-war camps to decrease the frequency of escape attempts).
3. Current federal, state, and local regulations result in the expenditure of untold dollars to correct the damage done to people who receive services in the human services system. Policies must be changed to ensure mental and physical health care practitioners are able to address quality of life issues (e.g., friends and social relationships) as part of their services, and, when necessary, take steps to ensure quality of life is brought up to minimum acceptable standards.
4. Mental and physical health practitioners must be trained to include broad quality of life measures in professional assessments and intervention plans. The experience of loneliness, number and types of friends, and quality and frequency of social interactions are all areas that should be evaluated.

CONCLUSION

The known effects of loneliness on physical health, mental health, and human behavior all indicate that loneliness is an aversive and punishing condition for a human being. Understanding loneliness as a causal aversive condition leads to a different perspective on the socially undesirable behavior resulting from this condition. For the sake of people's well-being, longevity, mental health, and positive social behavior, practices in the human services system that contribute to loneliness must be identified and altered. Having friends is not a luxury, but a necessity to life.

People are lonely because they build walls instead of bridges.

Joseph F. Newton

REFERENCES

Amado, A.N., Conklin, F., & Wells, J. (1990). *Friends: A manual for connecting persons with disabilities and community members.* St. Paul: Human Services Research and Development Center.

Baker, M.J., & Salon, R.S. (1986). Setting free the captives: The power of community integration in liberating institutionalized adults from the bonds of their past. *Journal of The Association for Persons with Severe Handicaps, 11*(3), 176–181.

Berkman, K.A., & Meyer, L.H. (1988). Alternative strategies and multiple outcomes in the remediation of severe self-injury: Going "all out" nonaversively. *Journal of The Association for Persons with Severe Handicaps, 13*(2), 76–86.

Chadsey-Rusch, J., DeStefano, L., O'Reilly, M., Gonzalez, P., & Collet Klingenberg, L. (1992). Assessing the loneliness of workers with mental retardation. *Mental Retardation, 30*(2), 85–92.

Hill, B.K., Lakin, K.C., Bruininks, R.H., Amado, A.N., Anderson, D.J., & Copher, J.I. (1989). *Living in the community: A comparative study of foster homes and small group homes for people with mental retardation.* Minneapolis: University of Minnesota, Center for Residential and Community Services.

Hojat, M., & Crandall, R. (Eds.). (1989). *Loneliness: Theory, research and applications.* Newbury Park, CA: Sage Press.

House, J.S., Landis, K.R., & Umberson, D. (1988). Social relationships and health. *Science, 241,* 540–545.

Luftig, R.L. (1988). Assessment of the perceived school loneliness and isolation of mentally retarded and nonretarded students. *American Journal on Mental Retardation, 92,* 472–475.

Lynch, J.J. (1977). *The broken heart: The medical consequences of loneliness.* New York: Basic Books.

Mount, B., Ducharme, G., & Beeman, P. (1991). *Person-centered development: A journey in learning to listen to people with disabilities.* Manchester, CT: Communitas, Inc.

Newton, J.S. (1989). *Social support manual.* Eugene: University of Oregon, Neighborhood Living Project.

O'Brien, J., & O'Brien, C.L. (1992). *Remembering the soul of our work.* Madison, WI: Options in Community Living.

Perlman, D., & Peplau, L.A. (1982). Loneliness research: A survey of empirical findings. In L.A. Peplau & S.E. Goldstein (Eds.), *Preventing the harmful consequences of severe and persistent loneliness.* Rockville, MD: NIMH.

Polansky, N.A. (1986). *Treating loneliness in child protection.* Washington, DC: Child Welfare League of America.

Schalock, R.L. (1992, May). *Viewing quality of life in the larger context.* Paper presented at the annual meeting of the American Association on Mental Retardation, New Orleans.

Sigelman, C.K., Schoenrock, C.J., Spanhel, C.L., Hromas, S.G., Winer, J.L., Budd, E.C., & Martin, P.W. (1980). Surveying mentally retarded persons: Responsiveness and response validity in three samples. *American Journal of Mental Deficiency, 84*(5), 479–486.

Skinner, B.F. (1953). *Science and human behavior.* New York: The Free Press.

Taylor, S.J., Asher, S.S., & Williams, G.A. (1987). The social adaptation of mainstreamed mildly retarded children. *Child Development, 58,* 1321–1334.

Tyne, A. (1988). *Ties and connections: An ordinary community life for people with learning difficulties.* London: King's Fund Centre.

Ulman, L.P., & Krasner, L. (1975). *A psychological approach to abnormal behavior* (2nd ed.). Englewood Cliffs, NJ: Prentice Hall.

Webster, D. (1979). *New collegiate dictionary.* Springfield, MA: Merriam-Webster.

Weiss, R.S. (1982). Loneliness: What we know about it and what we might do about it. In L.A. Peplau & S.E. Goldstein (Eds.), *Preventing the harmful consequences of severe and persistent loneliness.* Rockville, MD: NIMH.

Woodward, J.C. (1988). *The solitude of loneliness.* Lexington, MA: Lexington Books.

5

Natural Pathways to Friendships

Bruce Uditsky

The wonder and value of friendship has probably always been part of the human mystery. Philosophers, poets, songwriters, and lovers have struggled through time immemorial to capture the essence of friendship through expressions of rhetoric, poem, song, or passion. There is no question that friendship is integral to the human spirit and condition. It is part of what defines us as human; it is part of what is necessary to the expression of humanness. Furthermore, the value of friendship extends from the spirituality of its nature to its functionality—a functionality that covers the breadth of supports from moral to pragmatic. Yet, with all kinds of experience and knowledge, people's understanding of friendship remains tentative. Perhaps the greatest mystery surrounds the very personal, and as yet unexplainable, process as to how and when one person comes to call another a friend.

Recently, the subject of friendship has become a matter of some interest within the field of developmental disabilities. As a result, there has been a proliferation within the past 5 years of articles, books, workshops, manuals, reports, studies, techniques, and videos, all devoted to the promotion of friendship. Concurrently, and expectedly, friendship experts, facilitators, and projects have developed. In the rush to do the right thing, romantic illusion can rapidly displace critical reasoning, a recurrent phenomenon in this and many other fields. There have been many failed reforms of the past (e.g., group homes, segregated classes, workshops); in addition, even after decades of professed commitment to and understanding of persons with developmental disabilities, there has been a simple failure to notice until now the pervasive friendlessness and its devastating effects in people's lives. Both these failures should at least provide some tempering thoughts.

Questions exist as to why, with this history, human services professionals should trust themselves and more importantly why people with developmental disabilities should trust them to touch their lives in some of the most intimate and personal ways. Where within the history of the field does the knowledge base exist to justify the assumption of friendship expertise? Given the history of the field, what false myths, strategies, and promises are most likely to be created? This last question is not particular to the field of developmental disabilities or to the subject of friendship; it is rather a universal question applicable and necessary to developments within any field. Attempting to chart the course of probable falsehoods enables the development of possible safeguards against future perversions. For example, some efforts promise friendships as an outcome of the application of certain strategies. This is a false promise, however well intentioned, as the course of friendship can never be guaranteed or predicted. A safeguard issue arises as to how to protect the field from succumbing to such false promises and, more critically, how to protect persons with developmental disabilities and their families from being misled.

Every field exists as a set of conscious and unconscious cultural and historical factors. Any new idea that evolves or erupts within a field will always be bound in some ways to the culture of that field. As such, to maintain the merit and integrity of a new idea, an intense and ongoing critical appraisal is required. A meritorious concept will not only survive ongoing critique, but is likely to be improved as a result of it. The concern here is not with friendship itself, but with its promotion from within the developmental disabilities field, specifically the strategies promoted as the means to friends. It may be that true friendship and its timeless value cannot be separated from the pathways that allow for the possibility of friendship. Perhaps controlling the processes that lead to friendship may actually inhibit the full magic of friendship. For those questions that cannot be answered with certainty, which will be most of them, what then are the least dangerous approaches to the question of friendship?

SINGLE, SIMPLE, RAPID, FORMALIZED SOLUTIONS

What follows is not an exhaustive identification of historical and cultural factors with which the field of developmental disabilities is imbued. Rather, a number of examples are presented as illustrations of the conceptual issue of how current thinking on friendship is influenced by the past. There is a propensity in any field, and among human beings in general, to generate simple solutions to complex problems. In the field of developmental disabilities, examples abound regardless of the problem (e.g., deinstitutionalization, behavioral challenges, real homes). The solutions generated, in addition to their singularity, are inexorably tied to the reforms and even the problems of the past. Escape from this tendency probably requires a paradigm shift, which is discussed later in this chapter.

The approach to deinstitutionalization within the field of developmental disabilities provides a useful example of generating simple, past-based solutions to complex problems. Whereas each person entered an institution as an individual, uniquely torn from his or her family and community, deinstitutionalization often took place on a simplistic and deindividualized basis. The complexity of reestablishing the wholeness of family and community life was reduced to congregate living arrangements, often with strangers, in service-governed housing. Over time, the failings of these initially highly touted reforms became more and more visible. This visibility was sharpened by the continuing evolution of the values foundation upon which the reforms were based. The more individuals with developmental disabilities were perceived as equivalent to typical citizens in the totality of their humanness, the deeper the understanding of the limits of the latest reform.

The early days of the community living movement embodied the reductionist response to the complexity of a real home and true community belonging by concentrating on finding the right size service setting. Battles were waged and won, for example, reducing group homes to 10 or 12 people. When the numeric goal was achieved, but the promised lifestyles were not, the presumption appeared to be that the number was wrong. The answer was obviously 8, then of course 6, and so on until the real magic number could be found. The reduction in size had merit and does allow for improvements in lifestyles, but the complexity of a decent community life for societally marginalized citizens cannot be achieved through such a simplistic avenue. Furthermore, the strategy itself was routed within the very field that inhibited such a life. A paradigm shift would suggest that the knowledge and means to a valued community lifestyle might lie far more within the community itself than within a field whose historical roots and expertise lay outside the community.

The complexity of fostering or enabling a real home and sense of community obviously goes far beyond a belief in numerology. One can be isolated from community regardless of the size of the living arrangement. The independent community living movement provides yet another example of an overly singular concept to which many lives have been sacrificed, often resulting in loneliness and service dependency. Although these results are now understood within the field, questions still remain—questions that must force individuals in the field to look at the unconscious assumptions that guided its reform efforts. While leading interdependent and relationship-filled lives themselves, how did human services professionals arrive at reducing the complexity of community life for persons with developmental disabilities to independent living? Perhaps if the reform had been derived from the experience of community life common to everyone and not from the field's focus on continuums and skill development, the goals and methods would have been compatible with the dreams and needs of persons with developmental disabilities—that is, their dream and need to share in the life of community, not simply to be placed within a community.

Another feature of the propensity to simple solutions is to favor formal or technological solutions. Although the complex emotional and personal problems of individuals with a developmental disability are currently much less subject to the terror of aversive procedures than they once were, they are still reduced, in too many instances, to problems of technology (Uditsky, 1992). There has been a switch from aversive to nonaversive procedures, but within a technological paradigm. Some approaches, for example, promise liberation and solidarity by the repeated forced practice of meaningless tasks. The means to an ordinary lifestyle now require a broker trained in lifestyle planning technologies, as if the need for friendship cannot be discerned until an exhaustive list of strengths and needs are diagrammed with multicolored pens. Matters as complex as empowerment are reduced to individualized funding formulas and mechanisms. Empowerment is far more a function of relationships and community membership than having access to the funds to purchase many of the same services previously acquired under more traditional funding mechanisms. Individualized funding has done more to foster the employment and income of nondisabled individuals than to empower persons with a disability. It is not that individualized funding does not have merit, but again it should be within a context where it is a simple component of a more complex schemata, rather than a simplistic panacea.

The above brief critique is not an indictment of the field, but a reflection on the efforts of ordinary human beings to do better. For many, the means of resolution still lie in finding the right formal and simple solution that will work immediately. This precept is influencing the latest reform—the promotion and development of relationships, leading to some worrisome developments.

HUMAN SERVICES FRIENDSHIP TECHNOLOGIES

Given the powerful influences of the human services culture, it is not surprising to find friendship, to varying degrees, considered in the simplistic manner the field knows best. As a result, both old and new technologies now promise friendship. Relationships have become one more domain in the development of individualized service or program plans—one more goal to be measured and observed, a sort of add-on to existing service and programmatic procedures. For instance, it is true that those who are institutionalized desperately require friends and that friendship can contribute to personal well-being on many levels; however, rather than simply adding friendship as a service plan goal, it would be better to advocate for a very different life—a life in community with friends. Even if someone currently lives in the community, the encouragement of friendships must be seen as more than a simple programmatic add-on. It must be part of a broader values-based totality that calls for an inclusive community lifestyle, even when currently unachievable or extremely difficult. It is not enough to have friendship blocked into some programmatic schedule between menu planning and Special Olympics. Without care, it is very possible to turn friends into servants of, or an extension of, the agency—a new form of unpaid relief helping perhaps to justify community living by containing costs. In some parts of Canada friendships are written into individualized service plans for precisely these reasons. Efforts to develop friendships that are built on this agenda, even if subtly so, are likely to corrupt the friendship. Conscious and unconscious pressures may be exerted to have the friend fulfill the goal of cost containment.

Another difficulty emerges when friendship is viewed through a narrowly focused, if not overly romantic, lens. The complexity of friendship is often ignored in the mythological testimony to its inherent goodness. In encouraging the possibility of friendship, the reality is that it will bring pain, joy, or possibly both. For some people, friendship is not cemented until some mutual rite of passage is accomplished. Processes that overly control possible development of friendship may inhibit necessary and cathartic experiences that happen by chance. The real depths of some friendships are never known until they are tested; yet, some programmatic friendship efforts do everything to maintain friendships on a controlled artificial plane.

With friendship comes the possibility of rejection or betrayal. Friendship can bring pain, for example, when, through the friendship, the too often marginalized and vulnerable existence of an individual with disabilities is recognized. The pain can be increased further by the recognition of the limits of one's friendship in response to over-whelming or complex needs. A person with a disability may feel the pain of that limitation or the dilemma of a friend who is struck by the limits of his or her capacity to respond. For many community members without disabilities, there are usually sufficient positive relationhips and life circumstances to overcome the ordinary hurt and despair that can accompany friendship. This difference in relationships with persons with disabilities is not a caveat against friendship, it is a caveat about approaching friendship too simplistically and with too singular a conceptualization. Sufficient friendships cannot be measured numerically, and friendship alone may not be enough. At the very least, friendship should be approached honestly—that is, as good and bad; joyful and painful; and profoundly simple, yet utterly complex.

In many ways, current efforts to support friendship are extensions of earlier volunteer involvement strategies. There are simple, formal procedures such as matching nondisabled volunteers to persons with a developmental disability and more complex formal procedures such as "circles" or support networks. Matching is a relatively ancient strategy and the role of matchmaker has existed in many cultures. The process of matchmaking tends to be culture-bound; yet, even in those societies where it existed, it was not always the preferred or first strategy. It may rather have been a secondary strategy, used only when primary efforts failed, as it is perceived and understood today in contemporary western culture (e.g., singles ads). The applicable operating assumption is that formal and artificial strategies are weaker than informal and natural strategies. In services for persons with developmental disabilities, the need for matching may be more a function of segregation and limited knowledge of friendship-enabling pathways. The possibility exists, however, that a simple, singular strategy will be easily and readily embraced, even if it is a weak approach. This form of strategy almost invariably pushes out more powerful multidimensional strategies.

The circle of friends strategy is one example used here for purposes of illustration of this critique of formal, singular stategies. The concept itself may be no worse or better than other formal strategies. In effect, every new and promising idea should be critically appraised; such appraisal is even more important when fundamental human needs are involved. Given the unquestionable value of friendship and the lack of it in the lives of so many people with developmental disabilities, friendship-making strategies should be intensely scrutinized. The issues in the following critique can be used as a guide, at least conceptually, in the evaluation of many formalistic approaches.

The objections presented to the formalization and even bureaucratization of friendships should not be misconstrued as opposition to the necessary facilitation of such relationships. Facilitation may be very necessary, for any if not all of us, but it needs to occur within an appropriate paradigm.

Circles are one of the more widely known strategies to support friendship (e.g., circles of support, circles of friends) and are illustrative of a number of key points. The circle process is often, but not exclusively, applied to children and sometimes the formation of a circle is tied to a MAPS (McGill Action Planning System) session (e.g., Vandercook, York, & Forest, 1989). Typically in school settings, an adult circle facilitator asks a group of nondisabled children if they would be willing to join or create a circle of friends for a child with a disability. Often this is done in regular classrooms, either in anticipation of a student with a disability or when such a student is already a member of a class. The group usually meets regularly, in school or out-of-school, and discusses how their activities are going; circle members may also problem solve issues faced by the student with a disability and/or themselves. The group may be named for the student (e.g., Jared's circle of friends). Members of the group often assume a variety of roles under the tutelage of the facilitator. The expectation is that as a result of the group process a number of children will become genuine friends. Similar processes are also used for adults with disabilities. In effect, this approach is no more than a sophisticated variation of the friendship through volunteering strategy.

There are distinct and critical differences between the common expressions of typical community, such as "my circle of friends," and the circles of friends organized by human services professionals. There are also fundamental differences in the processes by which such circles form, one naturally and one artificially. In considering formal strategies for children, as an example, a number of helpful questions ought to be raised:

What does it mean for a child to be asked to volunteer friendship, to have the expectation of friendship placed upon him or her? What does it mean to a child to be the object of that volunteerism?

What does it mean to have friendships organized for a child that are administered by an adult, to have roles and duties assigned, and/or to be the object of a group rather than an equally valued member of a collectivity?

What does it mean for a child, adolescent, or teenager to make a commitment at the request of some adult, and what does it mean when circles and disability become conjoint terms?

Are circles more likely to prepare their participants for interdisciplinary team work or individualized program planning than for sharing lives together in ordinary ways?

What is lost when children do not have the opportunity to fall in and out of friendships normatively?

For children or adults, how long will formally facilitated friendships generally last?

How many of the amazing arrays of ordinary life strategies to facilitate friendships will be negated or neglected in favor of one simple, single solution?

Are such formal strategies more useful for bringing a group together to problem solve or advocate for change, rather than for encouraging real friendship?

How will these artificial networks survive life changes and changes in administrators or facilitators?

How many professionals see and understand their own constellation of friends in a simple and organized form?

Where in history and in the knowledge of community life has the power of formal friendship procedures been demonstrated?

What is the long-term success rate of strategies whose roots lie in the human services domain?

These questions regarding formal strategies are not meant to imply that valued and meaningful friendships are impossible if the means by which people are brought together is imperfect. In life in general, friendship is a possibility even from poor or bad beginnings. The power of friendship to overcome human weaknesses, however, is not a sufficient rationale for using weak or misguided strategies. The circles methodology represents a number of very important issues. Having recognized the value of friendships and their paucity in the lives of persons with a disability, professionals turn to the formal volunteer and formal group methods endemic to the field rather than to the wealth of knowledge that is present in the millions of relationships in ordinary community life. Friendship facilitators see children and their friends, but as they fail to see the subtle and powerful natural pathways that allow for the development of friendship, they are seduced by their perceptions of their own expert power—not expert in the realm of friendship necessarily, but in the realm of disability. Surely if it is held that people with developmental disabilities have the same human needs as those without disabilities, then it will be seen that the best means to friendship must be those that work so well naturally and informally. Clearly, professionals in the field of developmental disabilities have much to learn from children, who so much better exemplify the possibility of forging genuine friendships with persons with disabilities than the current adult generation. However, the best lessons to be learned from children are those which occur when they are simply being themselves. By watching parents or a day care scene, it is evident that friendship supports are fairly natural and consistent from both children and adults. Friendship for children with disabilities would be far better served if such natural methods were used to embed children with disabilities in the informal pathways that already work their ordinary wonders. The same concept can be used for adults by utilizing ordinary processes that contribute to friendships in the workplace or in the community.

FRIENDSHIPS, NATURALLY

Friendship, in all its mystery and wonder, is best understood and enabled from the knowledge base of community and the ordinary wisdom of the ages. The paradigm shift that must be considered is to move out of the context of developmental disabilities and human services, out of the context of simple or technological solutions to complex human problems, and into the disorganization, disarray, and incoherence of ordinary life. Such a shift means moving toward the unpredictable meandering pathways that weave their way in and out of relationships for all people. These pathways, given their continuity throughout life, are more likely to allow for the possibilities of friendships than the application of specific formal strategies.

An example of the concept of normative pathways and their power can be found when considering how children are initially supported in the development of a career or work identity. Before a child is born, parents may think about what the future will hold for their child. Although their vision is not necessarily well-focused, it assumes valued roles and identities, and possibilities and opportunities—that is, a path. From the earliest moments after birth, parents, relatives, and friends attribute personal characteristics to the baby's features. The shape of a hand may lead to projections, albeit humorously, of musical talents. Observations of play as the child matures lead to exclamations of a talent for engineering (building things) or renovating (knocking things over). The child is asked repeatedly what he or she wants to be as an adult (often as the adults are still searching for answers themselves). In addition, children are continuously encouraged and reinforced to act out roles and dress up as potential career models, such as doctors or teachers. The simple point is that there is a powerful and potentially universal process at work that supports a pathway toward work as an adult, however difficult it is to chart. It may not be a predictable pathway or one guaranteed to be successful, but it is a pathway that is well-known and intuitively understood. Similar pathways open the doors to friendships.

When young children are observed in play, adults can catch glimpses of the process whereby friendships are formed, but they can never enter into either the world of children or of the individual child. As a result, exact friendship formation remains a mystery. Children find their own pathway facilitated by adults, but adults cannot direct a child to either become or not become a friend of any particular child. Even with all the power of adults, such exact direction in this area is often outside the realm of that influence. Perhaps two children will become friends because they wear the same color shoes one day, perhaps they will become friends because a color feels or sounds the same to them; or perhaps there is no simple explanation for their friendship. Whether a child or an adult, the moment of recognition of friendship is still personal and only realized after, not before. People may wonder aloud if they are becoming friends, but the presence of friendship is determined by the heart.

For children, the normative pathways of childhood support and encourage opportunities to play together informally and formally (e.g., scouts, guides, clubs), sharing in the celebration of milestones, making discoveries together, and following each others' leads. These are the pathways that adults clearly need to support in such ways as making their home open and inviting to children, having toys that encourage interactions and are currently popular according to respective age grups, playing chauffeur, and supporting current clothing fads. The list can go on and is quite extensive as it is based on what many parents already know and try, often intuitively. These are processes learned culturally and over the millennia. What is often required for children (and adults) with developmental disabilities is the extension of the already present natural supports within the normative pathways.

Inclusive schooling provides another vehicle for normative pathways, especially when the educational methods used are ones which naturally support relationships. Schools that have peer support strategies in place for all children and where children learn in cooperative groupings are examples. Community inclusion for adults provides another pathway, such as finding the places in community that match one's interests and talents, leading to friendship possibilities through participation and belonging. Such experiences allow for the possibility of friendships and no more. As with everyone, only a few of many inclusionary community experiences may result in full-fledged friendships. Therefore, as many of such experiences as possible should be encouraged and, as much as possible, the pathways to community inclusion should be ordinary ones. For example, the means of joining a group, whether formal or informal, should match the processes typically followed. An informal group may gather out of a similar interest, such as soccer or travel, whereas a formal group may gather out of a common cause. With a variety of approaches, a number of pathways can be followed.

The intent of this chapter is not to delineate in detail informal and natural avenues that allow for the possibility of friendships, but to nurture a debate and a critical perspective that has been lacking. This pursuit of friendship-formation knowledge must be employed with humility and not exalted as the latest human services reform. Rather, such debate should be encouraged and provides the opportunity for continued learning. Professionals run a risk in bringing human services friendship practices and assumptions into the community domain. It is incumbent upon them to be the students of friendship, not the masters. They can learn and teach more by example, by living lives that allow for friendship, than by the dissemination of any one method.

It is possible to pick any age or community, observe the normative processes at play, and use this knowledge base to provide the additional or adapted supports a person requires to participate in and follow existing pathways. In this way, becoming friends, whether suddenly or over long periods of time, is as much a part of the friendship as the outcome itself. By being encouraged to follow as typical a pathway as possible, relationships can evolve on the tried and true basis of common cultural experiences and knowledge—au naturel!

REFERENCES

Uditsky, B. (1992). Non-aversives: A value based analysis. *Journal of Leisurability, 19*(1), 15–23.

Vandercook, T., York, J., & Forest, M. (1989). The McGill Action Planning System (MAPS): A strategy for building the vision. *Journal of The Association for Persons with Severe Handicaps, 4*(2), 205–215.

6

When "Staff" and "Clients" Become Friends

Zana Marie Lutfiyya

Relatively little thought has been given to the nature of warm and affectionate relationships between individuals with disabilities and the people who are paid to be with, take care of, or supervise them— that is, between staff and clients. Indeed, one of the more commonly held assumptions is that such "paid relationships" are inherently bad and by definition are not really friendships. By common understanding, friendships cannot be a bought or purchased relationship. It is believed that the knowledge that one is paid to spend time with another disqualifies the relationship from the "private" sphere and places it into a more public or "business" arrangement (De Freitas-Cardoso, 1987; Reiss & Daly, 1989; Rubin, 1985). This author has been a proponent of this view, especially as it applies to individuals with mental retardation and other developmental disabilities (Lutfiyya, 1988, 1990, 1991).

However, in the early 1990s, several researchers realized that in some cases the nature of the relationship between paid caregivers and people with disabilities (and sometimes with their families) is not as clear as it was thought to be (Fisher, 1991; Sures, 1991; Traustadottir, 1991). Although several informants with disabilities have stated that

Preparation of this chapter was supported by the Research and Training Centers on Community Integration (Cooperative Agreement No. H133B0003-90) and Community Living (No. H133B80048) (the latter through a subcontract from the University of Minnesota); by a grant awarded to the Center on Human Policy, Division of Special Education and Rehabilitation, School of Education, by the Office of Special Education and Rehabilitative Services (OSERS), National Institute on Disability and Rehabilitation Research (NIDRR). The opinions expressed in this chapter are solely those of the author and no endorsement by the U.S. Department of Education or NIDRR should be inferred.

The author wishes to thank Angela Amado, Ellen Fisher, Michelle Sures, Steve Taylor, Rannveig Traustadottir, and Pam Walker for their assistance in the preparation of this chapter. This chapter is dedicated with great affection to Catherine and Nicola Schaefer.

no paid person could really be a friend, others have challenged this view and have provided examples in which people with disabilities and their paid caregivers have formed mutually respectful and affectionate relationships with each other—they have become friends. Upon hearing that this chapter would be written, the director of a small respite service heaved a sigh of relief and said, "Finally, maybe it will now be okay for people to acknowledge that 'staff' and 'clients' can really be friends!"

This chapter describes and examines the phenomenon of friendship between "staff" and "clients," including the development of such friendships and the unique set of circumstances that these friends face. Some caveats are already in order: first, the actual existence of such friendships is rare (Amado, Conklin, & Wells, 1990; Lord & Pedlar, 1991). This chapter only describes those instances in which both people have clearly indicated that there is a mutually felt and acknowledged friendship. Those cases in which the relationship is described by an agency as a "friendship," but is not so defined by the individuals involved, are not described.[1]

Additionally, it is not suggested that close personal relationships between paid caregivers and recipients are substitutes for other possible relationships. This author believes that all human beings need a variety of personal relationships, including friendship with many different individuals. Thus, relationships with individuals who are not acting in a paid capacity are still essential for individuals with disabilities. The purposes here are to document the existence of close personal relationships and friendships between paid caregivers and receivers, to note that such relationships are deeply significant to those involved, to describe the types of sources for descriptions of such friendships, and to provide an analysis of the process of staff becoming friends with the people they serve.

ACCOUNTS OF FRIENDSHIP

Within the disability literature, there are several accounts of friendships between paid caregivers and people with disabilities. By examining these accounts, three distinct sources or types of accounts in which such friendships are described have been identified. These include accounts from parents, professionals who advocate for an indi-

---

[1]In some agencies, all of the clients are assigned a staff "advocate" or "friend." In others, a volunteer "special friend" may be recruited. In still other instances, some parents have made the assumption that the staff will naturally befriend their son or daughter. These types of relationships are not considered friendships in this chapter.

vidual, and paid staff who have personal friendships with people with disabilities.

Parent Narratives

The existence of friendships between paid caregivers and people with disabilities was probably first described in the "parent narrative" literature. This body of literature includes accounts written by parents (virtually always the mothers) of individuals with disabilities, describing the effect of their children on family life. Although the specific tones of such accounts vary, they are often meant to be, and are, perceived as being a source of inspiration to other parents. Such books often include the history of the parents' experiences: the reaction after realizing the child's disability and subsequent experiences in the service system (typically medical and educational establishments), which are usually frustrating and unpleasant. The standard conclusion to many of these narratives is that despite all of the difficulties and problems, the family has been enriched by the presence of their member with a disability (Buck, 1962; Park, 1982; Piper, n.d.; Schaefer, 1983).

Many of these accounts include descriptions of friendships with paid caregivers. Most often, the caregiver who became a friend was a babysitter or respite worker who came into the family home to take care of the person with a disability. In some cases, a recreation person became involved as a friend. This individual, typically young and relatively inexperienced as a professional, developed a personal relationship with the family as a whole and with the person with a disability in particular (Moise, 1980; Park, 1982; Schaefer, 1983).

In these situations, the mother (generally the writer of the account) tells how the friendship develops and the positive impact that it has on the family. This friendship may be one of the few positive relationships, if not the first, with a professional that the family has experienced. There are several reasons that may account for this phenomenon. First, due to age and inexperience, the babysitter or respite worker is not a full-time, fully socialized member of a profession and has not been inculcated by professional detachment. Second, it is not unusual in these situations that the family hires the individual themselves and is therefore not as dependent upon an agency for this assistance because the agency only pays part of the associated costs. Finally, it is much easier for a young respite worker to identify with and develop a relationship with an individual and his or her family than with an agency. Whatever the reason, this individual develops a bond with the person with a disability and his or her family.

Professionals Who Befriend and Advocate

Another type of personal relationship described in the literature develops between paid caregivers and people with disabilities when a staff person takes on the situation of another person as a cause (Traustadottir, 1991; Walker, 1993). These relationships often develop in fairly restrictive settings where the people with disabilities have very limited freedom and the direct care staff are also restricted (although not to the same extent). The paid caregiver identifies with the individual with a disability vis-à-vis the system. Out of this identification, the individuals involved develop an alliance and then a friendship.

In these cases, the paid caregiver moves beyond the staff role in order to champion the interests of the individual with a disability. The staff person protects, looks out for, and tries to ensure "preferential treatment," which in some settings may mean very basic items, such as food and clothing (Fisher, 1991; Sures, 1991; Traustadottir, 1991). The staff person may be accused by other staff of treating the person with a disability as a "pet" or spoiling them. In some cases, this staff person may still view the person with a disability as "childlike" and treat him or her in age-inappropriate ways (De Freitas-Cardoso, 1987; Goode, 1992). Although not specifically documented in the above examples, some staff people who claim a friendship with one of their "clients" may still mistreat other people with disabilities. In other cases, the efforts of the staff person were made only on behalf of a single person, their friend, but the impact extended to many others.

It was a physician's personal connection with a resident that helped prod him into unleashing the events that eventually resulted in Rivera's exposé of Willowbrook (Rothman & Rothman, 1984). Kaplan (1989), first a teacher and then a friend of Ruth Sienkiewicz-Mercer, assisted Ruth in the painstaking task of writing her autobiography so that her story would be available publicly. Perske (1988) provides us with the story of Ziggy and Clarence. Ziggy, a psychiatric nurse, helped Clarence find an expression for his musical talent and lobbied for Clarence's move from the institution to his own home in the community and the opportunity to play and study music at the local university.

A Citizen Advocacy coordinator (Bufis, 1992) has received dozens of requests over the years to recognize and extend an "official" status to paid caregivers who developed a friendship while advocating for a person within the service system. They hoped that such status would provide a legitimacy for the friendship and advocacy role that they had assumed.[2]

Inspirational Accounts of Friendship

Another source of descriptions about friendships between paid caregivers and people with disabilities comes from accounts written by professionals. These accounts differ from those in the previous section in type of authorship and nature of the relationship. Although most of the relationships in the previous section were described by people outside the human services system, these accounts include the professional's view of their own friendship with a person with a disability. The emphasis in the following accounts is on the impact that the person with the disability has made in the life of the nondisabled staff person. These are highly personalized accounts that describe how the people met and formed an attachment with someone within the sphere of the agency in which they were involved either as workers or clients (Edwards & Dawson, 1983; Klein, 1992; Schwartz, McKnight, & Kendrick, 1987). Generally, such accounts do not come from direct care providers or front line staff, but from administrators or program managers.

Another difference between these two types of staff accounts is the orientation of the staff toward their work. Rather than feeling oppressed in a regimented and bureaucratized system, some professionals have adopted the mission of assisting their friends with disabilities to participate as fully as possible in community life. In some settings, the staff are encouraged to develop warm relationships with the people they support and to do things together when the staff are not on duty (Walker & Salon, 1991). One natural extension of this is the development of friendships between professionals and people with disabilities.

The friendship typically represents a reversal of the official or public roles that the two people are expected to play. That is, the teacher, trainer, or professional cites the person with a disability as the one who instructed the individual writing the account, and who gave more to the relationship. The person with a disability may be a source of inspiration to the nondisabled friend in terms of both personal characteristics and professional work. In addition, the professionals acknowledge that it was the person with a disability, or client,

---

[2]Typically, within citizen advocacy offices, supporting a direct paid caregiver as an advocate is not practiced. This is based on the recognition that a staff person remains in a position of direct conflict of interest between the agency and the individuals who are served by that agency.

who was responsible for keeping the nondisabled person "rooted" in real life and important values.

For example, in one group home located in Washington state (Lutfiyya, 1986), the director of the facility in 1986, Kathy Easton, shared a friendship with one of the women who lived in the home, Joanna.[3]

> These two women do a lot of things together on Kathy's personal time, such as going to concerts, out for meals, visit with Kathy's friends and family. Kathy identifies with Joanna when she says, "Joanna and I are genuine friends. I like her, we have similar interests in music, watching people . . . we enjoy each other." (Lutfiyya, 1986, p.12)

Although Joanna does not talk much, it is clear to an observer that she is fond of Kathy. When asked if a picture could be taken of her, perhaps in her favorite place or doing her favorite thing, she chose to be photographed standing next to Kathy.

In addition, the other staff in this group home are encouraged to involve their own families and friends in the activities of the household. Therefore, the staff can spend time with their family or friends while on the job if they involve some of the residents. For example, one of the residents attends church with a staff person and her parents, brothers, and sisters. Another staff person described his job this way:

> It is sharing my life . . . sharing our lives together.
> Staff are supposed to share as much of ourselves as we can . . . even outside the group home. I can lead a normal life—I keep my own contacts and friends and it is great to share with [the residents]. (Lutfiyya, 1986, p.13)

The context for the possibility of close personal relationships and friendships is created and supported within this kind of atmosphere.

Meaning, Validity, and Accounts of Friendship

These accounts of friendships between paid caregivers and individuals with disabilities may be problematic for those outside of the friendship. The essential question of whether or not the relationship is a friendship may hover unanswered over the doubts that are raised. For example, do the young people described within the parent narrative literature have a relationship primarily with the person with a disability or with the family as a whole? Are the staff who advocate for an individual acting as "good" service providers or as friends? Is

---

[3]This name is a pseudonym.

the advocacy performed by a staff person an expression of friendship or merely a venue for the expression of dissatisfaction, a convenient way to get back at an employer? Skeptics might view some of the relationships as falling mostly within the realm of rhetorical posturing, akin to the integration credo of the 1960s that "some of my best friends are . . . ." Other, less cynical people may wonder if the nondisabled friend reports a friendship because he or she feels a social pressure (perhaps unconscious) to do so.

Outsiders to a particular friendship are often unable to understand the nature of the bond between people, although they acknowledge that such a bond exists (Fischer, 1982; Suttles, 1970). This inability to understand is particularly true for friendships that include a person with a disability (Lutfiyya, 1990). Rather than construct a template of friendship by which to compare and categorize relationships in this research, the findings here rely on the meanings of the relationship to the individuals involved. When people have identified themselves as friends, that joint definition is accepted as a valid one.

Within a context of mutuality and shared meaning, the essence of these friendships is quite clear for those who are involved in them. For example, Edwards (Edwards & Dawson, 1983) states that David Dawson is her best friend, "the most wonderful and faithful friend that I have." Despite the potential of other motivations, these accounts do point to the potential of genuine friendships between staff and people with disabilities, which are meaningful and therefore valid to the people involved.

THE PROCESS OF BECOMING FRIENDS

A review of the accounts of friendship between paid caregivers and people with disabilities reveals a process in the development of these friendships. The process includes identification with the other person and a mutual recognition of the other as a potential friend. A variety of critical events help the two individuals jointly define their relationship as a friendship. This transformation involves the transcendence by the friends of their "staff" and "client" roles. This section delineates this process of becoming friends.

In order for a friendship to develop, each individual must be able to identify something in the other person that reflects a kindred spirit. This recognition may be based on having a similar interest or common background. In some cases, the agency or most staff may define the individual with a disability as "noncompliant," "unlikable," or as having "challenging behaviors." Despite these descriptions, and sometimes because of them, the person with a disability may still be able to strike a responsive chord within one staff person. A friendship between a paid caregiver and a person with a disability thus begins with a recognition of some similarity that develops into an attachment. The two individuals undergo a process by which they jointly come to define their relationship as a friendship. Over time, the specific events may be lost or forgotten, but something more than the sum of the discrete interactions was created. As the people spend time together, they establish a history of activities and memories. This becomes the friendship, an abstract construction that carries meaning for each person involved.

The process of becoming friends is marked by what has been called a series of critical events (Lutfiyya, 1990) or "defining encounters" (Wiseman, 1986, 1987). Certain events take place that help the individuals examine and refine their relationship with one another. Critical events may help people recognize their friendship with each other and extend or limit the parameters of the friendship. Critical events can be any major life change that the individuals encounter or circumstances that are apparently beyond the control of the two individuals.

There seem to be two major types of critical events that affect the process by which staff and people with disabilities become friends. First is the transfer of the staff person (or, less often, the person with a disability) to another program or facility. The second type are events that involve the staff person's conflict of interest position as both a friend and an employee.

Physical Relocation

The high turnover rate of frontline staff within human services programs has reduced the possibility that friendships and other personal relationships can develop (Amado et al., 1990; Lord & Pedlar, 1991). Individuals have less time to get to know each other and develop a bond (De Freitas-Cardoso, 1987). Also, when a friendship has been established, a physical relocation of one of the friends may be enough to end the friendship. In a few cases, a relocation helps the two individuals confirm and strengthen their ties to each other (Lutfiyya, 1990). The two friends make and keep plans to stay in touch. In one instance, it was only when a paid job coach maintained her budding relationship with the person she was supporting after she left her paid role with him that the relationship was seen as a friendship by the person with a disability. He did not want to be friends with the job coach when she was paid. As the job coach later stated, "In the beginning, when I was in an official capacity with him, he had nothing for me" (Lutfiyya, 1990).

Such friendships with ex-staff may even be recognized by the agency and supported by invitations to the friend without a disability to visit or attend IHP meetings. When the relationship is not supported (sometimes agencies do try to limit contact between ex-staff and current clients), the two friends may face a formidable barrier.

Conflict of Interest

A second critical event that affects the process of paid caregivers and people with disabilities becoming friends arises from the inherent conflict of interest position of the staff person. This person is both an employee with a particular status within an agency and a personal friend to someone who is under the control of the same agency. The development of the friendship involves a transcendence of the traditional roles of "staff person" and "client." The two friends forego the expected ways of interacting with each other in favor of their friendship.

This transcendence often results in the transfer of at least some loyalty from the agency to the friend with a disability on the part of the staff person. In situations when this loyalty is tested or questioned, tension and difficulties often occur for the friends. The staff person may question the agency's policies and regulations, at least in terms of his or her friend with a disability. The agency may view the staff person's actions as insubordination and outside of the stated job requirements and responsibilities. Alternately, the friend with a disability may be placed in an especially vulnerable position in terms of the care and support that he or she receives, which can affect the actions of the staff person. The nature and extent of the friendship is shaped and defined through such tests of interest and loyalty.

Friends do not progress through this process of becoming friends and defining the nature of their friendship in the same ways. The process of creating and maintaining a friendship does not always follow a linear progression; that is, the friendship may not move in a straight path from two people getting to know each other to becoming closer as time passes. Some friendships can cool off and/or end, whereas others continue to grow. There can also be a range in the degree of closeness between people who are friends. In some friendships, ongoing contact is maintained with a level of closeness not much different than that which existed when the friendships were newer. Two people can define themselves as friends, categorize the type or degree of friendship that they have, and then maintain that same level of closeness for a long time. The possible categories include, but are not limited to, people who describe their relationship as: colleagues, confidantes, "chums," buddies and pals, companions, and intimates.

CONCLUSION

Friendships do exist between paid caregivers and people with disabilities and this phenomenon is gaining wider recognition and appreciation. However, it is important to recognize also that such friendships are the exception and not the rule. The well-established and powerful roles of "client" and "staff" form a rocky soil, making it difficult for friendships to take root and flower. Furthermore, as Lord and Pedlar (1991) point out, when such friendships do develop, it is not possible to fully explain why they do. Potential reasons include extensive long-term and constant contact and support (or at least noninterference) from the agency. A genuine interest in and attraction to a person with a disability and his or her situation, and in return, a recognition of an ally and/or protector, may also lead to the establishment of a friendship.

People with disabilities and paid caregivers can establish and enjoy genuine friendships with each other. As with all friendships, it is important to recognize and value these relationships. Today it is becoming more widely acknowledged in the disability field that friendship enriches the lives of individuals with and without disabilities. However, it is also important not to exaggerate the existence or significance of these friendships or to romanticize them. In addition, there are many instances in which individual staff members can and do provide excellent support to people with disabilities where mutual respect, but no friendship, exists; the quality of those relationships should not be disregarded.

Whether they have certain friendships or not, most individuals with disabilities live without adequate or guaranteed services, often in isolating and congregating settings with limited social networks or resources. As essential as friendships are, they should not be seen as an acceptable replacement for necessary support services. Many individuals with disabilities are still living in fragile and vulnerable situations with few friends and limited social networks.

REFERENCES

Amado, A.N., Conklin, F., & Wells, J. (1990). *Friends: A manual for connecting persons with disabilities and community members.* St. Paul, Minnesota: Human Services Research and Development Center.

Buck, P. (1962). *A bridge for passing.* New York: John Day Company.

Bufis, S. (1992, March). *Presentation to the board of Person-to-Person: Citizen Advocacy.* Syracuse, NY.

De Freitas-Cardoso, M.C. (1987). *A study on the existence of friendship between group home residents and nondisabled persons through an explora-*

tion of planned contacts. Unpublished doctoral dissertation, Madison, Wisconsin.

Edwards, J., & Dawson, D. (1983). *My friend David: A sourcebook about Down's syndrome and a personal story about friendship.* Portland, OR: Ednick Communications.

Fischer, C.S. (1982). *To dwell among friends: Personal networks in town and city.* Chicago: The University of Chicago Press.

Fisher, E. (1991). Unpublished field notes. Syracuse, NY.

Goode, D.A. (1992). Who is Bobby? Ideology and method in the discovery of a Down's syndrome person's competence. In P.M. Ferguson, D.L. Ferguson, & S.J. Taylor (Eds.), *Interpreting disability: A qualitative reader* (pp. 197–212). New York: Teachers College Press.

Kaplan, S.B. (1989). *I raise my eyes to say yes: A memoir.* Boston: Houghton Mifflin.

Klein, J. (1992). Get me the hell out of here: Supporting people with disabilities to live in their own homes. In J. Nisbet (Ed.), *Natural supports in school, at work, and in the community for people with severe disabilities* (pp. 277–339). Baltimore: Paul H. Brookes Publishing Co.

Lord, J., & Pedlar, A. (1991). Life in the community: Four years after the closure of an institution. *Mental Retardation, 29*(4), 213–221.

Lutfiyya, Z.M. (1986). *"Goin' for it": Life in the Gig Harbor group home.* Syracuse, NY: Syracuse University, Center on Human Policy.

Lutfiyya, Z.M. (1988, September). Other than clients: Reflections on relationships between people with disabilities and typical people. *TASH Newsletter,* pp. 3, 5.

Lutfiyya, Z.M. (1990). *Affectionate bonds: What we can learn from listening to friends.* Syracuse,NY: Syracuse University, Center on Human Policy.

Lutfiyya, Z.M. (1991). "A feeling of being connected": Friendships between people with and without learning difficulties. *Disability, Handicap, & Society, 6*(3), 233–245.

Moise, L. (1980). *As up we grew with Barbara.* Minneapolis,MN: Dillon Press.

Park, C.C. (1982). *The siege: The first eight years of an autistic child; with an epilogue, fifteen years after.* Boston: Little, Brown.

Perske, R. (1988). *Circles of friends.* Nashville: Abingdon Press.

Piper, B. (n.d.). *Sticks and stones: The story of loving a child.* Syracuse, NY: Human Policy Press.

Reiss, M., & Daly, K. (1989). *Building bridges: Stories from the Springfield Citizen Advocacy Project.* Springfield, MA: Authors.

Rothman, D.J., & Rothman, S.M. (1984). *The Willowbrook wars: A decade of struggle for social justice.* New York: Harper & Row.

Rubin, L. (1985). *Just friends: The role of friendship in our lives.* New York: Harper & Row.

Schaefer, N. (1983). *Does she know she's there?* (Updated edition). Toronto, Ontario, Canada: Fitzhenry

Schwartz, D.B., McKnight, J., & Kendrick, M. (1987). *A story that I heard: A compendium of stories, essays, and poetry about people with disabilities and American life.* Harrisburg: Pennsylvania Developmental Disabilities Council.

Sures, M. (1991). Unpublished field notes. Syracuse, NY.

Suttles, G. (1970). Friendship as a social institution. In G.J. McCall (Ed.), *Social relationships* (pp. 95–135). Chicago: Aldine.

Traustadottir, R. (1991). *Supports for community living: A case study.* Syracuse, NY: Syracuse University, Center on Human Policy.

Walker, P. (1993). "We don't put up the roadblocks we used to": Agency change through the Citizenship Project. In J.A. Racino, P. Walker, S. O'Connor, & S.J. Taylor (Eds.), *Housing, support, and community: Choices and strategies for adults with disabilities* (pp. 299–312). Baltimore: Paul H. Brookes Publishing Co.

Walker, P., & Salon, R. (1991). Integrating philosophy and practice. In S.J. Taylor, R. Bogdan, & J.A. Racino, *Life in the community: Case studies of organizations supporting people with disabilities* (pp. 139–151). Baltimore: Paul H. Brookes Publishing Co.

Wiseman, J.P. (1986). Friendship: Bonds and binds in a voluntary relationship. *Journal of Social and Personal Relationships, 3,* 191–211.

Wiseman, J.P. (1987). The development of generic concepts in qualitative research through cumulative application. *Qualitative Sociology, 10*(4), 318–338.

7

The Gendered
Context of Friendships

Rannveig Traustadottir

In the fall of 1991, the author of this chapter was invited to a house-warming party. Ellen, the hostess, is in her 40s and has spent much of her life in state institutions and other segregated group facilities for people with disabilities. For many years Ellen dreamed of having her own place where she could live by herself. Finally, her dream came true and she moved into a small apartment. For the first time in Ellen's life she has a place she can call her own, and she celebrated by inviting a group of people to a housewarming party in her new apartment. Between 25 and 30 people came to Ellen's party. These people were, with the exception of two, all women. This group of women consisted of Ellen's sister and niece-in-law; Ellen's friends (about half of whom have disabilities); and some of Ellen's previous and current case workers, most of whom also consider themselves to be her friend. The majority of these women assisted Ellen in preparing the party; they helped her plan the party, make the fliers to invite people, go shopping, and prepare the food. During the party, the women combined forces to make sure everything went smoothly and a few of them stayed after the party to assist Ellen in cleaning up.

Preparation of this chapter was supported by the Research and Training Center on Community Integration, Center on Human Policy, Division of Special Education and Rehabilitation, Syracuse University (Cooperative Agreement H133B00003-90) and the Research and Training Center on Community Living (Cooperative Agreement H133B80048) via a subcontract from the University of Minnesota to the Center on Human Policy, Syracuse University. The Research and Training Centers are supported by the U.S. Department of Education, Office of Special Education and Rehabilitative Services (OSERS), National Institute on Disability and Rehabilitation Research (NIDRR). The opinions expressed herein are those of the author and no endorsement by the U.S. Department of Education should be inferred.

The author would like to thank Steve Taylor, Zana Lutfiyya, and other members of the research team at the Center on Human Policy for their contributions to this chapter. Thanks also to Barbara Ayres for her insights and to Rachael Zubal for her assistance in the preparation of this chapter.

The party was a very enjoyable event for everyone involved— especially Ellen. This housewarming party highlights the issues addressed in this chapter: the overrepresentation of women in social networks around people with disabilities and the important role women play in terms of providing social support through their personal relationships with people with disabilities.

The emphasis on social networks and personal relationships with other community members is at the heart of current trends in the disability field. Efforts to understand and facilitate relationships and connections in the community have, since the 1980s, been written about with much depth and scope (Amado, Conklin, & Wells, 1990; Forest, 1989; Hutchison, 1990; Lutfiyya, 1990; Mount, Beeman, & Ducharme, 1988a; O'Brien, 1987; O'Connell, 1990; Perske, 1988; Strully & Strully, 1985; Taylor & Bogdan, 1989). This literature clearly indicates that, despite more than 2 decades of community-based services, most people with disabilities continue to be isolated, lonely, and have few friends—especially nondisabled friends (Bercovici, 1983; Center on Human Policy, 1991; Hutchison, 1990; Krauss, Seltzer, & Goodman, 1992).

Despite the wealth of literature and numerous efforts to explore how people with disabilities can become truly connected to other people in the community, there remain many gaps in our understanding of relationships and connections in the lives of people with disabilities. One of these gaps is understanding the gendered context of people's social networks and personal relationships.

A review of the literature on friendships between people with and without disabilities indicates an overrepresentation of women within social networks of people with disabilities. Although gender has not been the focus of attention or inquiry in studies of friendships between people with and without disabilities, many studies have reported gender-related issues among their findings. These studies indicate that from childhood on, women tend to be more accepting of people with disabilities and more likely to become their friends. For example, Voeltz (1982) studied the effects of social contact between children with severe disabilities and their nondisabled peers. Among other things she found "consistent sex differences in acceptance, with girls significantly more accepting than boys across the total sample and at each level of contact on nearly every dependent measure" (p. 386). Similarly, in a study of a school-based program established to promote friendship between students with and without disabilities, Kishi (1988) reported as one of her major findings that girls were more likely than boys to become friends of students with disabilities.

Studies of adult friendships similarly suggest that women are over-represented as friends of adults with disabilities. In a study of pairs of disabled and nondisabled friends, Lutfiyya (1989) reported that women seem to be overrepresented as friends of adults with disabilities. A recent Canadian study was "designed to understand friendships from the perspective of people concerned with developing and facilitating friendships for people labelled mentally handicapped" (Hutchison, 1990, p. 95). The people selected to be interviewed for this study all had experiences in friendships as facilitators, friends, relatives, or researchers. Of the 30 people interviewed for the study, the overwhelming majority were women. The study, however, did not explore gender as an issue in relation to friendships.

The same gender pattern can be found in the literature that focuses on efforts to promote and facilitate social connections between people with disabilities and other community members. For example, the majority of the people who are active in efforts referred to as "bridge-building," "circles of support," or "community building" are female (Mount, Beeman, & Ducharme, 1988a, 1988b; O'Connell, 1988, 1990; Shoultz, 1991). Although the literature reflects an over-representation of women in the social networks of people with disabilities—both as friends and as agents in promoting acceptance and inclusion of people with disabilities—the literature has not explored gender as an issue.

The purpose of this chapter is to examine the gendered nature and context of relationships, especially friendship, between people with and without disabilities. The analysis draws upon the aforementioned literature on friendship; on a long-term qualitative study of social networks and personal relationships in the lives of people with disabilities that has been conducted by a team of researchers at the Center on Human Policy, Syracuse University, during the 1980s and 1990s; and also on the author's study of women's caring work and relationship-building with people with disabilities (Traustadottir, 1988, 1991a, 1991b). The following two questions will be addressed: What accounts for the gender differences in friendships between people with and without disabilities? Why are women more likely than men to become friends of people with disabilities?

This chapter is organized in three sections. The first section examines women's and men's orientation toward people and relationships in general and explores if that orientation may influence and explain why women are more likely than men to become friends of people with disabilities. The second section describes gender patterns in friendships within the general population, and compares these with gender patterns in friendships between people with and without disabilities. The third and last section examines the influence of disability policy and the women's movement on friendships between people with and without disabilities.

GENDER DIFFERENCES IN
ORIENTATION TOWARD PEOPLE AND RELATIONSHIPS

Gender differences in friendships between people with and without disabilities, especially the overrepresentation of women in such friendships, may be related to the different orientation males and females have toward people and relationships. This section examines these gender differences and explores how these differences may influence friendships between people with and without disabilities.

Nurturing and Caring: Women's Orientation Toward People

Over the course of 3 years (1989–1991), this author conducted a study of the role of women in facilitating the acceptance and inclusion of people with disabilities into ordinary community life. This qualitative study used participant observation and indepth interviews as methods for collecting data. The women who participated in the study worked with people with disabilities as professionals or paraprofessionals, or they were friends of people with disabilities. One of the things learned from interviewing and observing these women is that women's decisions to become involved with people with disabilities seems to be firmly grounded in their orientation toward people in general.

At the outset of the study, all of the women were asked how they became involved with people with disabilities. Before the women gave the specific reasons or circumstances that led them to become involved with the field, most of them started out by saying that they had always been "people-oriented" and interested in caregiving. The answer from a female job coach at a supported employment agency was typical for how the women described this pattern. She said, "I've always been interested—even as a little kid—just in caretaking. It's always been an interest." A female college student who has a friend with a disability phrased her response in a similar way, "I've always loved working with children and teenagers, and adults, you know, just with people."

The majority of the women in the study described how they started taking care of children in the form of babysitting at an early age, and many of them were immersed in caregiving activities much of their lives. Thus, before these women were introduced to the possibility of working with people with disabilities, they already were, even as young girls, oriented toward caregiving and nurturing. These women were initiated into caring work at an early age and by the time they entered high school most of them had many years of experience in caring. What these women said about their early orientation toward caring and nurturing has a striking resemblance to Chodorow's (1978) and Gilligan's (1982) theories about how female gender identity and moral development is centered around activities of caring and relationship-building.

Explaining the Gender Difference

There seems to be a split between women's expressive attributes as nurturers, caregivers, and weavers of networks and relationships on the one hand, and men's possession of instrumental attributes and orientation toward autonomy on the other hand. The best known efforts to explain these differences have been provided by feminist scholars who trace the differences between men and women back to the sex differences in childhood personality formation (Chodorow, 1978; Gilligan, 1982). These scholars have outlined how female identity develops in the context of an ongoing relationship with the mother. Girls identify with their mothers and experience themselves as their mothers, fusing the experience of attachment with the process of identity formation. For boys, separation and individuation are critically tied to gender identity because separation from the mother is essential for the development of masculinity. Therefore, masculinity is defined through separation whereas femininity is defined through attachment (Belenky, Clinchy, Goldberger, & Tarule, 1986). This is, according to Gilligan (1982), one reason why males tend to have difficulties with relationships, whereas females tend to have problems with separation. Gilligan (1982) also writes that besides defining themselves in a context of human relationship, women also "judge themselves in terms of their ability to care" (p. 17). It is important to note that Gilligan emphasizes that caring is not "natural" to women, but is structured by social relations. Women are socialized to become sensitive to the needs of others and assume the responsibility for nurturing and caregiving.

Not all feminist scholars agree on the explanations outlined above. For example, DeVault (1991) argues against explanations that present women's nurturing and caring as an aspect of "womanly identity." Instead, DeVault emphasizes that caring and nurturing is socially organized and constructed as women's work, and it is the power of this social construction that draws women into and recruits them for caring work.

An examination of gender differences in orientation toward people and relationships helps explain the overrepresentation of women as friends of people with disabilities. Men's orientation toward people and relationships is likely to hinder connections with people with disabilities, whereas women's orientation toward people makes them sensitive toward the needs of others and susceptible for being recruited as friends of people with disabilities. A woman's decision to become involved in the lives of people with disabilities is clearly embedded in women's orientation toward people in general.

GENDER PATTERNS IN FRIENDSHIPS

Those who have studied friendships among people without disabilities agree that gender is perhaps the single most significant factor in explaining the meaning, content, and variations of friendships. This section examines the gender patterns found within friendships in the general population and compares these with the gender patterns in friendships between people with and without disabilities.

Friendships in the General Population

Many studies have documented the differences in friendships among men and friendships among women (Bell, 1981; Block, 1980; Fasteau, 1991; Lenz & Myerhoff, 1985; McGill, 1985; Pogrebin, 1987; Rubin, 1985; Sherrod, 1989). One of these authors goes as far as claiming that "there is no social factor more important than that of sex in leading to friendship variations" (Bell, 1981, p. 55). Gender seems to be a main organizer of friendships and most studies identify three major patterns: 1) friendships among women, 2) friendships among men, and 3) cross-gender friendships. Because of the significant differences between these three categories of friendships, most studies provide a separate account of each.

Friendships Among Women   Women typically describe their friendships in terms of closeness and emotional attachment—the feelings they have for their best friend, love, and affection. What characterizes friendships between women is the willingness to share important feelings, thoughts, experiences, and support. Women devote a good deal of time and intensity of involvement with friends. Friendships among women, more so than with men, are broad and less likely to be segmented. That is, women usually make a deep commitment to their female friends and their friendships usually cover a broad spectrum, whereas men's friendships tend to be segmented and centered around particular activities (Gouldner & Strong, 1987; Lenz & Myerhoff, 1985).

History does not typically celebrate female friendships, and there is a long-standing myth that the greatest friendships have been between men. The male friendship is usually portrayed as the most unselfish and perhaps the highest form of human relationship, whereas women's friendships have been devalued and seen as frivolous and superficial (Bell, 1981; Block, 1980; Fasteau, 1991; Rubin, 1985). Many people who have studied friendships believe that the traditional wisdom about female friendships as inferior to those of men is a reflection of a more general notion of female inferiority (Acker, Barry, & Esseveld, 1990; Bell, 1981; Block, 1980; Raymond, 1986). If women are seen as inferior, then obviously, and by definition, so is what they do—including friendship. A group of women friends is not seen as a team of colleagues, but as the "girls" trooping off to gossip, exchange recipes, and talk about the trivia of fashion, cooking, or dieting, over tea. Studies indicate that many of these stereotypes about women's friendships still exist.

Contrary to the myth about women's friendships, research shows that women have more friends—especially more close friends—than men, and women's friendships are usually characterized by closeness, emotional attachment, acceptance, and willingness to share (Bell, 1981; Block, 1980; Rubin, 1885). Many authors have reflected on these misconceptions about women's friendships. For example, Bell writes:

> I would argue that the historical beliefs in the inferiority of female friendships are wrong. The evidence clearly indicates that the friendships of women are more frequent, more significant, and more interpersonally involved than those commonly found among men. (1981, p. 60)

Friendships play an important role in women's lives and many women seem to consider close friendships with other women a necessity for their well-being. Therefore, women are more likely and willing than men to initiate contact and do the "work" of establishing and maintaining friendships (Gouldner & Strong, 1987).

Friendships Among Men   The great friendships recorded in history have been between men, and friendships among men have often been romanticized and idealized. Men's friendships have typically been described in terms of bravery and physical sacrifice in providing assistance to others. Hardly ever do these historical accounts celebrate interpersonal relationships characterized by closeness and compassion for other men. Bell claims that, "This has been so because masculine values have made those kinds of feelings inappropriate and highly suspect—they were unmanly" (1981, p. 75). Despite this historical romanticization of the male friendship, researchers have found that men have significantly fewer friends than women, especially close friendships or best friends (Bell, 1981; Block, 1980; Fasteau, 1991). In her study of friendships, Rubin (1985) found that "Over three-fourths of the single women had no problems in identifying a best friend . . . In sharp contrast to the women, over two-thirds of the single men could not name a best friend" (p. 62–63).

Although the majority of men may not have close friends, they do not conduct their lives in isolation. Block (1980) found that most of the men in his study had a variety of same-sex relationships, including what Block calls "activity friends," such as a weekly tennis partner or a drinking buddy; "convenience friends," in which the relationship was based on the exchange of favors; and "mentor friends," typically between a younger and an older man.

Whereas women's friendships are usually defined as self-revealing, accepting, and intimate, men usually shy away from intimacy and closeness. The idealization of the male friendship as the highest form of human relations stands in contrast to the reality found by many researchers. Block (1980), for instance, says that men's experiences of friendships "are filled with incidents of rivalry and betrayal" (p. 55). Eighty-four percent of the men in Block's study did not disclose themselves fully to other men. Instead, they relied heavily on activity such as playing, watching sports, or drinking, to connect with other males. Block also found that among male friends, support is rarely given graciously without strings.

Competition among men is identified by many authors as one of the major barriers to close friendships among men (Fasteau, 1991). Another obstacle is traditional masculinity and the stereotype of the "real man" as independent, autonomous, self-contained, emotionally invulnerable, and nonexpressive of his feelings. An additional obstacle to intimacy and closeness in men's friendships is the fear of homosexuality (McGill, 1985; Miller, 1983). Fasteau (1991) points out that a major source of inhibitions to express affection "is the fear of being, or being thought, homosexual. Nothing is more frightening to a heterosexual man in our society" (p. 81).

Some authors (Bell, 1981; Block, 1980) have found that in mixed-sex groups, women often facilitate a discussion that is more personal and intimate than when men are alone in groups. Fasteau (1991) claims that men often depend on women to start such conversations because then the men can "join in" without having to take the responsibility for initiating a discussion of personal issues.

The literature on friendship reports that a small but growing number of men express discontent with their friendships with other men (e.g. Bell, 1981; Rubin, 1985). The men who articulate this discontent wish their friendships with other men were closer and more intimate.

Cross-Gender Friendships Studies indicate that male–female friendships are less common than same-gender friendships. Especially for married people or couples, friendships across the gender line are much less common than among single people (Bell, 1981; Block, 1980; Rubin, 1985). Most studies indicate that this is primarily due to the possessiveness and jealousy that often characterize sexual relationships and coupled life (McGill, 1985). Rubin (1985) reports that social class also influences the frequency of cross-gender friendships. She found that college-educated, middle-class couples were much more likely to have close friendships across the gender line than people of other class backgrounds. Rubin also found that people who sustain their friendships after marriage tend to be professional people who married late. These people are likely to come to the marriage with a well-established set of friendships, sometimes including those of the opposite sex.

Studies on friendships state that a major strain in cross-gender friendships is created by sexual tension. "Sexual questions create more of a conflict than many other issues in male-female friendships simply because we value sex so highly today" (Block, 1980, p. 92). It seems to be the potentiality, rather than the actuality, of sexual involvement that creates the tensions around male-female friendships (Rubin, 1985).

In his study, Bell (1981) discusses what he describes as an emerging "new pattern" in cross-gender friendship. "Men turn more to women for close relationships, and relationships with other men are less stressed as the only 'real' friendships" (p. 112). Bell found that an increasing number of men report that their friendships with women are an important means of self-revelation and gaining a greater sense of self-worth. These men said that they regarded their female friends as equally important as their male friends "because of women's honesty, supportiveness, and willingness to listen" (p. 110). This group of men also tended to describe their attitudes toward their female friends in terms of feelings of closeness, love, affection, and warmth, whereas they usually did not describe their attitudes toward their male friends in terms of such emotional qualities.

Rubin (1985) found similar trends in her study. Some of the men she interviewed described how a friendship with a woman provided them with nurturance and intimacy, which generally were not available in their friendships with other men. The women in Rubin's study shared this view and most of them agreed that in their friendships with men, they were the ones who listened and nurtured. The vast majority of women, however, reported that their friendships with men were much less intimate than their relationships with other women. For their most intimate friendships, women turn to each other.

Friendships between People with and without Disabilities

There are at least two reasons why friendships between people with and without disabilities are seen as important for the person with the disability. First, it is generally assumed that such relationships will serve as the basis for some of the social, emotional, and practical support people with disabilities need in order to become truly integrated into the fabric of everyday community life. Second, many people regard social relationships with ordinary community members as the measure, or even the ultimate goal, of people's integration into community life.

Friendships between people with and without disabilities also seem to be organized by gender relations. However, instead of three major gender patterns, one pattern seems to be most common: friendship between nondisabled women and people with disabilities (men and women). Friendships that include nondisabled men as friends of people with disabilities to be much less common.

Friendships between Women and People with Disabilities   Although there are no conclusive studies available to determine the gender patterns in friendships between people with and without disabilities, the available literature indicates strongly that for the people with disabilities who have friends, women without disabilities are overrepresented in these friendships. The expectation that friends of people with disabilities will provide practical, emotional, and social support is probably one reason why nondisabled women are more inclined to enter into such friendships than men. The differences in men's and women's orientation toward friendships in general indicate that women would be more likely than men to provide such support. Women approach friendships in a way that is characterized by acceptance, intimacy, and support. Furthermore, women have traditionally been assigned the roles of helper, nurturer, and caregiver. Therefore, establishing a friendship with a person with a disability falls within the realm of women's traditional roles, as well as within the tradition of female friendships.

In a discussion of friendships between women with and without disabilities, Fisher and Galler (1988) point out that two areas seem to be of particular importance in developing a balanced relationship. These are the areas of "physical help" and "emotional reciprocity."

Fisher and Galler found that women with disabilities often allude to an unspoken bargain they strike with their nondisabled friends. Women with disabilities often need a certain level of accommodation or direct physical help from their nondisabled friends. Their way to balance the scale is to be especially attentive and supportive in the emotional sphere—for example, by being an extra-good listener and by providing emotional comfort to their nondisabled friend.

In this author's study of the role of women in facilitating the inclusion of people with disabilities into community life, a similar trend was found in friendships between nondisabled women and people with disabilities (Traustadottir, 1992). The person with the disability, either a man or a woman, attempts to balance the support provided by the nondisabled female friend through provision of emotional support, intimacy, and closeness. This kind of intimacy and mutual support is common in women's friendships, which makes women more likely than men to consider sympathetic listening, caring, and emotional support as important contributions to a friendship. These are qualities most women seek and value in their friendships, whereas many men would be uncomfortable with such emotional closeness.

Barriers to Friendships between Men and People with Disabilities   There are, of course, men without disabilities who have close friendships with people with disabilities, but these seem to be the exception rather than the rule. The reasons for this phenomenon are complex and there are a number of barriers that seem to hinder the establishment of friendships between nondisabled men and people with disabilities.

One of the major barriers to the development of such friendships seems to be the expectation that nondisabled friends of people with disabilities will provide support to their friend. This is particularly true if the person with the disability needs support of a very personal nature, for example, assistance in eating or going to the bathroom. Unlike women, men usually have little practice in providing such tending type of assistance. In addition, the taboos around emotional and physical closeness within male friendships can make it difficult for nondisabled men to provide such assistance to their male friends with disabilities. The fear many heterosexual men have of being thought of as homosexual may also be at work here. Physical and emotional closeness between men is often associated with homosexuality; therefore, heterosexual men may shy away from friendships with men with disabilities if they need support that requires this type of closeness.

The expectation that nondisabled people will provide a tending type of support to their friends with disabilities not only hinders friendships between men with and without disabilities, it also creates a barrier to friendships between nondisabled men and women with disabilities. In recent years, it has been increasingly acknowledged that women with disabilities are extremely vulnerable to sexual abuse (Asch & Fine, 1988; Cole, 1984; Musick, 1984; Senn, 1988). Support that requires physical and emotional closeness makes nondisabled men uncomfortable because it places them at risk of being accused of abuse. The need for such close support can also cause family members or friends of women with disabilities to be uncomfortable with the idea or potential of male friends. In discussions with nondisabled men, this author has found that the fear of being suspected of abuse is a major hindrance to the development of close friendships with women with disabilities. One man who has a male friend with a disability said, "I would not want to have a woman with a disability as a friend because I'd worry that people would suspect me of sexual abuse." Thus, the expectations around the provision of support creates multiple and complex barriers to the development of friendships between nondisabled men and people (both men and women) with disabilities.

Facilitating More Normative Friendship Patterns

If the general friendship pattern is compared with the pattern of friendships between people with and without disabilities, a significant difference is found. The patterns in general friendships are drawn by gender lines in such a way that friendships are most likely to be within gender, whereas people with disabilities (both male and female) are most likely to have nondisabled women friends. If culturally normative friendships between people with and without disabilities are to be promoted, there needs to be an awareness of the major characteristics of such friendships. Women's friendships are more likely to be focused on being together and men's friendships on doing things together. Therefore, attempts to promote friendships between people with and without disabilities need to take into account these gender differences. If friendships between women are to be facilitated, a successful approach is to emphasize emotional closeness and intimacy. If friendships between men with and without disabilities are to be facilitated and encouraged, shared activities should be stressed. There also needs to be an awareness of the traditional taboos around physical and emotional closeness among men. Yet, because of the growing discontent of some nondisabled men with traditional male friendships, this group of men may welcome the opportunity to become friends with people with disabilities because it would allow them to bring forward their more nurturing side.

It should also be mentioned that men with disabilities may be facing a particular problem in terms of their friendships. Men with disabilities are more likely to have nondisabled women as friends than nondisabled men. Thus, many men with disabilities learn how to be a friend through being women's friends. Because there are such gender differences in friendships, difficulties may be created if men with disabilities then enter into friendships with nondisabled men. Women with disabilities, who also are more likely to have nondisabled women friends, experience more gender-normative friendship patterns.

THE BROADER SOCIAL CONTEXT

Friendships between people with and without disabilities take place in a broad social and political context. In this last section, this context is examined as one way to understand why women are more likely than men to become friends of people with disabilities. For the purposes of this analysis, there are at least two issues of importance: 1) current disability policy, with its increasing emphasis on the inclusion of people with disabilities through informal care and social relationships; and 2) the contemporary women's movement, with its emphasis on sisterhood and solidarity among differently situated women.

Disability Policy and Friendships

The goal of current reform efforts within the field of developmental disabilities is the full inclusion of people with disabilities into all aspects of community life. Yet, many people with disabilities continue to be isolated, lonely, and have few friends. Studies have found that some people with disabilities who moved from institutions into community programs are almost as isolated from the community as they were when they were living in the institution (Bercovici, 1983; Traustadottir, 1991b). Despite almost 2 decades of efforts to establish community-based services, it appears that community programs have merely assisted people with disabilities to be in the community, but have for the most part not managed to enable them to become part of the community (Bogdan & Taylor, 1987). A major criticism of community-based services is the difficulties these programs have in enabling people with disabilities to participate fully in community life and connecting them with other community members. Thus, the emphasis on social networks and personal relationships with other community members is at the heart of current trends in the disability field, and disability policy has been increasingly directed at efforts to understand and facilitate personal relationships and connections to what are seen as "natural" community supports. These trends have resulted in growing emphasis on the importance of relationships in the lives of people with disabilities (Forest, 1989; O'Brien, 1987; Smull, 1989; Strully & Strully, 1985; Taylor & Bogdan, 1989). The increasing awareness of the limitation of the service system in connecting people with disabilities with ordinary community members has led to a call for a personal commitment on behalf of nondisabled people to establish social relationships with people with disabilities. Implied is the belief that such personal relationships and friendships will fill the gap left by the service system and serve as a basis for the supports necessary for people to participate fully in community life.

The belief that true inclusion of people with disabilities can only be achieved through supportive personal relationships with nondisabled people is beginning to have its effects within the field. In the research of this author, it has been found that people who work in the disability field, especially those who work in direct services (the vast majority of whom are women), are now being encouraged to establish personal relationships with the people with disabilities with whom they work. In addition, within some agencies it has become a measurement of a "good worker" whether he or she has made such a personal commitment. As a result, an increasing number of women have made commitments that go far beyond the formal requirements of their jobs (Traustadottir, 1991b).

The disability field has developed a new language to describe these workers and what they do—"committed and very involved." The language of "commitment and involvement" has not only been adopted by those who work within the field, it is also used within the institutions that train professionals. When the author was in the process of soliciting nominations for informants for a study of women's caring work and relationship-building with people with disabilities, many of the people interviewed used this language, including administrators, professionals, and college professors. The women who were nominated for the study and who were described as "very committed and involved" all had a friend with a disability, which was the main reason for describing them in this way. Often there was no mention of these women's performance in other areas. The language of "commitment and involvement" has become so widespread that it is now commonly understood to mean "committed to people with disabilities" and "involved with people with disabilities in a personal relationship." Having a friend with a disability has almost become the measurement of people's "political correctness." It seems as though "personal involvement and commitment" have become the most important qualities professionals and paraprofessionals in the field of developmental disabilities can have. This is in strong contrast to the "old" language of "professional distance" and "impartial treatment," which used to be considered among the highest professional qualities.

The pressure to be "committed and involved" has become so great that some human services workers have developed a language of friendship about their connections with people with disabilities. This author's observations, however, reveal that these connections often bear little resemblance to a close relationship such as a friendship.

Sisterhood and the Women's Movement

The women's movement has, at least for a certain group of women, provided a larger social context for the development of friendships among women. Many authors have described how this movement has influenced friendships among women, including Acker et al. (1990), Bassaro (1990), Bell (1981), Eichenbaum and Orbach (1987), Lenz and Myerhoff (1985), and Oakley (1981). The emphasis on sisterhood and solidarity among women is a part of the ideology of the women's movement. Among other things, this emphasis serves to encourage, support, and validate friendships between women and make women more aware of the value and significance of their female friends. The women's movement also emphasizes women's common experiences of oppression, and women have been urged to overcome the differences that divide them and build a broad-based social movement to work toward their shared interest of liberation. In writing about friendships between women with and without disabilities (including their own), Fisher and Galler (1988) point out that:

> In such a context, making friends with women who are "different" has been a logical outcome of the larger political commitment. Sometimes it also has been a test of political virtue, or a testimony to one's activist commitment. (pp. 173-174)

This emphasis on sisterhood has encouraged women to explore the possibility of friendships between differently situated women and across social barriers. This has also given friendship—a highly personal and intimate phenomenon in women's lives—a broader political context and meaning as one part of a struggle toward a more just and equal society.

Thus, two larger societal contexts for friendships between women and people with disabilities are provided by disability policy and the women's movement, giving these friendships a favorable social and political context. There are at least two reasons why men are less likely to be shaped by these larger contexts. First, men are much fewer in number as workers within the field of disability, making women the primary "audience" for the arguments in favor of personal relationships with people with disabilities. Second, while at least some women are influenced by the women's movement, men do not have a similar social context outside the disability field with which they can identify and that encourages them to establish personal relationships with differently situated people.

SUMMARY

This chapter examines friendships between people with and without disabilities in the context of gender, especially focusing on exploring and explaining the overrepresentation of women as friends of people with disabilities. Gender is a major organizer of friendships, both in the general population and in friendships between people with and without disabilities. However, when these gender patterns are compared, it becomes apparent that friendships between people with and without disabilities do not follow a normative friendship pattern. Instead of the culturally normative pattern in which friendships are mostly confined within gender, people with disabilities (males and females) who do have nondisabled friends are most likely to have nondisabled women friends. The reasons for this pattern are traced to women's orientation toward people in general and the characteristics of women's friendships. When women establish a friendship with a person with a disability, they are following a long tradition of women's relationships characterized by caring and nurturance. Additionally, larger social forces influence and shape women's lives in such a way that women are encouraged to establish friendships with people with disabilities, and these friendships are thus given a favorable social and political context.

REFERENCES

Acker, J., Barry, K., & Esseveld, J. (1990). Feminism, female friends, and the reconstruction of intimacy. In H.Z. Lopata & D.R. Maines (Eds.), *Friendship in context* (pp. 75–108). Greenwich, CT: JAI Press.

Amado, A.N., Conklin, F., & Wells, J. (1990). *Friends: A manual for connecting persons with disabilities and communty members*. St. Paul, MN: Human Services Research and Development Center.

Asch, A., & Fine, M. (1988). Introduction: Beyond pedestals. In M. Fine & A. Asch (Eds.), *Women with disabilities: Essays in psychology, culture,and politics* (pp. 1–37). Philadelphia: Temple University Press.

Bassaro, J.C. (1990). *Making friends, keeping friends.* New Canaan, CT: Mulvey Books.

Belenky, B.F., Clinchy, B. M., Goldberger, N.R., & Tarule, J.M. (1986). *Women's ways of knowing: The development of self, voice, and mind.* New York: Basic Books.

Bell, R.R. (1981). *Worlds of friendships.* Beverly Hills, CA: Sage Publications.

Bercovici, S.M. (1983). *Barriers to normalization: The restrictive management of mentally retarded persons.* Baltimore: University Park Press.

Block, J.D. (1980). *Friendship: How to give it, how to get it.* New York: Collier Books.

Bogdan, R., & Taylor, S.J. (1987). Conclusion: The next wave. In S.J. Taylor, D. Biklen, & J. Knoll (Eds.), *Community integration for people with severe disabilities* (pp. 209–213). New York: Teachers College Press.

Center on Human Policy. (1991). Social relationships. *Policy Bulletin No. 1.* Syracuse, NY: Author.

Chodorow, N. (1978). *The reproduction of mothering: Psychoanalysis and the sociology of gender.* Berkeley, CA: University of California Press.

Cole, S.S. (1984). Facing the challenges of sexual abuse in persons with disabilities. *Sexuality and Disability, 7*(3/4), 71–88.

DeVault, M.L. (1991). *Feeding the family: The social organization of caring as gendered work.* Chicago: University of Illinois Press.

Eichenbaum, L., & Orbach, S. (1987). *Between women: Love, envy, and competition in women's friendships.* New York: Penguin Books.

Fasteau, M.F. (1991). Friendships among men. In F. Ashton-Jones & G.A. Olson (Eds.), *The gender reader* (pp. 74–85). Needham Heights, MA: Allyn & Bacon.

Fisher, B., & Galler, R. (1988). Friendship and fairness: How disability affects friendship between women. In M. Fine & A. Asch (Eds.), *Women with disabilities: Essays in psychology, culture, and politics* (pp. 172–194). Philadelphia: Temple University Press.

Forest, M. (1989). *It's about relationships.* Toronto: Frontier College Press.

Gilligan, C. (1982). *In a different voice: Psychological theory and women's development.* Cambridge, MA: Harvard University Press.

Gouldner, H., & Strong, M.S. (1987). *Speaking of friendship: Middle-class women and their friends.* New York: Greenwood Press.

Hutchison, P. (1990). *Making friends: Developing relationships between people with a disability and other members of the community.* Toronto: The G. Allan Roeher Institute.

Kishi, G.S. (1988). *Long term effects of different amounts of social contact between peers with and without severe disabilities: Outcomes of school integration efforts in Hawaii.* Unpublished doctoral dissertation, Syracuse University, Syracuse, NY.

Krauss, M.W., Seltzer, M.M., & Goodman, S.J. (1992). Social support networks of adults with mental retardation who live at home. *American Journal on Mental Retardation, 96*(4), 432–441.

Lenz, E., & Myerhoff, B. (1985). *The feminization of America.* Los Angeles: Jeremy P. Tarcher.

Lutfiyya, Z.M. (1989). *The phenomenology of relationships between typical and disabled people.* Unpublished doctoral dissertation, Syracuse University, Syracuse, NY.

Lutfiyya, Z.M. (1990). *Affectionate bonds: What can we learn from listening to friends.* Syracuse, NY: Center on Human Policy, Syracuse University.

McGill, M.E. (1985). *The McGill report on male intimacy*. New York: Holt, Rinehart & Winston.

Miller, S. (1983). *Men and friendship*. Boston: Houghton Mifflin.

Mount, B., Beeman, P., & Ducharme, G. (1988a). *What are we learning about bridge-building?* Manchester, CT: Communitas.

Mount, B., Beeman, P., & Ducharme, G. (1988b). *What are we learning about circles of support?* Manchester, CT: Communitas.

Musick, J.L. (1984). Patterns of institutional sexual abuse. *Response to Violence in the Family and Sexual Assault, 7*(3), 1–11.

Oakley, A. (1981). Sisterhood. In A. Oakley (Ed.), *Subject women* (pp. 265–280). New York: Pantheon Books.

O'Brien, J. (1987). A guide to life-style planning: Using *The Activities Catalog* to integrate services and natural support systems. In B. Wilcox & G.T. Bellamy (Eds.), *A comprehensive guide to The Activities Catalog: An alternative curriculum for youth and adults with severe disabilities* (pp. 175–190). Baltimore: Paul H. Brookes Publishing Co.

O'Connell, M. (1988). *The gift of hospitality: Opening the doors of community life to people with disabilities*. Evanston, IL: Center for Urban Affairs and Policy Research, Northwestern University.

O'Connell, M. (1990). *Community building in Logan Square*. Evanston, IL: Center for Urban Affairs and Policy Research, Northwestern University.

Perske, R. (1988). *Circles of friends*. Nashville: Abingdon Press.

Pogrebin, L.C. (1987). *Among friends: Who we like, why we like them, and what we do with them*. New York: McGraw-Hill.

Raymond, J.G. (1986). *A passion for friends: Toward a philosophy of female affection*. Boston: Beacon Press.

Rubin, L.B. (1985). *Just friends: The role of friendship in our lives*. New York: Harper & Row.

Senn, C.Y. (1988). *Vulnerable: Sexual abuse and people with an intellectual handicap*. Toronto, Ontario, Canada: The G. Allan Roeher Institute.

Sherrod, D. (1989). The influence of gender on same-sex friendships. In C. Hendrick (Ed.), *Close relationships* (pp. 164–186). Beverly Hills: Sage Publications.

Shoultz, B. (1991). Regenerating a community. In S.J. Taylor, R. Bogdan, & J.A. Racino (Eds.), *Life in the community: Case studies of organizations supporting people with disabilities* (pp. 195–213). Baltimore: Paul H. Brookes Publishing Co.

Smull, M.W. (1989). *Crisis in the community*. Alexandria, VA: National Association of State Mental Retardation Program Directors.

Strully, J., & Strully, C. (1985). Friendship and our children. *Journal of The Association for Persons with Severe Handicaps, 10*(4), 224–227.

Taylor, S.J., & Bogdan, R. (1989). On accepting relationships between people with mental retardation and nondisabled people: Towards an understanding of acceptance. *Disability, Handicap & Society, 4*(1), 21–36.

Traustadottir, R. (1988, August). *Women and family care: On the gendered nature of caring*. Paper presented at the First International Conference on Family Support Related to Disability, Stockholm, Sweden.

Traustadottir, R. (1991a). Mothers who care: Gender, disability, and family life. *Journal of Family Issues* [Special issue on Gender and Unpaid Care], *12*(2), 211–228.

Traustadottir, R. (1991b). *Supports for community living: A case study.* Syracuse, NY: Center on Human Policy, Syracuse University.

Traustadottir, R. (1992). *Disability reform and the role of women: Community inclusion and caring work.* Unpublished doctoral dissertation, Syracuse University, Syracuse, NY.

Voeltz, L.M. (1982). Effects of structured interactions with severely handicapped peers on children's attitudes. *American Journal of Mental Deficiency, 86*(4), 380–390.

8

Affection, Love, Intimacy, and Sexual Relationships

Elaine Jurkowski and Angela Novak Amado

Put a lid on your urges.

Parents really don't understand that you grow beyond a point. I still hear these things, even though I am an adult, in my thirties. I am sure they don't tell my brother or sister to put a lid on their urges.

Sometimes the only information we ever get is from TV.

Joanne (Jurkowski, 1992)

The scope and depth of friendship extends broadly. Relationships and connections vary in amount of time spent together, intensity of emotional connection, degree of intimacy and trust, and reciprocity of sharing (Tyne, 1988). As friendship for persons with developmental disabilities receives greater attention and support, attention also needs to be paid to the importance of relationships that include love and physical affection. The most intimate end of the spectrum of friendship, relationships that include sensuality and sexuality, must also be addressed.

Traditionally, sexuality has been a topic politely avoided by parents, caregivers, and professionals; however, sexuality and sensuality are by and large still only associated with "sex." Although in recent years there has been an increase in sex education classes and more progressive attitudes, the training that is provided still tends to be biological; real and substantial support for intimate relationships has yet to be adequately addressed, whether with partners who do or do

---

All display quotes are from Jurkowski's 1992 ethnographic study and personal interviews. Although the quotes are used with the permission of the interviewees, all of whom were adults with multiple impairments, the names have been changed at their request.

not have disabilities. Even though there has been an increase in sex education materials, technical information, and classes on disease prevention, little attention has been paid to how persons with developmental disabilities experience their needs for intimacy and for sensual and sexual expression in their daily lives. More progressive attitudes have not addressed adequately the full expression of persons with disabilities as sexual beings, with the same needs for affection, lovemaking, and intimate relationships experienced by all people. In addition, sensuality and sexuality have not been explored as integral components of friendships between persons who have disabilities or with persons who do not have disabilities.

The tradition and aftereffects of the eugenics movement have primarily dealt with the sexuality of persons with disabilities through contraception and sterilization. The rise of the principle of "normalization" and full community inclusion has identified new challenges with respect to the sensuality and sexuality of persons with developmental disabilities, particularly as society moves toward greater respect for individual rights and equalization of opportunities. Yet, with these increased rights and responsibilities often come greater fear and apprehension, which still tend to be centered on the same concerns of pregnancy and, more recently, of abuse. With more fear can come strong motivation for new versions of control. However, from the perspective of persons with disabilities, intimacy and sexuality are real experiences in their lives; their perspective extends far beyond fear in a much broader life scope. Although at times these experiences may be confusing, they are nevertheless an integral and essential part of their lives (Heshusius, 1987).

Many of the issues regarding intimacy and sexuality involve relationships between persons with disabilities, as well as between these individuals and other community members. As individuals with developmental disabilities become more integrated into community life, meet more community members, and are supported in a greater diversity of friendships, other issues regarding sexuality must also be taken into account. First, people with disabilities themselves speak eloquently of the importance of sexuality and intimacy; these types of relationships should be supported. However, often due to this very importance, both confusion and vulnerability may occur. As a range of relationships develops, misunderstandings about the nature of those connections might arise in some cases; the limits of certain relationships might be misunderstood or overtures of friendship might be interpreted to have sexual overtones when they actually do not. Individuals may also have insufficient information and skills related to relationship building, and greater support for community connections may increase their vulnerability and potential for abuse. A volume on friendships and community connections would be incomplete without consideration of these important issues. Support for friendship should include support for the entire spectrum of relationships, including the most intimate and affectionate types of relationships. Both the factors of successful support and potential problems need to be addressed.

In this chapter, key issues regarding the sexuality of individuals with disabilities are explored, including how persons with disabilities themselves view the topic. Some sexual "subcultures" for individuals with disabilities that have been created as a result of the services system are described, as well as system factors that affect normal sexual development. The importance of sexuality education is delineated from the vantage point of enhancing quality of life and enhancing relationships, and as an important precursor to prevention of abuse.

Monat-Haller (1992) describes sexuality as a process that begins at birth. A person's sexuality does not pertain exclusively to his or her genitals, rather, it affects all of his or her senses and identifies the person as an individual. The process of sexuality identifies and formulates personality, as females and males. Sensuality, sometimes thought of as unrestrained sexual gratification, actually affects all of our senses: sight, sound, smell, taste, and touch. Both sexuality and sensuality are experiences essential to being human for all people. Although also essential to persons with disabilities, these experiences are too often minimized, ignored, or dealt with inadequately in services and programs designed to assist them.

THE DAILY REALITIES OF SEXUAL
EXPERIENCES FOR INDIVIDUALS WITH DISABILITIES

In terms of the day-to-day and real life experiences of persons with developmental disabilities, Heshusius (1982, 1987) has critically noted the discrepancies between how persons with disabilities experience their own sexual lives and how their experiences are treated by professionals who work with them every day. For instance, very little attention has been paid to even the very documentation of how persons with disabilities see their own sexuality; this lack of attention contrasts with the vast amount of literature on the perceptions of the population at large. Whereas the few studies that have been conducted have found that most persons with retardation definitely experience intimacy and sexuality as important and essential parts of their lives, the profession typically diminishes or distorts the importance of these issues and the expression of intimate behaviors.

In 1987, Heshusius summarized seven studies conducted in the previous 20 years that addressed the perceptions of sexuality by persons labeled as having mental retardation (Bogdan & Taylor, 1982; Edgerton, 1967; Henshel, 1972; Heshusius, 1981; Koegel & Whittemore, 1983; Meyers, 1978; Rostafinski, 1975). These studies included three participant observation studies, three interview studies, and one biographical account by the brother of a person with mental retardation. (Most of the persons observed or interviewed in these studies were individuals classified with mild or moderate levels of retardation; the experiences of those who are considered more severely impaired have yet to be fully addressed or understood.) These seven studies are very revealing and Heshusius's review is summarized in more detail here because of its comprehensive reflection of the personal views of sexuality on the part of persons labeled with mental retardation. Heshusius (1987) used qualititative research methods to summarize the studies by analyzing the number of observations in which persons expressed themselves about their views on sexuality. She documents the preoccupations with sexual matters in the minds of the persons observed and interviewed. An example of this preoccupation is that Henshel (1972) purposely tried to avoid the issue of sexuality in her interviews with persons with disabilities, but the persons interviewed persisted in bringing up the topic despite her efforts. The data in all seven studies revealed five distinct categories of attention and concern. Under each of Heshusius's categories are examples of statements or incidents illustrating that category:

1. *There is enjoyment of or desire for sensual and/or sexual contact.*
   "I like to go with him. I like to be with him. Something about him. I really don't know why I am so thrilled over him. . . . Maybe it's his body. He's not so musclely or anything but just the way he is—I don't know why. He touches me and I go into orbit." (Koegel & Whittemore, 1983, p. 236)
   "If you get the right, uh, movement, it can be real good." (Edgerton, 1967, p. 118)
2. *Touching, kissing, and nudity are fun and exciting.*
   A man intensely watching a girl who passed by wearing a halter top said to himself, "Hey, you sexy thing. . . ." (Heshusius, 1981, p. 67)
   After going to see a movie, Rob was asked if he liked it and he said there was a naked woman in it. "I liked it, I liked it . . . I

loved it!" Author: "But what was the story about?" Rob: "A naked woman . . ." Author: "What happened to her?" No answer. (Heshusius, 1981, p. 67)

3. *Sex is desirable, but belongs in marriage.*

Heshusius's (1981) participant observation study in a strictly supervised group home produced statements such as the following. The strong conservative attitude was not found in any of the other six studies.

"No, not until you are married." (p. 61)

When one of the men teased a woman about lowering her bikini top, the woman said, "We are not married yet." (p. 60)

4. *There is a feeling of ignorance about basic facts.*

"I didn't even know a single thing about sex." (Henshel, 1972, p. 70)

"They say when you first have an intercourse with a boy, you don't get pregnant. Is that true?" (Rostafinski, 1975, p. 12)

5. *Sensual and/or sexual contact generates fear or anxiety.*

"I don't like him to touch me. Makes me nervous." (Henshel, 1972, p. 198)

The first three categories of attention formed the overwhelming majority (86%) of all statements, far outweighing the occurrence of the last two categories. This high percentage could reflect a view of persons with mental retardation as pre-occupied with the physical components of sex. However, Heshusius summarized all seven studies as revealing that when persons with disabilites are asked what sex means to them, they overwhelmingly report that it is desirable, pleasurable, an essential part of life, and that it adds warmth, joy, and excitement to life. Their experiences reflect a view of sex as an integral part of life, and that the importance and meaning it has for them is not dissimilar from the meaning it has for most people. Heshusius found no data to support the view that people with disabilities see sex as any less desirable or meaningful than the population at large. In the 1980s and early 1990s, these findings also have been supported by self-advocates who have created the avenues to speak for themselves and to demand to have their concerns heard and honored. Many self-advocates have spoken eloquently of their desires for and the importance of all types of intimacy in a wide range of relationships (Jurkowski, 1992; Speaking For Ourselves, chap. 15, this volume; Watt, 1991).

This importance and desirability of sexual matters on the part of people with disabilities contrasts with the actual program structures common in their day-to-day lives. For instance, the following program practices are often still in place: segregated facilities for men and women, strict supervision around the clock, no privacy with regard to the opposite sex, little sex education or a lack of serious conversation on sexuality; and rules that limit physical contact beyond holding hands, sitting somewhat close, and light kisses. In Heshusius's naturalistic study of group home residents (1982), most of the residents were being taught independent or semi-independent living skills. The residents' conversations and attention were heavily concentrated on issues about sex and marriage. Their conversations about sexual matters and relationships were constant, especially about the importance of having a boyfriend or girlfriend, but also including marriage, children, affection, and companionship. At the same time, what the agency considered important and what the residents were being taught were self-help, household, and vocational skills.

When sex education is provided, it is often centered on sex as a distant concept or basic information, and it is focused on public behavior, including the facts of life, contraceptives, what not to do, avoiding disease, appropriate public behavior, and "coping responsibly" with sexual feelings. There is little address of private behavior or the enjoyment and beauty of lovemaking. "Sex education and communication about sex is not yet personal, intimate, experiential, and celebrative" (Heshusius, 1987, p. 52).

Whereas the literature on sex for the population at large uses a variety of terms for the sexual act, literature for persons with disabilities almost exclusively uses the terms "sexuality" or "sexual expression." Rarely is the term "lovemaking" used, perhaps because people have yet to think of "them" as lovers. Yet, what Heshusius's review of studies (1987) reveals is that when they talk about sex, they mean actually engaging in it.

It may initially appear that in the 1990s, group homes and small community residences have more modern policies or enlightened practices; yet, when the fundamental nature of those policies and practices is more closely examined, it can be seen that they often carry on the control and limitations of traditional institutions. Sexual expression is often limited to what can be supervised and therefore observed in public—what Elliott (1980) calls "public intimacy." Adults may be allowed to hold hands, kiss lightly, or staff may tease about a particular "boyfriend" or "girlfriend"; however, privacy with a member of the opposite sex, closed doors, and serious information about lovemaking are still all too often missing. Meyers (1978) recounted the story of his brother and the woman he eventually married. His brother said, "They wouldn't let us be alone together . . . It was as if they didn't trust us . . . Houseparents would criticize us if we held hands or if I put my arm around her." Meyers noted, "Their interest was affection, something few people were as yet willing to 'grant' them. What they were 'granted' was the right to remain in continuing adolescence, with little growth or progress" (p. 141). The attitude of perpetual adolescence is still reflected in the rules and expectations of many residential, day program, and other services. Yet, at the same time, the total life experiences of people labeled mentally retarded are influenced by the same constant sexual stimuli, images, and concepts that the rest of us experience, in television, movies, popular songs, and magazines. Persons who receive services are also subject to the sexual comments, jokes, and experiences of their own staff, and to having their experiences and behavior openly discussed by large audiences, such as interdisciplinary teams. They are treated as innocent teenagers in a world of adult stimulation and expectations. Heshusius (1987) notes:

> None of us would want to be forced into a position where our sensual behaviors are watched by all because we have no access to privacy, but it is good enough for retarded persons. Listening, however, to what they have to tell us, intimacy forced to play itself out in public, is not what they wish for . . . we cannot praise ourselves for doing a good job at sex education for adults when we provide information about sex but continue our endless variations of setting rules and restrictions that prevent them from becoming lovers if they so wish. (p. 55)

Many professionals have not even recognized that the enjoyable part of human sexual expression should receive as much emphasis as the responsible part. Healthy sex education should be a process that evolves naturally throughout one's life span; it should use a variety of sensations and activities that may not necessarily be limited to genital or safety issues, but also relate to relationships, companionship, tenderness, touch, warmth, and affection.

SEXUAL SUBCULTURES

In a services system in which the care of people with disabilities is provided by paid staff, the values of staff frequently are the controlling ones. As more and more persons are served in community settings, the roles formerly held by institution aides are being replaced by the roles of group home or support staff. Dependence typically remains essential to the survival of the consumer—dependence on staff, rules, paid services, and system-defined boundaries. Besides its effect on most aspects of life, this dependence also creates a host of "sexual subcultures" (Jurkowski, & Garwick 1991) faced by persons with developmental disabilities. These subcultures are stereotyped roles, defined by assumptions and generalizations about the sexual nature of the person with disabilities. They include the "sleep alone syndrome," the "pseudo sib," the "perpetual victim," "perpetual programming," the "eternal child," and "marriage only."

Sleep Alone Syndrome

Often the assumption is made that persons with developmental disabilities have no need for body contact or affection, and any attempt to legitimize such contact would result in procreation (Craft & Craft, 1983). The point is perhaps not so much the prohibition of the sex act itself or the denial of opportunities for physical affection, but rather that these prohibitions are also extended to the expression of the emotions that are commonly the precursors of sex (i.e., tenderness, emotional affection, and warmth through touch) (Craft & Craft, 1983). The person with disabilities, for example, may never have an opportunity to make a choice about a partner or marriage or be perceived as having lost anything, including this choice, since he or she is viewed as "asexual" (Cole, 1988). Because the person with developmental disabilities is often perceived as asexual, he or she is therefore perceived as always "sleeping alone." Unfortunately, this subculture denies individuals some of their basic needs for sensuality, such as touching, caressing, and tenderness.

> I never knew what it was like to get a good hug or kiss, until I was seven, and I stayed at my aunt's house for a sleepover. She kissed me goodnight. It was so weird. And so now I really am not sure what it would be like to have a boyfriend or a man who really cares about me, never mind about sex.
>
> —Mary Beth, 43 years old

Pseudo Sib

This subculture refers to the assumption that individuals with developmental disabilities live in care facilities similar to "one big happy family" with no sexual feelings toward any member of the same or opposite sex. Adams, Tallon, and Alcorn (1982) discovered in their survey of staff members who were in both institutions and community-based programs that there was a denial of sexual activity or attraction between people with disabilities. This begs the question: Are staff denying that individuals with disabilities have attractions to each other, or are they pretending that such attractions are nonexistent?

I kind of like Melissa, but they tell me she's like my sister, cuz we live together in the same group home. I'm confused because we're not related, we don't have the same parents.

—Donald, 25 years old

Perpetual Victim

Persons with developmental disabilities are often repeatedly victimized, frequently without the knowledge that they are being victimized. Their strong needs for love and affection often make them easy targets for prey (Kempton, 1977). In some cases, "incestual" intrusions may have been the only form of affection experienced by a woman with disabilities; therefore, she may have remained silent in order to maintain her place in the family or her friendship, or to avoid losing the person upon whom she is dependent for assistance. She may be unaware that the affectionate gestures are inappropriate (Cole, 1988). Many persons with disabilities who have experienced such exploitive situations do not realize it for many years or are not willing to tell anyone about it (Cole, 1986).

The effects of victimization are traumatic enough for anyone. However, persons with mental retardation and/or other developmental disabilities, unless they receive some counseling, may continue to be victimized; practice or exercise their sexuality in a noncaring, nonconsensual manner; or exhibit behavioral or psychiatric reactions.

I'm really not sure what it would be like to have a boyfriend or a man who really cares about me. I spent so many years being sexually abused by my older brothers, and I could not get away, cuz I couldn't walk or run, that I am really scared.

—Ann, 33 years old

Perpetual Programming

Persons with developmental disabilities are required by program staff to work on specific "functional" activities for years before they will ever have goals for relationships or meaningful social skills (Garwick & Jurkowski, 1992). Many challenged individuals may never master the spectrum of functional tasks required before they are given the opportunity to pursue developmental tasks related to socialization or even self-protection. Consequently, they are "perpetually programmed."

Functional activity checklists do not acknowledge sexuality, and many adaptive behavior scales do not include specific items related to friendships, socialization, or sexuality. Socialization skills are rarely taught in one's younger years or with full appreciation of the complex issues involved in relating. Skills such as learning appropriate distance or space, "asking for hugs," and understanding and identifying basic feelings are rarely ever identified as important. Goals related to specific ways to enhance one's self-esteem, decision-making, and relationships and bonding are rarely identified in individual program or education plans.

Eternal Child

A person with developmental disabilities is often infantalized "forever," with the assumption that he or she cannot learn or understand the demands of the adult world (Dupras, Levy & Trembly, 1984; Edmonson, McCombs, & Wish, 1979). Cole (1988) describes the plight of many young women with developmental disabilities:

> In many cases the families are intensely concerned about the sexual and emotional vulnerability of the daughter and hope that "nothing bad" will happen to her. They may, therefore, encourage her to wear youthful clothing and to maintain safety as a "little girl." These families can mistakenly assume there may be no sexual life ahead of her and protect her from this perceived bitter reality with youthful clothing and little girlish ways. The result can be, of course, that the young emerging woman may become societally handicapped in learning how to conduct herself as a sexual woman. She will be infantalized. (pp. 282–283)

The peers of individuals with disabilities, a key source of information for typical children, are likely to be equally ignorant. In addition, persons with mental retardation often lack the degree of literacy necessary to find out accurate information for themselves from written sources.

> We don't have the same opportunities to learn about sex and stuff. I can't read so I only ever learn from TV or pictures in magazines. It never really happens the same way in real life though.
>
> —Marie, 43 years old

Marriage Only

A study conducted by Coleman and Murphy (1980) of facilities serving persons with developmental disabilities led the researchers to conclude that staff conveyed mixed messages about sexuality. Despite staff attitudes that people with developmental disabilities should be made aware of information regarding sexuality and that staff should ensure safety against abuse, their behavior toward the issue of sex pushed for "masturbation" and "marriage only" for persons with disabilities. Furthermore, the study indicated that staff believed that individuals should only be made aware of information related to sexuality if they talked about marriage. In addition, moral judgments were placed upon persons with disabilities that denied them the opportunity for any affectionate or intimate (consensual) exploration until they were married. Persons with physical disabilities who required attendant care had fewer opportunities for exploration due to their dependency upon others for physical transfers (Jurkowski, 1992).

> So if I want a chance to cuddle with a man, they would have to transfer me onto the couch, or onto the bed. Unless my man wasn't disabled, or had a good back, then we could do it, together. . . . Attendants told me though, they would only transfer me if I was married.
>
> —Ann

At the root of all these subcultures and this cultural deprivation for persons with developmental disabilities is a variety of factors defined by Griffiths, Quinsey, and Hingsburger (1989), including a lack of a normal environment, segregation from the mainstream of activities, restrictiveness, privacy issues, one's sexual knowledge and expectations, vulnerability, and societal attitudes. In order for these subcultures to be overcome, for real assimilation to occur, and for individuals with disabilities to be supported in the lifelong learning and experience of sexuality, some intervention needs to occur with caregivers, parents, and professionals.

FACTORS AFFECTING NORMATIVE DEVELOPMENT

The life of a person with disabilities who is dependent on the paid services system is shaped by many factors. Several of these factors affect typical sexual development, promote the sexual subcultures, and affect the process of needed intervention.

Segregation

Many people with disabilities grow up in environments that do not provide culturally valued expectations or appropriate role models. Segregation even occurs for many individuals with disabilities who grow up in the community and in their own families. Despite the fact that the philosophical context of the disabilities profession promotes inclusion and community integration, individuals with disabilities may still experience segregation, 24-hour supervision, and a lack of privacy. The sociosexual patterns developed in these segregated and restricted environments may remain unaltered, even if individuals move to more inclusive settings or return to the community from institutions (Hingsburger & Griffiths, 1986).

Many children with disabilities may spend many hours at home because it is physically difficult or impossible to get around and be with friends. Isolated from their peers and uninformed about sex, they are often left to learn about their sexuality through the one-dimensional format of television. There they can observe many hours of unrealistic experiences, such as sexual acting out, innuendoes and sexual dialogue, and a frequent absence of specific or accurate information regarding birth control, pregnancy, risks, morals, or values. Children may develop misplaced and inaccurate images about women, sex roles, and behaviors from the media, whose culture generally describes sexuality through humor, double messages, and in sexist and exploitative ways (Cole, 1986; Massuda, 1990).

Restrictiveness

People with developmental disabilities who live in protected environments are often subject to close supervision. Policies in such facilities often prohibit or punish any activity that is perceived as sexual. In a survey of institutional staff conducted by Deisher in 1973, it was found that 50% of the staff would put an end to any kissing and petting between residents if the couple were heterosexual, and 86% would stop them if they were homosexual. In 1991, Jurkowski surveyed care staff within a residential care network and found that almost 20 years after Deisher's study, and in community facilities, policies still dictated that kissing and petting should be reprimanded. The residential policies did not indicate what type of follow-up should be provided for the individual with developmental disabilities, such as explanations of what is acceptable, inappropriate, nonconsensual, or exploitative. The practice of providing information to the person with developmental disabilities remained largely absent.

Restrictiveness may result in isolation and may overprotect the person with disabilities from information, experiences, or both. The end result is that individuals may have difficulty interacting with others, particularly around sexual issues. If the person has not acquired the "language of sex" in order to dialogue, flirt, tell stories, or "brag," then he or she may experience further isolation (Cole, 1988).

There are also practical implications of both segregation and restrictiveness that affect normal opportunities. These problems have been summed up by one person with multiple disabilities as follows:

You can't go on a date, you can like guys but there's problems like transportation, privacy, and going to parties.

—Julie

Privacy Issues

Young persons with physical disabilities or limitations in self-care skills often experience excessive touching due to health care tasks carried out by family members, personal care attendants, or other human services or educational staff. Cole (1988) suggests that cases are quite common of a child being handled so frequently that he or she may not even acknowledge or be aware of the separateness and ownership of his or her own body.

Cole (1988) also suggests that medical, professional, and other caregivers often do not stop to identify and negotiate necessary touching of a person with disabilities, sometimes resulting in further loss of autonomy. Caregivers assume such touching (e.g., physical prompts, personal care) is acceptable without recognizing the impact it may have; the individual may generalize such touching as being acceptable from anyone, not only from care professionals.

Massuda (1990) describes the issue of inappropriate touching in a qualitative study she conducted with women with disabilities across Canada. The following are excerpts from her research:

"A doctor touched her breasts with both his hands and his cheek 'to hear my heart beat.' " (p. 23)
"Once when I was in the hospital, one of the evening visitors from a men's service club asked if he could see my legs. He lifted up the blankets —looked and then put his hand between my legs—then left quickly." (p. 24)

Ironically, although these individuals knew this type of touching was uncomfortable, when they reported the incidents they were not believed by their caregivers.

Beginning at puberty, some young ladies with disabilities may need assistance in menstrual hygiene care; conspicuousness and a loss of privacy are then added to this sensitive, personal event. In addition, a person with disabilities may have trouble distinguishing appropriate touch from inappropriate touch, further adding to the possibility of being a strong candidate for sexual exploitation (Cole, 1986).

Often, individuals with disabilities do not have access to physical resources that allow privacy. Coleman and Murphy (1980) found that of the institutional facilities they surveyed, only 15% indicated that there were any private residential areas made available to residents with mental retardation.

Griffiths et al. (1989) suggest that in most care facilities the only sexual expressions that can be enacted in private are auto-erotic or homosexual in nature. Consequently, individuals never learn about the gentle persuasive feelings of touch, nor do they easily learn to replace auto-erotic behavior with relationship building. Both homosexuality and heterosexuality, without safe sex practices or an understanding of one's own sexuality, can also lead to concerns regarding the transmission of AIDS.

It is ironic that persons with disabilities have experienced explicit handling of their bodies for physical care or medical reasons, but, at the same time, have often experienced a total void in sexual expression or experience. In addition, many have never spoken or been spoken to directly about sexuality (Cole, 1988).

Sexual Knowledge and Expectations

Watson and Rogers (1980) found that persons with developmental disabilities have significantly less knowledge about sex in comparison to typical groups. Griffiths et al. (1989) suggest that sex education for persons with developmental disabilities is limited, tends to be technical training of a biological and protective nature, and fails to offer information within the context of a social and caring relationship with an appropriate partner. They also suggest that individuals with disabilities gain their knowledge of sexuality from their limited observations of their relationships with nondisabled people (i.e., staff, parents, and advocates); their own sociosexual experiences, which may be atypical and abusive; and television. They suggest that this dearth of normal experiences contributes to the development of unrealistic expectations and the possibility of persons with disabilities becoming targets for abuse and violence.

It can be difficult to protect persons with disabilities from exposure to undesirable "sex education" gleaned from R- and X-rated films, television, magazines, and pornography. This distorted exposure as well as the limitations in opportunities to express sexuality contribute to the frequent inaccurate understanding of images about sex roles, messages that portray exploitation, and sexism (Cole, 1985; Massuda, 1990). One result of these misunderstandings can be a lack of understanding of realistic boundaries on the part of many persons with disabilities.

Craft and Hitching (1989) emphasize that persons with mental retardation need knowledge that will give them some protection against exploitation. He also argues against the unrealistic demands and expectations of society for responsible sexual behavior from people who have never been taught what constitutes responsibility and irresponsibility in sexual matters.

Sociosexual Skills

Programs for persons with disabilities have largely been targeted toward the development of domestic and vocational skills (Griffiths et al., 1989). Less attention has been paid to teaching the interactional skills important for developing and maintaining satisfying social relationships. Although there has been an increased emphasis on teaching social skills to persons with developmental disabilities, the focus usually has been on single behaviors such as eye contact, rather than more complex social interactions. Furthermore, these programs have been typically ineffective in generalizing these skills to other environments.

Griffiths et al. (1989) explain that a person's ability to understand and develop sociosexual skills affects his or her range and ability to express individual sexuality appropriately. Although research indicates that sexual development for persons with disabilities broadly follows the same pattern as typical development (Deisher, 1973; Gordon, 1973; McNab, 1978), there may be some particular or individualistic difficulties. Problems of persons with disabilities may include poor discrimination of time, place, or partner, and behaviors such as inappropriate touching, public masturbation, and disrobing.

Given these five factors and many others, it is of little surprise that people with disabilities who have actually succeeded in getting married, living together, or establishing an intimate relationship have often had to do so *in spite of* service professionals and the system. Typically, success has come, if it does at all, only after long periods of fighting for their rights and their "love" (Schwier, chap. 9, this volume; Meyers, 1978). The gap is cavernous between what is important to people and what "support" is actually provided to them. Although people with disabilities are often blamed for their behavior or problems, the discrepancy between what is important to them and what "services" are being provided deserves examination as the very root and source of the behaviors or problems (see also R.S. Amado, chap. 4, this volume).

ABUSE AND EXPLOITATION

When sexuality is viewed as exclusively involving sex, the range of intimacies that are related to healthy sexual development and that evolve through friendships and relationships are not taken into consideration. Viewing sexuality purely from a "sex"-oriented perspective leaves individuals ill-equipped to deal with the many challenges that relationships and friendships pose. Some of those challenges, especially for vulnerable individuals, can entail abuse and exploitation.

A discussion of friendships and relationships cannot occur in isolation from a discussion of sexuality and sensuality issues as integral components of abuse prevention.

Abuse and exploitation can be seen as a problem that may increase with greater independence and more community integration, an issue that has been addressed by both professionals and caregivers (Cohan & Warren, 1987; Lakin & Bruininks, 1985; Pincus, 1988; Sobsey, 1990). Although caregivers clearly want to provide typical opportunities, including friendships and the enhancement of quality of life, Hall and Morris (1976) concluded that with the thrust on offering "normalized" choices and opportunities for individuals with disabilities, there is also a greater risk that people with mental challenges will be abused and exploited or exercise poor judgment as a result of inadequate awareness of the consequences resulting from their actions.

As opportunities for friendship are expanded, fear of abuse sometimes becomes a grave concern for the caregiver (Jurkowski, 1992). Abuse and exploitation of individuals with disabilities are documented and are a growing problem, especially as persons with disabilities become increasingly integrated into the mainstream of society (Aiello, 1984; Brookhauser, Sullivan, Scanlan, & Garbarino, 1986; Chamberlin, Rauh, Passer, McGrath, & Burket, 1984; Chorimer & Lehr, 1976; Davies, 1979; Doucette, 1986; Massuda, 1990; Sobsey, Gray, Wells, Pyper, & Reimer-Heck, 1991). Studies indicate individuals with disabilities are more prone to abuse than others (Yoshida, Wasiluschuk, & Friedman, 1990). In Sobsey's 1990 study, 77% of abuse cases were for reasons of impaired judgment or knowledge, lack of assertiveness, inability to communicate mistreatment, or too much trust in others. These vulnerabilities, therefore, become a focus for consideration as caregivers and advocates strive to enlarge a person's circle of relationships and friendships. There are also growing health concerns due to sexually transmitted diseases and AIDS, and the increasing link between behavioral disorders and abuse (Chaimowitz & Moscovitch, 1991; Griffiths et al., 1989).

Sobsey et al. (1991) studied actual interventions and treatment for abuse victims with disabilities. Ironically, counseling was provided in less than 15% of the cases and actual educational programming or teaching was given to less than 5% of the victims.

SEXUALITY EDUCATION

A host of misconceptions, attitudes, and behaviors needs to be addressed before effective avenues will be created that naturally allow individuals with disabilities to create and develop intimate friendships. Support, education, and information need to be provided to address the whole context of life, not simply the crises that occur or the prevention of crises. One of the key misconceptions that needs to be tackled is that the concept of "sexuality" is generally confused with the act of lovemaking (i.e., intercourse or "sex"). Parents, caregivers, and professionals often perceive intercourse as an off limits and taboo subject. It is common that the topic is not dealt with, the person with developmental disabilities is viewed as an "eternal child," and then the teaching of all concepts related to sexuality becomes prohibited.

Parents and professionals often do not view individuals with disabilities as having the same needs, desires, and psychosexual developmental stages as their nondisabled counterparts. Because of this lack of recognition, issues regarding sexuality often have to be addressed in reaction to the crises that occur when the issues are not addressed in a straightforward manner. Crisis-oriented sexuality education can be avoided through a process in which issues related to sexuality become an integral part of the training process, and sociosexual skills are incorporated into the continuum of skills addressed within the realm of activities of daily living.

In addition to the level of discomfort experienced by most parents, caregivers, and agency staff regarding sexuality, often an argument is made about the general lack of human and financial resources for training; basic needs related to food, clothing, and shelter seem to take priority. However, given the vulnerabilities faced by persons with disabilities, sexuality education programs become a critical component of skill development. It has been documented that staff development training in the area of sociosexual skills positively influences caregivers' perceptions of interventions around sexuality. Rowe, Savage, and Dennis-Delanney (1987) argue that skill development for parents and care-providers requires ongoing consultation and training. This training must be addressed as a child evolves through his or her own growth and development. The necessary skills to address must not be limited to the traditional scope of sexuality education (anatomy, physiology, and contraception), but also include self-esteem, self-identity, relationships and relationship building, decision-making, and positive health behaviors. Work on relationship building and friendship also needs to integrate sensuality and sexuality realistically.

Sexuality is essentially a lifelong process of gleaning information and developing values and attitudes about one's sexuality and behavior. Many nondisabled persons gather information from a variety of sources both formally and informally, including their families, peers, school, community and religious institutions, literature, and the media (Planned Parenthood Federation of Canada, 1989). For many individuals with disabilities, their sources of informal and formal information are generally minimized or distorted because of lack of supports, lack of mobility, illiteracy, and poverty. Consequently, the need for teaching and discussion in areas related to sexuality is more critical for this population compared to nondisabled people.

Many special education curricula are designed to instruct students about functional skills. Typically absent is information about understanding some of the basic skills related to students' social and sexual development and the development of meaningful friendships. Current sex education and abuse prevention programs for the target group of persons with developmental delays generally aim at the notion of genital intimacy and sexual assault; they usually fail to integrate key or critical components for enhancing meaningful friendships and caring, emotionally intimate relationships.

Intimacy falls at one end of the continuum of relationships and friendships. Everyone has needs for both intimacy and sexual gratification. Given these needs, programs for persons with developmental disabilities should not only address the facilitation of friendships and relationships, but also build and develop skills for meaningful contacts for intimacy, sensuality, and sexuality.

Education that keeps pace with actual social and sexual development should begin in infancy, moving through the preschool level, childhood, adolescence, and into adulthood. Instruction needs to incorporate the development of one's self-esteem, identity, decision-making, relationship-building, and abuse prevention. Given the need to develop a knowledge base that will precipitate typical behaviors and expectations (Griffiths et al., 1989) and the need to develop interventions that will promote self-protection (Kempton, 1983; Sobsey, 1990), specific education is needed. Jurkowski and Garwick (1991) have developed a series of goals to be addressed as steps toward tackling the challenge of building a person's awareness of his or her own sexuality. Their recommended goals and aims, which incorporate the concerns and work of many professionals in this area, are as follows:

1. Improve the self-esteem and self-concept of the person.
2. Encourage age-appropriate, typical behaviors and opportunities.
3. Lower anxiety, guilt, stress, and self-criticism.
4. Improve one's ability to express preferences and make decisions.
5. Improve one's communication skills, particularly in "taboo" areas (including accuracy of information, frequency, and honesty, all of which may prove to be useful in cases of future difficulties).

6. Expand one's vocabulary and store of information (especially the correct names of body parts).
7. Expand one's awareness of the range of human relationships possible and the different levels of intimacy (i.e., friendships, dating, long-term relationships, and marriage).
8. Create and improve one's awareness of anatomy, reproduction, and contraception; improve health and physical well-being; promote positive health behaviors.
9. Lower the probability of sexual contact aggression or dangerous sexual activities by stressing positive alternatives.
10. Decrease the likelihood of unplanned pregnancy, vulnerability to abuse, AIDS, and sexually transmitted diseases.

Teachers and agency staff can be a valuable resource for parents. When considering the sensitivity of issues related to one's sexuality and the overwhelming needs parents may experience relative to their child's disability, teachers and staff can contribute significantly to the awareness and development parents may need in order to provide their child with accurate information geared toward the child's level of understanding. Educators and professionals can also act as a buffer for misinformation and myths that both persons with disabilities and their families face.

THE CHALLENGE AHEAD

I would like to get married to the right guy . . . I want to have a wedding day. I would hire my own staff, and have them assist with my needs . . . It's just not that easy, because I need my support staff right now.

—Mary Beth, 43 years old

The way sex education has been conducted is passé and obsolete. What is vital and alive is education on relationship building, sensuality, and intimacy as functional skills built into the compendium of activities of daily living. Intimacy and "making love," for many of us, began with touching, holding hands, learning about meaningful embraces compared to "hormonal hugs," and sharing secrets and confidences. Meaningful intimacy leading to sexual intimacy with our partners did not just happen; it was built following a series of trial and error relationships, and blossomed with our understanding of closeness. Many adults consider intimacy equal to or more important than intercourse; therefore, these feelings also need to be supported for individuals with developmental disabilities. Teaching individuals about healthy sensual expression and allowing them permission to explore their sexuality through a variety of ways (e.g., meaningful relationships with friends, having close friends as well as lovers) are far more valuable and important than just education about "plumbing." Skills such as self-stimulation are gratifying only on a physical level. Learning the skills to express caring and some degree of emotional intimacy broadens gratification to oneself and to others and enhances relationships with friends. It is important to begin this education as early as possible; early intervention is the key to rehabilitation, integration, and maximization of opportunities for integration. However, even for adults, education should be initiated to support the development of meaningful relationships with an appropriate level of intimacy.

The challenge ahead lies with the evolution of the understanding of individuals with mental retardation and disabilities as not just human beings, but as sexual and sensual beings with desires and needs developing from birth. Inclusion and community based activities will never be totally integrated until parents, professionals, and caregivers learn to facilitate that understanding. The successful meeting of this challenge requires recognition that sexuality and sensuality are critical skills to develop within the spectrum of skills for socialization and daily living. The challenge is as Dickerson (1982) stated: "To dare to raise adults, and to celebrate the person's sexuality" (p. 12).

REFERENCES

Adams, G.L., Tallon, R.J., & Alcorn, D.A. (1982). Attitudes toward the sexuality of mentally retarded and nonretarded persons. *Education and Training of the Mentally Retarded, 17*(4), 307–312.

Aiello, D. (1984). Issues and concerns confronting disabled assault victims: Stategies for treatment and prevention. *Sexuality and Disability, 7*(3/4), 96–101.

Bogdan, R., & Taylor, S.J. (1982). *Inside out: The social meaning of mental retardation.* Toronto: University of Toronto Press.

Brookhauser, P.E., Sullivan, P., Scanlan, J.M., & Garbarino, J. (1986). Identifying the sexually abused deaf child: The otolaryngologist's role. *Laryngoscope, 96,* 152–158.

Chaimowitz, C.A., & Moscovitch, A. (1991, March). Patient assaults on psychiatric residents: The Canadian experience. *Canadian Journal of Psychiatry, 30,* 107–111.

Chamberlin, A., Rauh, J., Passer, A., McGrath, M., & Burket, R. (1984). Issues in fertility control for mentally retarded female adolescents: Sexual activity, sexual abuse and contraception. *Pediatrics, 73*(4), 445–450.

Chorimer, N., & Lehr, W. (1976). *Child abuse and developmental disabili-*

ties: A report from the New England Regional Conference. Boston: New England Developmental Disabilities Communication Centre.

Cohan, S., & Warren, R.D. (1987). *Fellowship report: Child abuse, disability and family support: An analysis of dynamics in England and the United States, with references to practices in other European countries.* New York: Hunter College of the City University of New York, Programs in Education.

Cohan, S., & Warren, R.D. (1990, May/June). The intersection of disability and child abuse in England and the United States. *Child Welfare, LXIX,* (3), 253–262.

Cole, S.S. (1986). Facing the challenges of sexual abuse in persons with disabilities. *Sexuality and Disability,* 7(3/4), 71–88.

Cole, S. (1988). Women, sexuality and disabilities. *Women and Therapy,* 7(2/3), 277–294.

Coleman, E.M., & Murphy, W.D. (1980). A survey of sexual attitudes and sex education programs among facilities for the mentally retarded. *Applied Research in Mental Retardation, 1,* 269–276.

Craft, A., & Craft, M. (1983). *Sex education and counselling for mentally handicapped people.* Baltimore: University Park Press.

Craft, A., & Hitching, M. (1989). Keeping safe: Sex education and assertiveness skills. In H. Brown & A. Craft (Eds.), *Thinking the unthinkable: Papers on sexual abuse and people with learning difficulties* (pp. 29–38). London: FPA Education Unit.

Davies, R.K. (1979). Incest and vulnerable children. *Science News,* 116, 224–245.

Deisher, R.W. (1973). Sexual behavior of retarded in institutions. In F.F. de la Cruz & G.D. La Veck (Eds.), *Human sexuality and the mentally retarded* (pp. 145–152). New York: Brunner/Mazel.

Diamond, L.J., & Jaudes, P.K. (1983). Child abuse in a cerebral-palsied population. *Developmental Medicine and Child Neurology, 25,* 169–174.

Dickerson, M.U. (1982). New challenges for parents of the mentally retarded in the 1980s. *Exceptional Child, 29,* 5–12.

Doucette, J. (1986). *Violent acts against disabled women.* Toronto, Ontario, Canada: DAWN (DisAbled Women's Network).

Dupras, A., Levy, J.J., & Trembly, R. (1984). Path analysis of parents' conservatism toward sex education of their mentally retarded child. *American Journal of Mental Deficiency, 81*(2), 162–166.

Edgerton, R.B. (1967). *The cloak of competence.* London: Cambridge University Press, Berkeley: University of California Press.

Edmonson, B., McCombs, K., & Wish, J. (1979). What retarded adults believe about sex. *American Journal of Mental Deficiency, 84*(1), 11–18.

Elliott, G.D. (1980, July). The enemies of intimacy. *Harper's,* 50–56.

Garwick, G.B., & Jurkowski, E. (1992). Evaluation of HIV prevention and self-protection training programs. In A.C. Crocker, H.J. Cohen, & T.A. Kastner (Eds.), *HIV infection and developmental disabilities: A resource for service providers* (pp. 171–179). Baltimore: Paul H. Brookes Publishing Co.

Gordon, S. (1973). *On being the parent of a handicapped youth.* New York: New York Association for Brain-injured Children and The Association for Children with Learning Disabilities (95 Madison Ave, New York, NY, 10016).

Griffiths, D.M., Quinsey, V.L., & Hingsburger, D. (1989). *Changing inappro-*

priate sexual behavior: A community-based approach for persons with developmental disabilities. Baltimore: Paul H. Brookes Publishing Co.

Hall, J.E., & Morris, H.L. (1976). Sexual knowledge and attitudes of institutionalized retarded adolescents. *American Journal of Mental Deficiency, 80*(4), 382–387.

Henshel, A.M. (1972). *The forgotten ones.* Austin: University of Texas Press.

Heshusius, L. (1981). *Meaning in life as experienced by persons labeled retarded in a group home: A participant observation study.* Springfield, IL: Charles C Thomas.

Heshusius, L. (1982). Sexuality, intimacy, and persons we label mentally retarded: What they think—what we think. *Mental Retardation, 20*(4), 164–168.

Heshusius, L. (1987). Research and perceptions of sexuality by persons labelled mentally retarded. In A. Craft (Ed.), *Mental handicap and sexuality: Issues and perspectives* (pp. 35–61). Kent, England: DJ Costello Ltd.

Hingsburger, D., & Griffiths, D. (1986). Dealing with sexuality in a community residential service. *Psychiatric Aspects of Mental Retardation Reviews, 5*(12), 63–67.

Jurkowski, E. (1991). *An assessment of agency policies and practices related to socio-sexual education.* Huron, SD: Report to [the] Huron Adjustment Training Center.

Jurkowski, E. (1992). *The impacts of disability.* Unpublished manuscript, Community Health Sciences, Faculty of Medicine, University of Manitoba, Winnipeg.

Jurkowski, E., & Garwick, G.B. (1991, May). *Normalizing friendships, relationships, community inclusion and sexuality.* Presentation to the American Association on Mental Retardation, Washington, DC.

Kempton, W. (1972). *Guidelines for planning a training course on human sexuality and the retarded.* Philadelphia: Planned Parenthood Association of Southeastern Pennsylvania.

Kempton, W. (1977). The mentally retarded person. In H.L. Gochros & J.S. Gochros (Eds.), *The sexually oppressed* (pp. 239–256). New York: Association Press.

Kempton, W. (1983). Teaching retarded children about sex. *PTA Today, 8*(6), 28–30.

Koegel, P., & Whittemore, R. (1983). Sexuality in the ongoing lives of mentally retarded adults. In A. Craft & M. Craft (Eds.), *Sex education and counselling for mentally handicapped people.* Baltimore: University Park Press.

Lakin, K.C., & Bruininks, R.H. (1985). Social integration of developmentally disabled persons. In K.C. Lakin & R.H. Bruininks (Eds.), *Strategies for achieving community integration of developmentally disabled citizens* (pp. 3–25). Baltimore: Paul H. Brookes Publishing Co.

Massuda, S. (1990, June). *Meeting our needs: Access manual for transition houses.* Toronto, Ontario, Canada: DAWN (DisAbled Women's Network).

McNab, W.L. (1978). The sexual needs of the handicapped. *Journal of School Health, 48*(5), 301–306.

Meyers, R. (1978). *Like normal people.* New York: McGraw Hill.

Monat-Haller, R.K. (1992). *Understanding and expressing sexuality: Responsible choices for individuals with developmental disabilities.* Baltimore: Paul H. Brookes Publishing Co.

Pincus, S. (1988). Sexuality in the mentally retarded patient. *American Family Physician, 37*(2), 319–323.

Planned Parenthood Federation of Canada. (1989). *Family life education: Keys to success.* Ottawa, Ontario, Canada: author.

Rostafinski, M.J. (1975). Subjects related to sex as viewed by retarded people. In M.S. Bass & M. Gelof (Eds.), *Sexual rights and responsibilities of the mentally retarded.* Washington, DC: American Association on Mental Deficiency.

Rowe, W., Savage, S., & Dennis-Delanney, J. (1987, September). *The effects of training in human sexuality for individuals working with developmentally disabled persons.* Presentation at the annual meeting of the American Association of Mental Deficiency, Region IV, Edmonton, Alberta, Canada.

Sobsey, D. (1990). Too much stress on stress? Abuse and the family stress factor. *News and Notes: Quarterly newsletter of the American Association on Mental Retardation, 3*(1), 2,8.

Sobsey, D., Gray, S., Wells, D., Pyper, D., & Reimer-Heck, B. (1991). *Disability, sexuality, and abuse: An annotated bibliography.* Baltimore: Paul H. Brookes Publishing Co.

Tyne, A. (1988). *Ties and connections: An ordinary community life for people with learning difficulties.* London: King's Fund Centre.

Watson, J., & Rogers, D. (1980). Sexual instruction for the mildly retarded and normal adolescent: A comparison of educational approaches, parental expectations and pupil knowledge and attitude. *Health Education Journal, 39*(3), 88–95.

Watt, J.W. (1991, October). *Talking openly about sexuality.* Presentation at the Conference on Community, "And Justice for All," Ellensburg, WA.

Yoshida, L., Wasilushuk, D.L., & Friedman, D.L. (1990). Recent newspaper coverage about persons with disabilities. *Exceptional Children, 56*(5), 418–423.

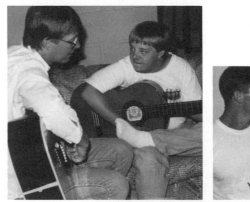

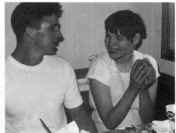

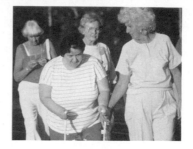

II

STORIES OF FRIENDSHIPS

Stories are important and often the best teachers. As Ivan Illich told Leopold Kohr in the preface to *The Breakdown of Nations*, "Like a Rabbi or a Mullah, you avoided putting forward theories and told stories instead. All your life you have spoken and written like one who knows that arguments can end merely in conclusions and only stories make sense" (Illich, 1986, p. vii). John McKnight and others have pointed out that story-telling calls forth commonality and the true sense of community; while systems thrive on counting things, community networks thrive on stories about real people. Perhaps the real truth, the real lessons, are only or best learned from stories. As the heart of a human being is centrally located, so are stories central to this book.

Over the years, Karin Melberg Schwier has collected and published many stories of people's lives through interviewing and listening. She begins this section in Chapter 9 by presenting many types of friends telling their own stories; the stories of these various relationships include those between persons with disabilities and community members, people who are married to each other, and other testimonies. Kathy Bartholomew-Lorimer has done significant work in attempting to build community both in Louisville and through John McKnight's Community Building Project in Logan Square, Chicago; in Chapter 10, she tells three stories of the ups and downs in attempting to build community over a period of 7 years and shares many useful lessons for persons attempting the same work.

The next three chapters tell stories of particular friendships. Joe Shapiro got to know Jim, who lived in a state institution, when Joe was a college student 16 years ago; after becoming a reporter for *U.S. News and World Report*, Joe investigated disability issues nationally. Part of that investigation was finding Jim again after 16 years, and gathering others together to try to free Jim from the institution. Their story in Chapter 11 is one of how an "outside" friend can often see things that are invisible to those on the inside, and of how a friend can advocate and move mountains that are seemingly immovable to others. Jane Wells, in Chapter 12, tells the stories of three women, Jane, Mary Ann, and Sue, who have changed their respective roles from advocate, client, and stranger to that of three friends, and of the remarkable changes in all three as they have shifted their relationship over 5 years. Jeff and Cindy Strully discuss the lessons of friendship that they are learning as their daughter Shawntell moves from high school and the friendships she developed there to go off to college; in Chapter 13 they discuss this shift in all their lives and apply what has been learned from supporting friendship in school systems to services for adults.

Betty Pendler provides a mother's perspective in Chapter 14 on the issues of sexuality that affect friendship, and offers advice from her experiences with her own children to other parents and to professional staff on how best to talk about and support friendships that include sexual expression. Finally, Karl Williams has captured in Chapter 15 the words of many self-advocates and their friends about the nature of their friendships and relationships; he interviewed and has recorded conversations between persons with disabilities who belong to Speaking For Ourselves (a self-advocacy group in Pennsylvania) and their "partners" who are friends and supporters. The words of people themselves can provide profound understanding of the nature of such friendships—the mutual give and take, the deep meaning to both parties, and the real heart.

Of course these stories and experiences are only some of those that could be shared. Across the country and in many towns people are coming together to get to know each other, have fun, and help each other. Such friendships are what keep the heart of community beating.

REFERENCE

Illich, I. (1986). Foreword. In L. Kohr, *The breakdown of nations* (pp. vii–x). New York: Routledge & Kegan Paul.

9

Ordinary Miracles
Testimonies of Friendships
Karin Melberg Schwier

There is something about being naked in the shower at the YMCA. It is one of the great equalizers to stand there shampooing and shaving with lawyers, shop clerks, journalists, at-home moms, professors, secretaries, university students, and accountants of all sizes, ages, and definitely all shapes. Some have Ph.D.s and some have tattoos. But in the shower, and in the pool, they are all there to enjoy the company of each other, their bodies, the feel of the water, and the pursuit of fitness. At the YMCA, it is just a fact that not everyone is at the same level of fitness. Yet, people are respected and encouraged for showing up to try.

During the 5 years since my husband and I joined the YMCA, I have met an interesting assortment of people. During the aquafitness classes, complete with plastic bleach bottles doubling as "floatation devices," a variety of women lurch their way around the pool amidst good-natured kidding and laughter. During classes such as "Swimming for the Truly Terrified," the "not-quite-so-terrified" naturally accept the responsibility for gently calming the raw nerves of the "really terrified." Soon the gasps are replaced by shaky laughter and babysteps of self-confidence. During lane swims, people are a little more focused, but there is still time to offer advice and encouragement or at least call out a friendly, "Hi, how are you doing?" All the while, everyday, everyone is in the same pool. Sure, the faster and more experienced swimmers go to the fast lanes or the deep end, and the ones who use the verb *swim* as optimistically as they can venture

---

All quotes were taken from personal communications with the author, 1989–1992.

around the shallow end or cling to flutterboards. But no matter where you are in the pool, there is an opportunity—and an expectation—to say hello, chat a bit while you adjust goggles, meet for coffee upstairs, or just talk about careers or families while you stand in the shower afterward.

I have met another writer, a broadcast journalist, a master's student with the challenge of cerebral palsy, a young man with a mental disability who is trying very hard to learn the mechanics of lane swims without crashing into other swimmers, a woman with a fascinating tattoo of a peacock across her entire back, a grandmother who travels and buys a souvenir t-shirt from every port of call, and a young mom who swam lanes up until the day before each of her four children were born. The YMCA experience has not only made me a healthier person physically, but my growing and ever-changing network of connections has nurtured the emotional me inside this body. Each meeting has happened individually and casually, the way many friendships and even business contacts are born. The opportunity exists, along with the expectation, that people reach out and tap into it. Ironically, that opportunity and especially the expectation do not exist for some people who need them most.

Compare the YMCA experience with the following scenario: At a riverbank fair this summer in our city, my husband, Rick, and I dropped our bikes and found a vantage point for people-watching. Local bands played, children devoured hotdogs and stared skyward at balloons tied to their wrists. People dressed up like soldiers and Indians to commemorate the native uprising. There were tug-o-wars, watermelon eating contests, and music.

In the midst of the noise and color, eight middle-age and older men, all with obvious disabilities, were steered up to the hotdog stand nearby. The two staff seemed very tense about keeping the group together and encouraged the men to "hold their buddy's hand." The day was sunny and warm. The younger staff person had on bright shorts and a matching tank top, her hair was caught up in a ponytail, and she wore sunglasses. The other, an older woman with grey hair, wore peppermint green slacks, a white blouse, and a light windbreaker. All eight men, squinting in the sunlight, wore black or dark brown pants, blue ball caps, and identical blue jackets emblazoned with the name of the sheltered workshop they obviously attended. The group of them huddled together reminded me of an awkward blue raft, lashed together to prevent the pieces from being pulled away in the current.

Hot dogs in hand, the raft bobbed around and churned through the crowd, navigated along the route by the staff, one stationed at port, the other at the stern. The sea of fairgoers generally gave a wide berth to the raft and it finally came to a stop on the grass. One or two of the men smiled broadly and said something to passerby; one held up his hot dog. The staff distracted the smiler by pointing to the band and asking if he needed a napkin.

What chance, my husband and I wondered aloud, do those eight men ever have of striking up a conversation with someone, let alone creating even a casual friendship? We watched them solemnly anchored there in the park on that sunny July day, looking silly and overdressed. Eight old men, clinging to each other's hands in the midst of a crowd teeming with potential friends.

We thought of other people we know who not only manage the limitations of their own disabilities, but also battle the obstacles that their label and the service system have strewn in their path. We talked of our own son, of the friendships and connections he has made in the community, some orchestrated by us, others not. Some last, others do not. When we moved to a new neighborhood, I wrote an ad for the community association newsletter, inviting teenagers to meet Jim (no "special" friends, please, just *regular* ones). Jim has been involved in a leisure buddy program through the city parks and recreation department. As a professor at the university, Rick keeps an eye out for potential connections. Jim regularly makes the purchases at local shops in our neighborhood, and lately has taken to insisting that we stay in the car. If we are shopping for jeans or shoes or a potato peeler, we encourage him to approach the clerk and ask for assistance. One summer, two brothers (good looking, athletic types) and Jim had a ball going to the waterslides, just roaring around in the car; it was the summer of Jim's 16th birthday and the brothers gave him his first driving lessons—in *their* car, not ours, and *way* out in the country! Because of the way Jim looks, people sometimes back away and miss out on getting to know him. Our role is to keep stirring the waters and as the opportunities bubble to the surface, it is Jim's job to reach out and cup them in his hands.

• • •

I would like to introduce you to some people, some people worth listening to. The words of the people you are about to meet are elegant in their simplicity and honesty. As a journalist, I am conscious of accuracy as I relate the thoughts and feelings of people with mental disabilities. I want to make sure the words are *theirs,* not merely my interpretation. They speak to the essence of friendship and respect for other people. They explain their sadness with those who seem to have so little time. They are proud of their own achievements and they remind us how important we are to one another. Their words are a testament to the unspectacular and ordinary miracle of friendship and caring.

Somewhere along the way, we decided we knew best. We didn't ask how they see the world. We've forgotten what human beings really need from each other. Or perhaps we believe something so simple can't be the answer. It's not so hard really, just to listen.

(Schwier, 1990)

RAINA AND MABELE

Raina, 67, and Mabele, 68, get together every Thursday at four o'clock. Mabele gets the coffee going and arranges the reading materials on the kitchen table. Raina impatiently rides the bus home from the sheltered workshop so she can "freshen my face up" before she heads over to "my good friend's house." For Raina, who has a mental disability, these weekly get-togethers mean that she is learning to read. For Mabele, the visits mean she is able to teach. For both, there is the quiet joy of sharing each other's company. Raina spent most of her life in an institution.

Raina

"No one ever ask me about my readin' before and my poems. I'd like it if my poems were in a magazine. I had a grade two reader when I was a little girl. I can still say poems outta my head, I went to grade two. I was sick all my life. I took in every disease goin' around, my mom said. I was unlucky. But now I'm lucky! I see my good friend Mabele once a week and we learn to read together. I do homework and Mabele checks it and then we work on the next part at her house. I like her. She's a real nice lady. I like Mabele awfully well. She dresses so nice with blue eyes and grey hair and I think she's five feet two in her stockin' feet. I'm five foot two, too! I read to her and she helps me with the big words. We have coffee and she gives me cookies and candy. She makes her own cookies, Mabele does. Her husband is nice, too. We like poems and she gets a real kick outta the ones I tell her outta my head. Like this, my favorite: 'Love is such a funny thing, it's somethin' like a lizard. It winds itself around your heart and nibbles at your gizzard.' Ain't that a good one? I read to Mabele every week. I count the . . . syllables . . . and sound out words for her. She says I'm doin' real good. I feel smarter all the time."

BRENDA AND DON

Brenda and Don's tumultuous life together began long before the birth of their son, Trevor, and the long tentacles of problems ignored or denied continue to creep into their lives today. The couple, both of whom have a mental disability, have been through a 2-year custody battle for their child and, although he has been returned to them, the family is still desperately trying to hold itself together. Don lived for years in a large institution. Nearly beaten by a social services system primed to look for fault and inability rather than designed to nurture and teach, the family may never fully recover.

Don

"I felt like I had to be strong for Brenda because she really needed me to be the man, you know, but sometimes I didn't feel so strong inside. My family didn't think we should get married. They figured I could do better, that's what they said, but I didn't think so. There were people who said I was slower and shouldn't get married and that didn't make me feel too good. We met at the workshop. Brenda came in one day and ask where the bathroom was and I showed her. Then I called her about a week later. I guess we what you call dated, but mostly I hung around the farm a lot, mostly at suppertime! After we was married, we had to really have it out a few times about sharing the work and that. We had a few arguments like. I told her she has to help me so it's not all left to one person to do the work. That's what marriage means is sharing of stuff."

Brenda

"Don's family never wanted me around. They was always trying to break him and me up and they did lots of cruel and mean things to run me off. I feel better about myself now that I know how to keep my house clean and cook and wash clothes. Don and me share, but it took me a long time to get over being lazy. I never did anything at home with my mom. When the baby came along, I was still learning not to be spoiled and lazy. I wanted them to just send me home from the hospital and they wouldn't so I told one of them that I hit Trevor. I thought they'd get mad at me and send me home, but they took

Trevor instead. They watched us with him and we couldn't feed him or change him or dress him. It felt like everyone was waiting, you know, for us to make a mistake so they could, you know, say 'See, they aren't fit to have a baby.'

"The whole time in court, I sometimes felt scared about getting close to Trevor. He was living at the foster people's house, but sometimes we could see him if somebody watched us. I didn't want to love him a lot because what if they just took him away in the end? He always used to go to Don when he was little, until one day he came over to me and hugged my leg and held up his arms to me. Dora, the lady from Home Care, told me to stop what I was doing and pick him up. So I did. He never done that before. I want to be a good mommy and we know we can call people for help. I love Don, but I don't want him to touch me sometimes. I got hurt one time from guys and I don't like it. But the one person I know I could really count on during bad times is my husband, Don. He was always strong. I think marrying him was one of my best ideas."

DALLAS

In a small rural town, people's routines soon become familiar to everyone. So when tall, lanky Dallas, 43, who has a mental disability, shuffles into the local cafe, they know the man coming in the door on his heels will be his uncle. The routine is played out with such weekly punctuality that if it doesn't happen, people inquire about Dallas's whereabouts.

Dallas

"My uncle, he and me have a thing going. Every Saturday morning. He picks me up at ten o'clock sharp. My Aunt Elaine, she sends along some little goodies for me to enjoy to eat. Then my uncle and me go for coffee. We talk about important things. We say hello to everyone at the cafe. Then he takes me back home. It's a little routine we got going. Every Saturday. Me and my uncle. It's important."

FRANCIS AND RICK

At first glance, Francis, 31, and Rick, 41, do not look like they would have much in common. Francis works at McDonald's after making the break on his own from a sheltered workshop. He lives in a group home with seven other men and rides home with his sister on weekends to visit his elderly parents who live in a tiny rural farming community. Francis, who has Down syndrome, does not read or write and, even after a lot of rehearsal, cannot sign his name without help. When he makes a purchase, he trustingly holds his wallet open to the cashier. Rick, a father of three, is a university professor with a doctorate in education. Through Rick's wife, both men discovered a common obsession—the World Wrestling Federation (WWF). They meet now and then at Francis's McDonald's for a cheeseburger to discuss the latest dramas in the ring; they attended a live Grand Slam performance. On one occasion so far, a colleague of Rick's, also a university professor and a WWF fan, came along. After, over a beer, the three regaled each other with recounts of the evening. A few weeks later, Rick's colleague mentioned Francis in a conversation at the college faculty lounge. Without thought, he said, "Francis is a retarded kid whom Rick has befriended." After a few seconds of reflection, however, he changed his stereotypical description to "Francis is a young man who's a wrestling aficionado; he's a friend of Rick's." Carefully trying to manage a stutter, Francis talks of his friendship with Rick.

Francis

"I'll tell you one thing right now. I love wrestling. So does Rick. He knows almost as much about WWF as me. I know all about it because I study it. I called Rick to ask him if maybe we could go to Grand Slam when they came to town and he said sure. I said all right! Then, in about another week, I called him again and said I got an idea. I said maybe we should go out for supper before we go to WWF. So Rick's wife picked me up at McDonald's after work and we went and had a barbecue. I wore my good Hulk Hogan t-shirt and I have something else just like Hulk Hogan, that's my cross. We discuss wrestling a lot, me and Rick. I been following it for a long time now, ever since I went to that Maple Leaf Gardens and saw WWF. That Ted Dibiase is a bad guy, I don't like him. And someone else I don't like either is Scary Sherri. A guy at McDonald's likes wrestling, too. His name is Lorne and he is the fix-it guy. If anything needs fixing, we call Lorne. He takes his three kids to wrestling. They all yell at the wrestlers. I do, too. So does Rick. I yell 'give him one' and then I yell 'thank you!' Then I yell, 'Give him another one!' I'll tell you one thing right now, we can hardly talk after. The other seven guys in my house and the house mother, Marj, all went to the fair, but Rick and me went to wrestling. That's better anyhow. Marj is retiring. And guess what else I have to tell you? I'm going to take a class and get my own place. I hope I pass. Rick said that was great and maybe we can have a party when I pass and get my own apartment. And another thing. Once I get my nephew married off next year, then I will get married. Rick is married and he says it's good when you marry the right girl. I got one all picked out, but I got to pass my class first and get my own place. I haven't told Mom and Dad yet. I will tell Mom when she's sitting down. I'm going to visit my sister next month, but my godmother is going to tape the next WWF Summer Slam off TV. Rick and I will get together and watch it. I got his phone number at work and he said I can call him and if he's not there, I can give a message to his secatary. He's a good guy, all right. He gave me some wrestling magazines and he even showed up at McDonald's where I work on my birthday as a surprise and gave me a good wrestling magazine. We even had a cake with a sparkly thing on it. I'll tell you one thing, we got something great in common, that's for sure."

MARTIN AND CHERYL

Martin, 48, and Cheryl, 38, are getting married next year. They met 2 years ago in an adult special education class when Martin was "assigned to Cheryl to help her with her mathematics and making change at the store." As their friendship grew and evolved into romance, the couple found themselves facing formidable obstacles: family and social workers. Martin lived for 20 years in an institution. He did not become a man in his own eyes until he was 42 and he finally had his Bar Mitzvah; he did not have one on his 13th birthday because staff felt it would upset routine. Today, Martin, who has a mental disability and epilepsy, works as a maintanance worker for an emergency rescue station and Cheryl continues to take classes and look for work. She would like to work in a daycare; she loves children, but the couple has decided against having their own.

Martin

"My mom and brother and worker are afraid to let me get married because of my temper. I sometimes get into argaments. I tell them I disagree with what my mom and brother said. I know Cheryl for 2 years and have disargaments with her, but we settle it down like adults. We talk about it. I never, ever raise my fist at her. So if we were married and had disargaments, why would I harm her? We sat down with my parents and Cheryl's parents and our workers and they talk and talk. I want to get on with my life with my fiancé, but how can I when there is so much intraference with everything we do? Even though we are having a hard time, we cannot give up. In the last meeting, I was so proud of my Cheryl. She listened for long time, then she says, 'I want to tell you, Mrs. Levine, your son and I always got along together, but I understand where you are from and what you are trying to say, but I do love your son and I do want to marry him sometime next year in May and you shouldn't worry. We will be all right together.' That Cheryl, she is something!

"Even with all the trouble and hard times we are going through together, to show our parents we was meant for each other, that our marriage will work out fine. She is a real kibbitzer, that is a Jewish word for somebody who kids around a lot. I just want to say as long as our parents allow us our freedom and don't always intrafere and disturv us just cause we have a slow learnin' disbilty, our marriage will go very well. I know we will have to help each other with our problems. There is a fine difference between advice and telling us what to do. I believe we can do it, and I know our lives will be different than it is now. Marriage is a great big sponsibility for both of us, but it will be better than living seprate from each other. We will show the parents what we are all about, and that we are not little children and that we have come a long way."

SALLY

After graduating 5 years ago from high school, Sally, 26, lives at home with her parents, delivers flyers, and walks the dog every day. Sally has Down syndrome. She volunteers twice a week for bingo at a senior citizens' complex, and every Tuesday evening she "works out and runs" in a Special Olympics team with former classmates from the special class at her high school.

Sally

"I don't think I'll ever get an apartment because Mom says she and I are together for ever and I will look after her when she gets old. Maybe I'll get a job someday; Mom says she has to find it for me because no one else is gonna. I have a friend over sometimes. She used to be in my class at school. Sometimes she stays overnight and we put on music and listen to it and sing. We watch Much Music and sing. We look at all my magazines like the *National Inqueer* and the *Sun* and *Teen Beat*. Then we have pizza or sometimes we get Kentucky Fried Chicken. I used to go to a youth committee meetings. Some of them go to school at university and we'd have pizza and watch movies and party. It was fun and we'd all stay overnight. I am the only Down syndrome.

"Sometimes they said they were coming to pick me up and then they didn't. I got dressed up and waited, but they didn't show up or phone or nothin'. I am very upset and I cried. One guy I like a lot from that. One time at a meeting I got very mad because I love one of the guys and he told me not to. His name is Brian. He must be 20 or maybe 19, and I love him. He said he would send me a birthday card last year, but he never, so I am still waiting every day when the mail comes. He musta forgot. I write him letters, but I don't tell Mom or she'll get mad. One time I phoned him, but Mom found out cause it was long distance, and told me I can't call him no more. I got in trouble one time at school, me and another guy I like, David. He is Down syndrome, too. We was in the bed together at school, but I never get pregent in my stomach. Mom said that could happen to me, but then I would have a baby and me and him would get married cause he would want to have a baby, too. I heard Brian has a girlfriend already, but I don't believe it. I love him and he is going to send me a birthday card and he is gonna write his name in it and I have a spot for it in my scrapbook."

JOE AND RON

Joe spent 18 years in an institution highlighted by intermittent "escapes" and corresponding punishments. In 1986, he was suddenly discharged. Today, 39 and unemployed, he lives with three dogs and two cats. He exists on poverty level social assistance in a low-income, high-crime neighborhood, and is careful never to mention his years in the institution because "people think I am crazy for bein' in there and won't be my friend no more." Joe, who has a physical and mental disability, relies on Ron, 42, a neighbor, for help now and then. He considers Ron one of "my real best pals."

Joe[1]

"I don't wanchoo to tell no one I was in there. If my friends knew I was in there, they wouldn't wanna be my friends no more. It's like a nuthouse. If you are sick and you chop somebody up, you go to the nuthouse. Okay, this was like that. I don't want nobody to know, okay. They won't be my friends no more. When I was a little kid, I had a dog. I love dogs. In the intuition, you can't have no dogs or nothin.' I got dogs now I'm out. I got two dogs that are brother and sister. I gotta watch they don't, you know, *do it,* cause if they *do it,* the pups come out stupid. I heard people is like that, too. I do stuff. I useta drink a lot. But now I am careful. My friend and me went to the bar and I told my friend I hadda go home cause I got a roast in the oven and if we stay in the bar, my roast would be on flames and my house, too! I like dogs bettern cats, I don't know why I got a cat. She just show up. She always is gettin' predkant. One time I was walkin' down the street and

---

[1]Adapted from Schwier (1990).

a guy walkin' by yell at me, 'You nothin' but a goddam goof, you re-tard.' I got me my friend Ron next door. He is bouncer in the bar so Ron says if I get any trouble with people, I should tell him. Ron is big and he looks like he's mean, but he is not to me. If people are both-erin' me, you just get me next door even if it's in the middle of the night, he tells me. That Ron, he looks out for me! He help me build a fence and he's gonna help me build a dog kennel for my dogs. Some-times Ron and me talk over the fence. He says I got nice dogs and says I take good care of 'em. It's good to have a nice neighbor. I tell him I watch his house for him if he goes somewhere. And he watches my house in case someone try to wreck it. That's what friends do, you know, they watch each other's stuff. Maybe I tell him someday about the intution, but maybe not. I don't want to chance him not likin' me no more."

ORDINARY LINKS

One of the most striking things about all of the connections in this chapter is that most people involved do not have that much in com-mon. Perhaps these linkages do not have to be startling in their com-plexity and the points of departure that lead to friendships do not have to be significant.

The "you two have so much in common and therefore will be great friends" myth is a barrier that can drown the tender growth of or-dinary friendships. Assumptions and fears about people with dis-abilities and misconceptions about what they can offer have created isolation. But when the seeds of acquaintance are nurtured, even oc-casionally, gifts such as compassion, a sense of humor, a common in-terest, a hidden talent, the ability to listen, and other undiscovered wonders can flourish.

The mechanics of that nurturing are simple, so simple we worry that it could not possibly be the answer to having more caring com-munities. Having coffee, talking on the telephone, seeing a movie, including one another in celebrations, getting together to wash the car or the dog, or to go for an evening walk along the river are the things of which friendships are made. Some of these connections are planned and regular; some are casual and intermittent. When they happen, it is as though something tight and hard deep within us slowly unfurls, spreading a warmth in us and through us to others.

We must respect relationships that exist between people who both have disabilities. Although we must promote and encourage connec-tions between people with disabilities and those without if we ever hope to have a complete community, we cannot diminish the quality of the relationships in which both people have disabilities. Too often, lifelong friends are torn apart during moves from institutions or group homes; men and women with disabilities are kept apart and their love is denied; or connections are simply forgotten, creating wounds that may never heal. Often, there is so much that can be done to re-connect people who were once deeply involved with each other. Beyond that, people's lives and relationships have been so ignored and trampled upon already that we must not disregard or sever relation-ships, therefore adding to their pain and loss. People with disabilities must be supported and encouraged to develop relationships with a vast and interesting assortment of people on a variety of levels, to ex-plore the excitement of making new friends and sustaining those they choose to maintain.

The relationships we have with the people who drift in and out of our lives and with those who are with us for a long time are all unique. Having a friendship or a connection with someone with a different intellectual ability does not have to mean an all-absorbing lifetime commitment. It can be an ordinary relationship. A damaging perception tells us a connection with someone who has a disability should somehow be "special" or "extraordinary"; both are adjectives hard to live up to in everyday life. Most people with disabilities also expect their relationships to evolve differently from person to person. The rewards of two friends who meet for a monthly lunch date can be as meaningful and satisfying as those enjoyed by two who share more frequent contact. The loss occurs when a relationship withers before it has begun, before there is a chance to see the possibilities.

Most relationships are not healthy or positive all the time. Experi-encing the lows is part of the changing dynamics between growing and developing human beings. Some relationships grow toward dis-solution, regardless of someone's intellectual ability.

A friend of mine, who spent years in an institution, struggled with the words to describe an ache he is afraid will never diminish. "It's a . . . a . . . reptation. People think what I am like before they even meet me," he says. "They decide before they see if there's anything here they might like in me after all."

Organizational advocacy can mean change in slow, lumbering steps. People do not have that much time. Individual change can come much more quickly and meaningfully one connection, one cup of coffee, one telephone call, one aquafitness class, one shared laugh at a time.

Friendship is a thing most necessary to life, since without friends no one would choose to live, though possessed of all other advantages.

Aristotle

REFERENCE

Schwier, K.M. (1990). *Speakeasy: People with mental handicaps talk about their lives in institutions and in the community.* Austin: PRO-ED.

Community Building

Valued Roles for
Supporting Connections

Kathy Bartholomew-Lorimer

In the work of building community, sometimes people with disabilities and community members come together very strongly. The stories of these particular relationships shout the message of connection and commitment. They are the stories that seem to be told most often about community building, the stories everyone keeps hearing. They are the stories that may be called "successes" and that, unfortunately, will seduce us into believing that the only valid community-building efforts are those that end in these loud "successes."

During the 8 years I have worked in community building, many of the stories have been much more quiet, not quite so easy to understand. They are about little things that often happen in brief moments. In addition, they are not always stories about things that work out. This does not make them any less real or important; they contain the stuff that life is made of.

I share the following three stories because, in my opinion, they represent the challenge to find valued roles and relationships in community. It is my hope that these stories offer more than a vision of "success," that they can also be stories to learn by.

The first part of each story was written between 1984 and 1987 when I was working as program director at Options for Individuals, Inc., in Louisville, Kentucky. I am currently a consultant with the Options program. Each story reflects what happened in 1987 and what is happening today, 5 years later.

The names of people and community sites in this chapter are pseudonyms.

The author thanks the associates, staff, and executive director, David Block, of Options for Individuals, Inc., 102 E. Oak, Louisville, Kentucky 40203.

Options for Individuals, Inc., is an adult day service. The agency supports 25 people with developmental disabilities in a variety of ways in community settings. The focus of Options has been to create personalized space for individuals within the community and to build relationships. This work is done by first getting to know people and identifying each person's unique interests. Then, staff look for places where people can contribute and become a part of the everyday life in the community.

Staff explore local areas and neighborhoods around people's homes and identify places that hold the potential for individuals to be included and to contribute in some way. Options staff become familiar with the owners or regulars at a community site, determine if they would be open and interested, and invite them to welcome a particular individual with disabilities. Careful consideration is given to the individual's interests, potential contribution, and interest of the community members. Staff usually accompany the individual initially, but it is expected that when possible the community members will be able to support the individual on their own. It is also hoped that the community members will come to know the individual, develop closer relationships, and that eventually many environments of mutual appreciation and interdependence will be built.

The three stories in this chapter are not stories of grand successes, but rather of real ones. They tell the story of the hard work of supporting community between individuals with and without disabilities. Once that work is begun, failures and disappointments may occur. Rather than grand successes, perhaps community-building is primarily constituted of many small moments of connection.

There are many lessons to learn from these three stories. That community members can be not just tolerant but even welcoming of individuals who may be difficult to get to know and challenging to include. That perhaps one of the most important reasons to work on including individuals is the opportunity for community members to open their eyes and hearts. That the right amount of support for a person requires a delicate balance that may go up and down over time. That casual acquaintances are as much part of building community as long-term, deep friendships. That after much hard work, it may be necessary to face painful realities that a situation is just not working. That even though we have worked hard and relationships have lasted for a number of years, they may come to an end and it is all right to be sad when they do; the work of building community may consist of having to often start over to seek out new connections. That surrounding an individual with community members brings that person a different life. And, that the ordinary moments when people share daily life together make all the work worth it and are what is the heart of community.

NANCY

Nancy lives with her father in Louisville. She is a woman of great diversity. She needs to be understood and respected in order to get close to her. If you are close, she will give you respect, too. She is probably admired the most for her spunk and spirit. People almost always comment that she "lets her feelings out"; that is appreciated because a lot of people are not able to do so. She likes to be in charge— sometimes it is done in a helpful way, other times she gives orders. She hates to be told what to do. If you say, "Come on, Nancy, get your coat and let's go," she will ignore you and maybe even walk away. But if you say, "I'm leaving, Nancy. I want you to go, but you decide," she will be right behind you, ready to go. If you make life fun, Nancy joins in, which allows all of us the opportunity to learn to enjoy life more, too. She is a teaser and is drawn to people who have a playful nature. We (staff at Options for Individuals, Inc.) have learned that Nancy even draws this out in people. She says, "It's cold," and throws her head back and laughs so heartily that it becomes contagious. Before you know it, you are laughing, too.

Nancy likes hair. She says, "your hair," and touches it. She has been going to Miller's Beauty Supply twice a week for almost 2 years. At first, a staff person went with her. She had a routine of things she did for the beauty shop. Nancy does not always like to do things just because someone says, "It's your job." She likes to be helpful to a particular person who says, "Will you bring me a towel, please?" She likes to help Janet, one of the hairdressers; she hands Janet clippies while she sets hair. Sometimes Nancy hands them too fast, "Here, here," and sometimes she forgets altogether. But it does not seem to matter. Nancy likes to feel she is needed and Janet likes to include her. A lot of the customers know her, too. Sometimes Nancy comes in and sits by herself listening to music.

Currently Nancy goes to the beauty shop without a staff person. This is significant because it means that the people at the shop have to find ways for Nancy to be included. They all say that she has grown since they first met her. Yet, they can ask her to assist them and she will say, "Leave me alone," and walk off. Nancy does not mean to be rude, she just does not always know how to react to personal attention. Usually someone can say, "Well, when you get ready, I could really use your help." Nancy requires respect and if you tell her she is needed or that she is really a good person, she will almost always come around, and "help you," as she says. It is like the people at Miller's say, "She can be a very nice person when you treat her like all the others. And that's how she likes to be treated, like the others. It has opened our eyes to someone different than us and that she is one of us, too."

Nancy's wish to be helpful has drawn her to helping children. She started helping at Western Day Care Center about a year ago. "Ms. Nancy," as she is called, plays music for the children. Western is a warm and caring place and Nancy has learned about gentleness and kindness there. She has learned to say "please" and "thank you" and speak softly. She goes without a staff person twice a week. Nancy is very comfortable with the people at Western. She likes to go and does not like to leave. She feels important there and she feels needed.

When I talked with the director and staff at Western, I heard the expression of commitment and appreciation for Nancy. It is not that Nancy is always pleasant or that she always does as you ask. In fact, sometimes she disrupts things. She moves at her own pace, which may mean you have to change yours. We talked about Nancy and all her ways. We laughed when the conversation turned to her sense of humor. The word "sunshine" is a magical word. It can turn a dark mood into laughter. When she is upset or in a dark mood, someone will say, "Nancy must not see any sunshine today." She will struggle not to smile, but she never can stop herself and the spell breaks. It is as though the positive side of Nancy is so powerful that the rest is insignificant. The people at Western say, "In the beginning she seemed to only mimic what the other teachers said. But we learned that Nancy could express her own thoughts and feelings. Nancy's contribution has come mainly from her presence here."

It is hard to describe how I feel at times like this. It is like this is all coming together before my eyes. They see and understand that this simple woman has a gift. I wonder once again why it is so easy for some people to see while others are so blind.

Nancy has learned to be a teacher in other settings as well. Nancy's mom tells a story about Nancy attending a wedding. She is not one to sit for long periods of time, so her mom was apprehensive about taking her. She sat through the whole thing and only spoke out once when some children were getting noisy. She said, "Hush," and when they did, she said, "Thank you."

This is a story about a woman with many sides to her personality. Sometimes she is charming and sometimes not. It is a story about people who accept her as she is, and despite her moods and willful ways, genuinely like her and want her to be with them. This is not the way we typically envision the path to social acceptance. Some people might think Nancy needs to change to be acceptable. The truth is, Nancy has changed. She has been around people who treat her fairly and with respect. She is given choices and she has responded by being a more pleasant person. The key to Nancy is knowing this and perhaps changing the way we might wish her to be, to accepting her as she is. Nancy helps us all learn more about acceptance. This is her greatest contribution.

Nancy Today

Nancy no longer goes to Miller's; it closed. It is disappointing when things end, for whatever reason. Staff want to see lifelong, committed relationships grow, but a lot of relationships are more casual and often they do not last forever. This, too, is part of the reality of community-building work. People are challenged to appreciate and to keep building all types of relationships as they ebb and flow over the natural course of life.

Nancy does still help out at Western Day Care Center. She has been there for 6 years, since 1986. She went to Western without staff support for several years. However, she was involved in a specific incident and the director of the daycare decided that Nancy needed more support than they could provide on their own. Options then sent a staff person back to Western to support Nancy. This support will continue until the people at Western again feel that they themselves can provide the support Nancy needs.

Such reconnection is not unusual. Staff support is removed and community support of individuals is requested whenever possible. However, it is important to continue to support by stopping by and seeing how things are going (even if day-to-day staff support is not needed). It is not over when the staff person leaves. In a number of situations it has been necessary for staff to return to day-to-day support. The person may go through a difficult time or the place may go through a difficult time. Whatever the reason, it is important to be flexible and to be able to offer support when it is needed.

JOHN

John lives at home with his family in Louisville. Staff have had a hard time getting John involved with other people. It is hard to know what John likes and he does not seem to respond much to people. He keeps his fingers in his ears a lot, like he does not want to hear. He likes to roll his wheelchair, wave his arms, and yell loudly. I guess for him it is an expression of freedom. But he is loud, and in public places it can be embarrassing. The truth is, he probably will not stop. Staff have learned that people can become tolerant of much of this type of behavior if they grow accustomed to it and understand. The alternative is that John does not go anywhere because he might yell out, but that does not seem either fair or right.

John is a free spirit. When no one is watching, he will go in the bathroom and squirt water, open lotion bottles and dump them. He will flick your lights off waiting for a reaction, and if you do not give one, he will flick them back on and roll away.

John has a knowing look—a way of looking at a person that appears as though he understands precisely what is going on but chooses not to participate. He loves freedom. If he starts to roll away in his wheelchair and no one goes after him, he looks back and starts rolling faster and faster. We have often wondered what he would do if we could allow him his freedom.

Once when he was sitting with Carol (a staff member) and she asked someone his name, John was heard to say, "John Jones." John does not talk.

One afternoon John and I went out. It was raining when I got out of the car to get his wheelchair. As I got to his door, he reached over and locked the door. I pecked on the window and said, "Open the door, John," but he looked straight ahead as if nothing was happening. I banged and yelled, "Open the door." He turned and looked at me as if to say, "Do you have a problem, lady?" That is John. He does his thing and most of the time his thing is not the thing you wish him to do.

John has two places he goes. One is Smith's Food Service in his neighborhood. We chose it because it is big and open and people hang around the trucks and talk. It is a place he can yell and people are not bothered. He helps by breaking down boxes. He also goes to United Sporting Goods—a stable place chosen because John likes stores with aisles where he can wheel around and look at things. He likes to try on hats. He helps at the store by stuffing gym bags with paper. He is supported by staff in both places. What he does in both of these places is not very interesting or meaningful to him, but it gives him a reason to be there regularly and provides him with the opportunity to be with people.

Until recently, however, the people were not really connected with John in either place. The people spoke to him, but that was about all. They usually did not come too close to him. Bernie and David (staff members) say it is hard for them, too. It is easier to bury themselves in tasks and say,"Come on, John, here's another box." It is more difficult to engage in conversations and draw John in. So, they stand back and ask, why are we doing this? Perhaps the answer is that people need each other. It is as true for John as it is for anyone. It is important that he has people in his life who know him and like him. How this is expressed is individually determined, but the possibility exists that they might do what people typically do for each other—stop by, ask how things are going, spend a few minutes, ask a few questions, take an interest in his life, remember him on special occasions, and miss him if he does not come. Small things such as these are important for everyone.

On John's birthday, he took a cake to Smith's to celebrate. People stopped by and wished him happy birthday. At United, they gathered to share his cake and they sang happy birthday. They asked where he lived, how he spent his time, and other questions. They took an interest in him for the first time. David told John's mom and it really made her happy. She said when the Smith's trucks go by, the men always wave at John on the porch—a simple thing that matters so much.

John Today

John no longer goes to United. He did not seem interested in the place. He no longer wanted to stuff gym bags. Furthermore, it seemed that the people at United were taking a little but not really much of an interest in him. When supporting community building, making a decision to stop going is never easy. John does not say, "I don't like this any more." He tells us in much more subtle ways. Having a relationship with John is necessary to knowing what he is trying to communicate.

These realities can be painful to face. Staff ask themselves if there is anything more they can do, but ultimately, they have to accept that they cannot force relationships. They can open the possibility, try to influence what happens (without interfering too much), but over time they have to look at what has happened and ask, "What is John getting out of this? What are the people at United getting out of this?"

John still goes to Smith's. He has been going for about 5 years. He no longer breaks down boxes by hand. He puts them in an automatic box smasher and pushes the button. (Automation calls us all to change.) He is still supported by staff and he has become acquainted with five or six people in casual ways. The staff believe that he has definitely made a place for himself.

RON

The last story is about Ron. Ron lives at home with his parents in Louisville. This story is taken from the journal I kept during the

3 years I worked at Options. Various days over the course of the 3 years are described.

•••

I went to French Pantry today to see Ron. This place is wonderful. It is a bakery and seems European in atmosphere. Yvette is a waitress who is French. Her English is broken. She says, "Bonjour," "Merci," "Au revoir." She obviously likes Ron. He watches her and smiles. She gets right in his face and enthusiastically talks to him. She told Joy (a staff person who accompanies Ron) once that Ron made her happy.

Another waitress came in and waved at Ron, then came over and greeted him. Said she saw him last week with a man, asked if he lived nearby. . . . A man rode by on a bike and Joy said they always talked to him.

The man at the fruit market across the street was really nice, too. He was a little uptight when they first started going in, but now he is warm and knows Ron by name.

Ron ate a tart and drank a cup of coffee (with Joy's assistance). He did seem glad to be there. I can see as I've seen so many times, this is going to be beautiful. It's always unique. Sometimes people come together in a quiet way and sometimes with a band playing. Ron is so full. But it's the people at the Pantry I notice. They are so pleased to know Ron.

Ron dresses very nicely. He wears a buzz hair cut and he is very pale because he doesn't get out much. He uses a wheelchair to get around. He needs assistance to do almost everything. He bites up and down and shakes his head back and forth most of the time. But he does look when something is interesting and he watches people.

I saw an image of Ron or people like Ron sitting on a ward at Wedgewood (a state institution) or sitting in a classroom or activity center doing the same thing. The difference is what is around him now. Here he is surrounded by other people in a nice place and some of the people look forward to seeing him, give him attention and are learning a little bit about one man with disabilities. They bring quality to his life.

•••

Joy said French Pantry was great for Ron. They ate a croissant. The people were nice and friendly and Ron loved it. Then she told about all the places they went. The things Ron saw and touched and smelled and how responsive he is. But no wonder, he has never done anything like this.

Joy said maybe his mother could meet them for coffee some morning. And we agreed that would be a good thing to work toward. Imagine having this woman who has rarely been in public situations with her son, who is uncomfortable with the thought—going into a little bakery where people say, "Hi Ron," and show that they like him for who he is. Imagine how she would feel.

• • •

When Joy talks about Ron's morning in his neighborhood, it's a series of one merchant after the other coming to know who Ron is and enjoying his presence. "There's Ron." "You're out for a walk again." "How are you Ron?" "How's your friend?" This is so nice for Ron and he smiles in anticipation of his croissant at French Pantry.

• • •

Joy said Ron is so alert on their neighborhood outing. He looks around and actually laughs out loud and when they go into French Pantry, the French waitress runs over saying, "Ron-Ron."

• • •

I went to see Joy at French Pantry with Ron. She's had a lot of illness in her family and I was asking how her mom was doing. She said the longer she lives she realizes that all we have is today and we need to learn how to live it. She said being with Ron reminds her of that because he enjoys his day so much. She said, "I almost envy him. He gets more out of life than most."

• • •

I went to see Ron at French Pantry. He sits with his head back and shakes it around and every time he looks at Yvette she smiles and talks to him and he smiles at her. The other waitress touches him each time she passes. Nobody looks at him like he doesn't fit. It is hard to describe how it feels to see him in the midst of it all. In these moments I know why I do this. People are hungry to give to each other in all kinds of different ways.

• • •

Joy said on Ron's birthday the waitresses sang happy birthday and gave him champagne and orange juice. Ron had a mimosa. And every time I tell it, people just smile. Ron loved it.

• • •

David (a new staff person) went with Ron to French Pantry. He said people stepped in and told him what Ron likes and interpreted Ron's actions to David. This is so great to see.

• • •

We asked the people at French Pantry what they thought other customers thought about Ron. One of the waitresses said, "Perhaps they
see him as one of the Wednesday morning regulars." Ron is a regular.

Ron Today

Ron still goes to French Pantry. He has been a regular for 7 years, since
1985. One waitress who left several years ago maintains contact with
Ron through cards, and a gift at Christmas. Ron's life is enriched by
his relationships at French Pantry. What people cannot always know
for sure, but can sometimes catch a glimpse of, is how much the lives
of customers and employees of French Pantry have been enriched
by Ron.

CONCLUSION

When I think of the last 8 years, I feel like I have had a romance with
community building. I am thinking of an analogy to romantic love—
when you find the magical person, everything around you suddenly
has meaning. Over time, however, you start to see the flaws. Eventually, you come to a crossroads and you either leave because it is not
perfect, or, you start the hard work of real love. In community-building work, people must see beyond the human flaws and still find the
magic.

This has been a powerful lesson for me. One cannot pretend that
the flaws, difficulties, and disappointments do not exist and that it is
all perfect in community. People can always choose to end the stories
about relationships in community life before the part of the story
when things get difficult or fall apart. Or, they can avoid telling these
kinds of stories altogether. But, it is important that they tell whole
and real stories. The strength of honesty must be built upon. Commitments to do community-building work have to be made out of a
deeper understanding of the way it really is, not simply out of a sensa-
tion of excitement and romance.

Community building is a way to pay attention to the ordinary as
well as the spectacular. It is a way to engage and celebrate the human
experience. It is not just about "successes," it is about life. The things
that do not work can teach as much as the things that do. This work
challenges all people to learn and grow.

Relationship building is a life-long process. It is a way to know people and to be known over time. It is not an outcome to be achieved,
but an experience of life.

It is about hope. The hope is not just for people with disabilities,
but for all of us and for our communities. People are rarely challenged

to be related to those individuals who are different from them. Communities need opportunities to experience diversity in small and personal ways, have stories to tell, have images of community as a whole, create new images of contribution, believe in each other, and have hope. Communities need community-building practices to be healthy and strong.

11

Believing in a Friend

Advocating for Community Life

Joseph P. Shapiro

Some day, my friend Jim may become the first person to ever fly out of a state institution.

The flying machine is stowed away in the storage room under the cottage where he lives. The parts are hidden among the wood and wheels Jim keeps there. I tell him to show the room—a magical laboratory where he keeps his inventions and works-in-progress—to anyone who visits him and then he will be able to walk out of the institution before he has to fly out.

For Jim's 31st birthday, I helped arrange a visit by two of Jim's sisters and a brother. It was the first time anyone from his immediate family visited him at the Faribault Regional Center, the state hospital in southern Minnesota where he has lived since arriving in 1966, the week before his 7th birthday. The moment that forever changed the family's understanding of Jim came when I suggested that he take us down to that narrow concrete storage bunker, dimly lit by the sunlight that pushes through a small pigeonhole of a window just at ground level.

Jim is a wizard with tools. If given a pair of bald tires, some scrap wood, and junk metal, he will build a sophisticated go-cart. Actually, those in Jim's storage room are perfectly proportioned models of Grand Prix Formula One racers, with sleek lines, steering mechanisms, and real tires bolted to axles.

But most wondrous of all is Jim's graceful flying machine. An aide in the household where Jim lives once showed him a picture from the *National Geographic* of the Gossamer Condor, the bicycle-pedaled glider that had flown in 1979. Jim, from memory, was building one in the basement. There, for his family, Jim pulled out the magnificent 10-foot wingspan of light cardboard, girded by a wire frame to hold the sail. His sister picked up the bicycle pedal he had enclosed in a wooden frame and Jim explained that he needed to find a way to make it lighter. He kept his right hand tucked in his pocket and pointed with his left, as if he were a college professor speaking from a lectern in the Science Hall auditorium.

I watched the stunned looks on the faces of his siblings and his Aunt Evelyn, who also came. "Jimmy, can you fix that bicycle?" asked his brother, pointing to a broken one in a corner. Only several weeks before, when Jim's aunt convinced the two sisters to meet Jim on one of the institution's outings to Minneapolis, the sisters had told aides they expected Jim to be a "vegetable." That was an entirely reasonable expectation, given general public perceptions of retardation and the fact that officials at the institution originally told Jim's family that he was "profoundly retarded" and had an IQ of less than 30. But now Jim's siblings were trying to figure out if he could work in a bicycle repair shop. It was an entirely correct way to be thinking about him.

I am a journalist. In 1990, I took a fellowship and a year's sabbatical from my job at *U.S. News & World Report* in Washington to write about disability rights issues. In the course of my reporting I was impressed by community living programs, supported employment, and self-advocacy by people with mental retardation. My thoughts had turned back to Jim. It had been 16 years, since 1974, that I had last seen him. I was a student at Carleton College in Northfield, Minnesota. Jim, then 14, lived at what was then called the Faribault State Hospital for the Mentally Retarded. Jim was on a list to get out. He would live either with a foster family or in a group home.

With a dozen friends, I had started a transition program for Jim and others like him at Faribault. The thinking was that before Jim left the institution he needed to know what it meant to live in a house. He needed to eat family style around a dinner table, instead of a noisy cafeteria. He needed to sleep in his own room, instead of in a barracks with 3 dozen beds in a row. So, my friends and I got the college to give us an old, rambling three-story Victorian home. We each "adopted" one kid from Faribault and, shuttling to Faribault and back in a donated turquoise Cadillac with hightail fins, we brought them for overnight visits. One might say we figured that a house full of college students was a close approximation of a group home. Only the college students, of course, acted out more and exhibited more bad behaviors that needed correcting.

In the course of my writing, I thought about how public attitudes had become so much more generous in 16 years and I wondered if the promise of living in the community had been kept to Jim. Did he have a job? His own apartment? Maybe even a wife. I knew all this was possible.

I started my search for Jim by calling directory assistance in Minneapolis and asking for his telephone number. But the quest ended back at the institution, on the same wing of the same cottage where he lived 16 years before. Jim never left Faribault.

Before flying out to Minnesota to see him, I thought about the last time Jim and I were together. Jim was fascinated by wheels. He always carried one, along with toy cars, in his pockets. On his last visit to our house, 16 years before, Jim brought an Erector Set kit to build a go-cart big enough to ride. I, along with my housemates, puzzled over the complicated instructions. Between us there were Phi Beta Kappas, National Merit finalists, and magna cum laudes. Yet, we could not figure out which bolts screwed into what metal plate to keep the cart sturdy. After waiting patiently for us for well over an hour, Jim tired of our ineptitude. He threw a small tantrum. We had tried our best, I explained to him. Then I left him on the porch to cool down. When I came back a few minutes later, Jim was sitting on the go-cart he had assembled correctly by himself.

When Jim and I were reunited in August 1990, he was still fascinated by cars. He still carried a wheel, a model car, or something round, sometimes a Frisbee, with him. We went to the County Fair. We rode the bumper cars. Somehow, Jim knew how to drive and was skillful at speeding around the rink, avoiding being hit. We sat in the grandstand at the track and watched the sprint car races. We went to the movies to see Tom Cruise as a race car driver in *Days of Thunder*.

No label fit Jim. The institution called him "moderately retarded." This supposedly was a generous reprieve from Faribault's initial and long-lingering diagnosis: "profoundly retarded." When Jim was admitted to the institution in 1966, the testing child psychiatrist concluded, "The final diagnosis was mental deficiency, idiopathic severe." The IQ score under 30, although discredited, has been passed along through the years and remains a permanent mark on his records. Perhaps no one illustrates better than Jim why labeling people by "levels" of retardation is not only misleading and undignified, but dangerous as well.

A better description of Jim is that he is sometimes brilliant. He is mechanically gifted, perhaps even a mechanical savant. Similar to many other left-handed people, Jim has a sharp spatial memory. It is true that he is not very verbal. That would explain why he would have fared so poorly on an IQ test in 1966. But Jim is highly inquisitive and very curious. One expert who has spent time with Jim says that, if tested today, he might be considered simply to have a "severe learning disability." Jim understands what goes on around him, even if he does not always acknowledge it verbally. When I told him I wanted to write about him in a book, Jim's response was neutral and vague. "A book," he repeated, and that was it. But on my next visit to the institution, he greeted me holding a "present" in a crumpled brown paper bag: it was two notepads, like the ones he had seen me write in. Most of all, Jim is an engaging man—quick to smile; warm around others (except, seemingly, his peers at the institution, from whom he kept his distance), instantly likeable, and fun to be around.

Staffers at the institution described him differently. Instead of celebrating his strengths, they seemed to harp on shortcomings that needed fixing. They complained, for example, about his occasional flashes of temper or bad moods. It is true that Jim sometimes seems to chafe under the restrictions of the institution. He seems to understand that he does not belong there. Everything Jim does at Faribault is regulated. When he wakes up he is handed his "token recording sheet" for the day. When he completes a listed task, such as getting dressed, shaving, or making his bed neatly, in what is called a "complete" and "compliant" way he gets a smiley face or a check on his token sheet. These are counted toward privileges such as getting sodas or spending free time in the woodshop. As a condition for continued use of his storage space, for example, Jim has to keep his basement area neat. The agreement specifies that he has to sweep the area each week and keep no more than 12 tires and 4 bike frames there at any time (although the household staff thought the contract was stricter and let him keep only half as many). At a weekly inspection, a staffer is to find "no dirt or debris on the floor."

Despite near constant grumbling from the household staff, anytime I saw Jim's storage area, it was impeccably tidy. He even figured out how to cover the basement drain with heavy electrical tape so that after heavy rains water would not back up into the small room and soak his projects. Looking at the small, clean room, I realized I would not fare nearly so well if counselors and social workers paraded through my home each week to see that I had dusted properly and not kept piles of mail and paper lying around.

One of Jim's worst behaviors is said to be his "threats." Not surprisingly, these revolve around cars. When Jim gets angry he might say, "I'm going to throw rocks at your car" or "I'm going to take the wheels off your car." This is just the way Jim curses. But, threats or curses, they are duly noted in Jim's "daily progress notes." One of my favorites came from the counselor whose simple entry stated: "Ate breakfast with Jim. Threatened to take the wheels off my car. Called it rusty, an accurate statement." Jim's counselors could proudly tell me how many of these so-called threats he had made. There were nine in March, then 52 in April, and only three in May. But nobody could tell me what it was that had bothered Jim so much in April. Nobody had even tried to figure it out.

Jim's mechanical skills won him a reputation around the Faribault campus, but it was a negative one. There was one particular incident that led to intense monitoring of Jim's behavior. One evening, when a Faribault social worker backed her pick-up truck out of the parking lot, one of the rear wheels fell off. Jim had been angry with the woman and he had been seen in the parking lot. And only Jim, it was assumed, could figure out how to loosen the wheel on a pick-up truck. He was forced to make restitution out of his monthly paycheck for damages to the truck. For the following year, he was placed on 24-hour restriction if he left the cottage without notifying anyone, or for other infractions.

One result of the pick-up truck incident was that whenever someone saw what appeared to be new damage to their car, Jim got blamed. Charges were made against him in one incident, but dropped when an investigation made it clear that Jim could not have been involved.

Similarly, if a workman misplaced a tool, it was often concluded that Jim had stolen it. It was assumed that Jim then hid these tools in the woods surrounding the institution. Aides had somewhat hazy recollections of Jim returning tools when asked or, on one occasion, being found wearing a workman's boots (Jim's own shoes always seemed to have holes in them). But there were no reports in the "daily progress notes" of any such incidents over the previous 2 years. On the other hand, I did know that many things were stolen from Jim over the years. He had to obtain a locked storage room and a key to his own closet in the bedroom he shared with three other men. When I would send Jim something—photos from a recent visit, a wheel, or a tool—I would call and ask if he received it. "I've still got it," was Jim's inevitable reply. Property, to this man who grew up with little privacy, was something that was passing and temporary. I heard so much about Jim's alleged stealing that, concerned, I approached Ben Weeks, the man who ran the woodshop. The reports, he said, were exaggerated. He had never known Jim to steal tools.

Weeks also added that although most people on campus assumed that he had shown Jim how to put together the go-carts and various inventions, Jim made these things by himself. Later, Jim's job coach on the lawn crew at the institution said she assumed that I, as a college student, had taught Jim how to use tools. Yet, my idea of a home improvement project is screwing in a light bulb. If Jim's mechanical skills seemed to cause mischief, then it was assumed he acted on his own. But if he used those skills to do something creative and useful, it was assumed he had needed help.

For years, Jim saw his friends and peers leave the institution to go to this mythical place called "the community." But he had little idea of where it was or what it meant to live there, beyond the trips he had taken to the house I started at Carleton. On my first trip back to Minnesota I took Jim to see group homes and community work sites. Staffers from an innovative supported work program called Opportunity Services took us to a restaurant and a factory where they placed workers. And, of course, they took us to an auto body shop. In the back room, where the new tires were stored, Jim was in heaven. He bent over to touch the tires. He petted them, as if he were petting a dog. He breathed in the smell of new rubber, he thumped the sidewalls to hear the deep, full echo from within. The next day, I told the cottage social worker about Jim's thrill at being in an auto body shop. The social worker had one reaction: "Did Jimmy steal anything?"

But nothing more underscored the negative view of Jim than all the excuses that officials came up with for keeping Jim at Faribault. He could not live in a group home, this social worker explained, because there would be no place to keep all his tires and wood. (When, concerned, I expressed these objections to Nancy Gurney of Opportunity Services, she laughed: "That's easy to solve. We can buy him a $100 tool shed from Sears.") If he lived in the city, his Minneapolis-based social worker said, people would take advantage of him and talk him into wrongdoing. For these two social workers, if there was anyone seen as failing more than Jim, it was his family. As people at the institution saw it, Jim's parents gave him up and did not care enough to keep in touch; the institution was there to help him.

When I got Jim's records, I learned much more about Jim and his family. (Getting the records took every ounce of my reporter's skills. When I got to Minneapolis, the home county caseworker who had promised me the files reneged at the last moment. But I had already planned for such a disaster by trying to figure out how the system, and any avenues for appeal, worked. Kay Hendrikson, the sympathetic public guardian for wards of the state, gave me crucial standing as an "official friend.") Jim came from a large family. He was the middle of nine children, all closely spaced together. The parents, an anonymous caseworker wrote decades before on a mimeographed sheet I found, were "inadequate or ineffectual," intermittently employed, and struggling to care for their large family. By the time Jim was 2 years old, it was clear that he was different. As soon as he could walk, I was told, he would find his way down the steps into the basement where he would unscrew the wheels and knobs on the furnace.

At age 3, I later learned, his mother found him under the kitchen sink trying to detach the drain pipe. At age 4, he began running away from home. When, at age 6, he darted into traffic, getting hit by a car, social workers came and removed him from the family.

I debated whether to call Jim's family. If involved again, they could, after all these years, prefer that Jim stay out-of-sight and out-of-mind in the institution. And, even though they had long ago given up guardianship, their wishes, by state law, could derail my attempts to get Jim into his own apartment. But I knew, most of all, that Jim missed his family. At the end of my first visit, I told Jim I was leaving to go to Minneapolis, where I would catch my flight back to Washington. "Minneapolis," Jim said in his short staccato way of speaking. "My mother. Five or six years." I knew what these cryptic fragments meant: His mother lived in Minneapolis and it had been, he was precisely correct, 5½ years since he saw her last. That, the Minneapolis case manager told me, was a rare 20-minute holiday visit when Jim, as the case manager put it, "ripped up the house." More precisely, the case worker revealed when asked, Jim was alleged to have pulled down a curtain in the living room. The visit to the mother's house was disastrous, the case manager claimed, and, as a result, the mother cut off contact and asked for no more visits.

But I did call the family. I started with Jim's Aunt Evelyn who, I knew, sent cards and then reestablished contact with Jim 3 months before I did by coming to Faribault to visit on Family Day. It was her first trip to the institution and she was impressed, finding it a much more pleasant place than she expected. From Evelyn, a kind and loving woman who treated her nieces and nephews like the children she never had, I got a different picture of Jim's parents. Jim's mother was not so much neglectful or a bad parent, but overwhelmed. She felt guilt and embarrassment over the loss of her son. Jim's parents found that their family had grown too big, too fast. There was no child care and little money, nor was there a social services system offering any other help beyond institutionalization of Jim. Even after Jim's accident and costly hospitalization, his parents did not want him taken away. But social workers insisted it was for the best and removed him briefly to a boarding home before sending him to Faribault.

The family, as much as Jim, were considered failures. Their son was taken away and they were deemed unfit parents by a dizzying parade of doctors, child psychologists, social workers, and a courtroom judge.

I also learned from Evelyn that Jim's family shared his love of wheels and cars. The oldest brother was a mechanic with his own auto body shop. The oldest daughter was a bus driver. Another brother was an engineer. And then Evelyn mentioned that seeing Jim, clutching his orange Frisbee, reminded her so much of Jim's Uncle Fortune. "You've heard about his Uncle Fortune, of course," she said. I confessed that I had not. "Oh, Jim's Uncle Fortune," she declared. "He won a medal in the Olympics. He was a discus thrower."

So on my second trip to Minnesota, on Jim's birthday weekend in October, I drove Evelyn back to Faribault to see Jim again. And, at her suggestion, I readily invited his sisters Peggy and Julie and brother Rob to come down, too. The trip to the dingy storage room forever changed their view of Jim.

Harder, perhaps, was to get people at the institution to see Jim in a new way. Clearly, they felt they provided Jim with a caring environment. It was one, they argued, that would be hard to match in the community. He had acres of woods on campus that he loved to explore, sometimes on the bicycle he bought with the money from his job on the lawn crew. He had his storage room and, until a few months before our reunion when it was moved off campus, access to a woodshop.

The cottage Jim lived in had a reputation for being one of the most pleasant on campus. It was a place where, coming back one night from one of our outings, a staffer was waiting with gooey Rice Krispie bars she had made. It was a place that the aides had tried to make feel a little less institutional by stenciling the cinderblock walls with a trim of ducks and cattails. But I felt Jim deserved the chance to be part of the community. He told me he wanted to live in a group home. He had been telling the staffers in his cottage, for many years, that he thought he wanted to try one. Also, a medium-security state prison was now taking over many of the buildings on campus. The barbed wire around the prison buildings could be seen beyond Jim's window. Eventually, the institution would be downsized from some 500 residents to less than 100. Jim was almost certain to leave at some point, but it might not be for another decade.

My task was to build a consensus that it was time for Jim to leave. Like any investigative reporter, I set out to learn everything I could about the system: Who controlled it, who could push it, what made it work, what made it fail, what programs were available, why they were used, or why they were resisted. I made scores of phone calls, to any expert I could find, inside the system or outside, asking how they would approach getting Jim into his own apartment. At the invitation of Colleen Wieck, the director of the Minnesota Governor's Planning Council on Developmental Disabilities, who would prove an invaluable guide through the state system, I attended a session of "Partners in Policymaking." The program brought together parents of young children with disabilities, and sometimes the older children themselves, in self-empowerment training so that they could confidently advocate for their needs when dealing with politicians and government officials. These activist parents urged me not to settle for second best for Jim.

It was the director of the Partners program, David Hancox, who told me how families in Minnesota were now successfully using a process called "Personal Futures Planning" to help people with mental retardation set long-term goals. The Personal Futures Planning team I put together included more than a dozen people. Besides Jim and me, there were staffers from Faribault, the state ombudsman's office, service providers, Jim's social worker, state officials, a self-advocate, and members of Jim's family. The point was to build a group of friends who not only cared about Jim, but who had the knowledge and ties to get the system to work for him.

The Futures Planning team would plan for his future by putting Jim—his wants, his needs, his desires—first. It was for these meetings that I returned in October 1990. But the first session, held on Jim's birthday and the day after the visit from his family, went poorly. I had invited only a few people from the institution, the ones who I felt were caring and who would be positive. Instead, Jim's whole social services team showed up. Instead of being a friendly, personal session, it turned into one of the impersonal annual reviews that Jim had come to hate because he knew it was a yearly exercise in listing his shortcomings. "I hate meetings," Jim told me. This was supposed to have been different. I had even picked a neutral site in the oak-paneled coference room at the 19th century vintage Faribault City Hall.

Marijo McBride, of the University of Minnesota's Institute on Community Integration, had agreed to be our facilitator. She opened by reconstructing Jim's history, taking notes on poster paper set on an easel. A stick figure, representing Jim, was drawn in the center. Others who knew him—service providers, family, friends—were drawn into the circle at varying distances from the center, depending on how close they were to Jim.

But things began to degenerate when the cottage psychologist started talking about how Jim had a mean temper. McBride noted that Jim seemed extremely sociable. "When you wear one of his tires around your neck, you don't think of him as very sociable," the psychologist responded, speaking generally and of no specific incident. Another staffer said Jim would steal tools or other things needed for his inventions. And the psychologist added that Jim was a "pack rat" and therefore unsuited for living in a place of his own. "A gymnasium might last a week," the psychologist pronounced. "He'd fill it."

Throughout this wild fault-finding, Jim appeared not to be listening. He sat in the middle of one of the four long conference tables that was joined together in a large square and played with a small metal toy car. But after a while he looked up and glowered at Deb Lenway, the counselor who knows Jim best and who was his strongest champion at Faribault. Her offense, apparently, was that it had fallen upon her to get Jim, always suspicious of a meeting, into her car and bring him to the session. "You're dead, Deb," he muttered angrily, "I'm going to break your car." He continued expressing his displeasure, speaking almost under his breath, and shooting withering glances at Lenway.

I was forced to hustle Jim out of the room and back to the institution. "I don't go meetings anymore," he said petulantly in the car. "I hate meetings. Meetings are boring." I cursed myself, fearful that my efforts to help were about to collapse in hurt, anger, and recrimination. I worried that I had betrayed Jim. But I was particularly fearful that Jim had made a bad first impression on his new case worker.

I was disappointed that Jim's previous social worker of several years had taken no steps to get Jim out of Faribault. He denied me access to Jim's records. When I got them I understood why: Jim's individualized service plan, although required annually by law, had not been completed in several years. Nor had the screening been completed that was required before Jim could be considered to move into his own apartment. When I returned home to Washington from my first trip back to Faribault in August, I formally requested that this planning be carried out. I asked that Jim's home county apply for a special "enhanced waiver," a one-time only offer of money to relocate people from Faribault. When the county balked at using the waiver, I took it upon myself to track down the state director of the program, Alexandra Henry, and get the answers that would satisfy the concerns of the county officials.

I realized that the social worker had an expanding caseload and, perhaps with no one pushing for Jim, it was easy to let Jim's needs drop to the bottom of his list. Because he claimed he was too busy to complete them, I requested the assignment of a new social worker. Again, I would not have even thought of asking for a new caseworker. But, in all my phone calling, a state worker advised me it was a right that existed for Jim. This request would prove to be a crucial turning point for Jim.

Within weeks, a new social worker was assigned to Jim's case.

I liked Steven Schmit immediately. He was young, energetic, and creative. He was intrigued by my stories of Jim and by what he read in Jim's file. Unlike Jim's previous social worker, he did not insist that Jim could not make it outside the institution. In fact, Jim, he told me over the phone, should be out of Faribault.

So I worried that Jim's outburst, at the first meeting with his new social worker, would alter Schmit's generous thinking about him. There was no need for concern. Schmit was experienced enough to understand, just as I had, that Jim was only responding to the unfair criticisms that he was hearing.

Things seemed to work out better once I rejoined the group for the last hour of the meeting. McBride did a good job of keeping things positive. Together, the group seemed to take a good first step toward identifying Jim's preferences and setting goals for him. Among the goals were to accelerate family contacts; help Jim continue to develop his mechanical skills; eventually move him into the community and find a job for him, perhaps in a bike shop, an auto body shop, or a junkyard; and get Jim into a house or apartment of his own.

Things went even better at our second meeting, which was held 2 days later in St. Paul so that family members could attend. The new location had the unintentional effect of keeping down the number of participants from Faribault to the few supporters of Jim I had wanted in the first place. Jim was excited to see his aunt, sister Peggy and, at the end of the meeting, another brother, Dennis.

I also asked Irving Martin to be there. He is a self-advocate, active in People First of Minnesota. A large man, with a loud, hearty laugh and genteel manners, Martin had recently been in Washington, where I first met him, to witness President Bush sign the Americans with Disabilities Act. Martin worked at the dietary center of a nursing home, helping to prepare and distribute food. Everyday after work he went to Mickey's Diner, what he affectionately called a "high class greasy spoon," for an afternoon cup of coffee and to talk politics and current affairs with the restaurant's regulars. But what Martin called the "highlight of my life" was being able to address the congregation of his church, explaining to them what it meant to have mental retardation.

It was Martin's common sense and wisdom that again changed Jim's family's definition of retardation. At the first planning meeting, the cottage psychologist had claimed that if Jim were to live outside the institution there was a good chance of his getting into trouble stealing and possibly "ending up in jail." But at the second meeting, Martin rose to say it was important to let Jim learn from his own mistakes, and that he was sure to grow once he left the institution. "I myself am retarded," Martin said to preface his remarks. "My way of thinking is that you take one step at a time. If he takes one step at a time, with lots of room for mistakes, he'll be okay. There is not one person in this room who has not made mistakes in their life, and why can't he? People learn from their mistakes."

Things seemed to go more smoothly at the second session. It was here, after Martin's words, that the team began to talk about Jim leaving Faribault as a given, no longer as a big risk. McBride put a chart on the easel that identified "Desirable Images of the Future." We agreed to keep building on Jim's reconnections to his family and that Jim should be encouraged to make other friends, find a job that reflected his mechanical ability, and have access to a woodshop. Somehow, almost imperceptibly, the session reached a new level. Jim won supporters, instead of having doubters. The group process, despite my initial doubts, truly worked. It was positive and upbeat. At its core was an unshakeable agenda of putting Jim's needs first. McBride skillfully prevented the sessions from becoming an explicit indictment of anyone. That allowed the Faribault staffers to become less defensive. The presence of family, when no family had been around before, added substantial weight to this new direction of building a circle of support for Jim in the community. Jim seemed to catch the shift in mood, too. He was no longer bored or angry, and became involved in the discussion. At one point, McBride asked Jim what he would like in his house. "How about a cat in the house?" Jim asked in his slow, soft voice. He, too, began to feel empowered.

I was anxious to watch the growth that would come with choice and independence. The night between the two Personal Futures meetings, Jim and I went to Owatonna, a town 15 miles away from Faribault. We went shopping. That meant going to auto parts shops, tire stores, and farm implement dealers. We looked at car tires, tractor tires, motorcycle tires, and all-terrain vehicle tires. For dinner, we ate hamburgers and cherry Cokes at Costa's Chocolate Shop, sitting on orange vinyl benches at a booth in the back, past the glass display counters of handmade chocolates. Across the street was a bank building designed by architect Louis Sullivan, with a large arching doorway. It was the type of beautiful architectural detail that one often stumbles across in otherwise plain Minnesota towns.

At dinner, Jim mentioned that Robin, a woman who had lived at Faribault, now resided in Owatonna. The first time I heard of Robin was at the first Personal Futures meeting. She was listed as one of Jim's friends—the closest thing he had to a girlfriend. "Jim, if we can find Robin, would you like to visit her after dinner?" I asked. "Yes," he said smiling. At an outside phone booth, while the sun was going down and a swirling wind sent the temperature plummeting, I buttoned up my coat and fed quarters into the phone booth in search of Robin. I did not know even her last name. But I put my reporter's skills to work and a half hour later we were at the front door to Robin's group home.

It was clearly a "girl's" apartment, a nice four-bedroom apartment for Robin and her roommates, decorated in pinks and sky blues, with straw bonnets and dried flowers on the walls. There were yellow stencils of a woman in a bonnet with a goose on the wallpaper. A large television sat against the wall in a small living room that also doubled as a kitchen and dining area. When we walked in, I could not figure out if Robin was present. Four women said hello, but no one made any special greeting. Jim kept close to my side. "Is Robin here?" I asked out loud. One of the women, with a pleasant, round face, short hair, and pretty eyes, wearing a blue sweatshirt with a goose printed on it, raised her head and smiled.

Jim and Robin sat on a loveseat while the rest of us watched a TV movie. Robin placed an orange plastic bowl of popcorn between her and Jim. At first they made only halting, awkwardly shy conversation. But soon Jim was talking away—talking more and faster, it occurred to me, than I had ever heard him talk to anyone. From time to time, Robin would excuse herself to take a trip to her bedroom. She would come back with something to show Jim: a new coffee pot she had bought, a new pair of shoes from her sister. Soon Robin moved the popcorn bowl from between them. I sat in front of them. But occasionally I would turn around. Jim kept an eye trained on me. But from my stolen glances I could see that, when he thought I was not looking, he would timidly run a finger along Robin's knee.

I wondered if the staffers at Faribault would be annoyed with me. But I figured Jim, at 31, was old enough to be "dating," or whatever this was.

After seeing Jim at Faribault and at the Personal Futures meeting, Jim's sisters and brothers talked excitedly to their mother about their talented brother. She sent word that she wanted Jim to visit for Thanksgiving. Evelyn sent a letter to the institution asking that arrangements be made, as was routinely done, to drive Jim to the Twin Cities.

On Thanksgiving morning, Jim's mother baked two apple pies for her son. Dinner started, but Jim never arrived. Later, staff at the institution would apologize to the disappointed family. Evelyn's letter had gotten lost, they said, and they were unaware of the family's desire to see Jim. But I knew that this excuse was untrue. I had made two telephone calls the week before Thanksgiving to make sure the car arrangements were made. I had gotten a bureaucratic shrug. It was in the pipeline, I was told. I did not have the time to march Evelyn's request from person to person to make sure the car pool worked. Evelyn was too polite to do more than write her kindly letter of request.

There would be a reunion on Christmas Day. The family video shows Jim sitting quietly in a chair in his sister's living room, beaming with joy, as he watched his boisterous family kidding and exchanging presents. Jim happily soaked it all in, as if his being there for Christmas was a regular occurrence. But the kind of miscommunication and bureaucratic slow pace that had sabotaged a Thanksgiving reunion seemed to delay efforts to get Jim out of Faribault. Another year, another birthday, and another Christmas would go by and Jim was still waiting anxiously for a placement in the community. Even with a team dedicated to getting Jim out of Faribault, the system was too large and too unwieldy to be responsive, with any kind of urgency.

The plan for Jim seemed simple enough: to let him live and work in the community. A county close to Jim's family in the Twin Cities and nearby Jim's favorite mall and tire store had agreed to include Jim in a new community home to be designed for three men. There would be two staffers on hand for the three men; on weekends there would sometimes be one-to-one staffing. Jim would have a private job coach, too. That guaranteed that there would be someone to help him expand his skills using and maintaining lawn mowers, or working in a gas station, a tire store, or somewhere else of his choice.

The second of the three men for the new home was already living in that county, at home with his parents. But finding roommate number 3 proved frustratingly elusive. The search would go on for more than a year. One man was found and I was summoned back to Minneapolis to introduce Jim to his new roommates. Jim was thrilled. But then the parents of the third man got cold feet and pulled their son out. At one point, Jim had the chance to move into a six-person house. But it meant sharing a room. Over dinner one night, I explained his options. He could get out of the institution right away, but share a bedroom. Or he could wait several months longer, but be ensured of having his own bedroom for the first time in his life. This came at a time when Jim was particularly anxious to leave Faribault. He was quiet for several seconds and then told me his preference. "My own room," he said quietly.

Making his frustration bearable was the fact that Jim now had a circle of friends. McBride, Wieck, and Schmit were frequent visitors. Wieck took Jim to her family's farm in northern Minnesota for Thanksgiving. The previous spring, McBride had driven to Faribault for Family Day. The parents' luncheon speaker was a state senator who spoke passionately about the need to block any plans to close the institution. "That's my husband," the woman sitting next to Jim said proudly, leaning over him expecting to commiserate with McBride. "It's terrible that anyone would think of closing down this wonderful institution." It was at that point that Jim offered the woman his hand in a handshake and spoke up, saying publicly for the first time: "I'm moving to a group home."

Yet, our promises to Jim of "just a few more months" kept spreading out to still "a few more." Jim seemed to trust us, despite our empty words. "Tell them to hurry up," he instructed me. Midway through this process I had been at a conference where I heard Michigan advocate Gerald Provencal talk about the double-standard of time we apply to people with disabilities. "We're far more tolerant of the passage of their time than we are of our own," Provencal had noted. Just because Jim had spent a lifetime in an institution did not mean he had another year to waste. "If you're in a Club Med, time flies," said Provencal. "If you're in a day room, it is agony."

Things brightened for Jim. For the first time, he had advocates, he had a circle of friends outside the institution, and he had contact again with caring family. All these people were fighting for him. They knew the system and everyone wanted to see it work for him. And, yet, Jim was still a disposable man. His status as a man with disabilities made him a little less worthy. He was a little less of a priority to the bureaucracy that was supposed to help him. Similar to people with disabilities everywhere, he had a little less value and got a little less respect than everyone else.

EPILOGUE

Once it became fact that Jim was leaving Faribault, staff at the institution began to speak of him in a new, positive way. He was re-tested 3 months before he moved. Now the man who supposedly needed to stay at Faribault because he was "moderately mentally retarded"—and who had been labeled "profoundly mentally retarded" most of his life—was found to be "mildly mentally retarded." Even that newly generous label seemed to underestimate him. At the discharge planning meeting 2 weeks before his move, staffers at the institution told newly glowing stories about Jim's capabilities. People in town would call the institution and ask for Jim by name to mow their lawns. He was so responsible, the lawn crew job coach explained, that Jim would be left at a house with his lawnmower while the rest of the crew went to some other job. When they would return an hour or so later, Jim invariably would be sitting on the stoop wait-ing, lawnmower at his side, having done the job to perfection.

Jim left Faribault in May of 1992 and moved to an old farmhouse on 10 acres of land in the exurbs of Minneapolis. He shared the small house with two other men, but had the entire second floor to himself. Jim adjusted with great ease and happiness, as if he had always been meant to be there. Freedom for Jim meant falling asleep at night while listening to his new clock radio, his clothes still on and the overhead light brightening the room. That had been impossible in a life of three or more roommates. Freedom meant eating lunch with the men without disabilities on the work crew at the state park. No-body seemed to mind that Jim did his job, riding a small tractor and grading the softball fields, faster than the man without disabilities who had the chore before him. Freedom also meant borrowing a tool from a neighbor, then getting on his bicycle and riding a few blocks to return it. Freedom meant having a barn where he could retreat, at any time of day, to hammer and saw. The cars he built got bigger and more elaborate. But Jim left his marvelous flying machine at Faribault, per-haps for someone else to plot an escape.

12

Making It Up as We Go Along

A Story About Friendship

Jane Wells

The growing body of literature focusing on friendships among persons with and without disabilities offers hope as we struggle with the consequences of isolation. Stories of friendship between students attending the same school (Strully & Strully, 1985), of co-workers spending time together after work, and of paid staff taking action and making commitments beyond the requirements of a job description (Lutfiyya, 1990) are a source of encouragement for others seeking to build a vision of the future that includes a network of friends and people who care for each person with disabilities.

Factors that seem to have an impact on the strength of personal connections include the amount of time people spend together, the intensity of emotion that is invested in the relationship, a sense of intimacy based on trust and sharing confidences, and reciprocity (Tyne, 1988). The role that a person assumes or is given can also affect the nature of a relationship. For example, the fact that one person is the employer and another is the employee has an impact on the way they interact. Clearly defined roles can also determine ways in which people communicate, determine boundaries, and dictate authority and control.

On occasion, when a person with a disability meets with friends and family to develop a vision for the future, the dream includes living in a home of his or her own with a nondisabled roommate. Paid roommates are not uncommon in supported living services provided by human services organizations. There are also a number of examples of individuals with and without disabilities living together in intentional communities (Taylor, Bogdan, & Racino, 1991). Members of such intentional communities, which are often based on a religious ideology, describe the work they are doing as "lifesharing."

This chapter tells a story of different kinds of roommates and a different type of "lifesharing." It is a story about Mary Ann, Sue, me, our families, and our friends who are sharing life in a rather unique way. It is also a story about changing roles and redefining relationships from "advocate" to "friend," from "client" to "friend," and from "stranger" to "friend." Our experiences include working within and outside of the human services system, making commitments that require faith and risk, and learning about friendship as we "make it up as we go along."

JANE: FROM ADVOCATE TO FRIEND

Making It Legal

In the beginning, Mary Ann and I had an "arranged" relationship. I had been working with individuals with disabilities in group home settings for 10 years. When working with people every day, I did not take time to consider the nature of my relationships. Part of the job was to spend time with people. I had a "defined" involvement; my role in each person's life was related to instruction, supervision, assistance, planning, and documentation, the kinds of things that can be left at work at the end of the day. With each new job, I had good intentions of maintaining contact with the people I left behind, although I knew it would be difficult and unlikely.

In retrospect, perhaps some of the energy that might have been given to a personal relationship was channeled into volunteer involvement in advocacy organizations. I spent time talking with others about how things should be; what the local, state, and federal government should do; and how communities should respond. Although the issues that affect persons with disabilities dominated my work, not one person with a disability was a part of my life.

During a late night discussion with co-workers about how complicated our lives had become, we confronted an ethical dilemma: how does someone earn a living talking about the lives of persons with disabilities unless he or she is willing to make a personal commitment to someone who experiences a disability? I had no immediate or simple response, but continued to keep asking myself this question trying to find an answer that could work for me.

Shortly thereafter, a friend provided me with an opportunity to become personally involved. She was working for the state Arc (formerly the Association for Retarded Citizens) as an advocate, and had been contacted by a county case manager who was trying to find someone to get involved with Mary Ann, one of the individuals on his caseload. Mary Ann was going to inherit a large sum of money from her mother's estate and the case manager wanted to take advantage of what he saw as a unique opportunity. Recent discussions in Minnesota and around the country about consumer-owned housing prompted him to wonder if she could use the inheritance to buy a house. Mary Ann and I were "introduced" so that I could act as her advocate and possibly become her guardian.

We first met at the group home in which she lived, an intermediate care facility for persons with mental retardation (ICF/MR) for 12 adults. The day we met, her hair was in pigtails and I thought she was about 20 years younger than her actual age. Our first "outing" was lunch and a visit to a pet store. The first time that she spent the night at my home, I wondered what we would find to talk about and how we would fill the hours until I took her back to the group home the next afternoon. She told me at breakfast that she did not want to go back and that she would just stay with me.

Over the next year or so, we saw each other infrequently, perhaps once every 3 months. I investigated the possibility of becoming her legal representative, first just as "guardian of the person" and not "guardian of the estate." As her personal guardian, I would not be responsible for managing her assets, but would be responsible for making all other decisions about her life. I looked into ways that her estate could be managed, and it was suggested that I contact a fiduciary company that was familiar with this kind of situation. However, when I learned that the fiduciary company would take what I thought was a high percentage of her assets as a fee for managing them, I knew that her money could be spent for things more important to her. It seemed to me that whoever would be responsible for spending her inheritance should not only know about money, but more importantly, should know Mary Ann. I decided that I was willing to become her substitute decision-maker for all aspects of her life, including financial decisions, and decided to pursue becoming her guardian.

I talked to Mary Ann about what it might mean if I were her guardian and asked her if she wanted me to help her in this way. We talked about the death of her mother (whom she never really knew because she was institutionalized as a young child), and what it might mean to have money to buy a house. We made slow but steady progress through the legal system, and in the summer of 1987, we went to court. After the proceedings during which I was appointed Mary Ann's conservator, she gave me a hug and said, "Now you can keep me." My first role, as a legal representative appointed and approved by the court, was now well defined. My relationship with Mary Ann, as someone who would "keep" her, was just beginning.

Rethinking Personal Advocacy

At the time, my understanding of advocacy was completely rooted in the service system. I knew the system inside and out and was willing to use my personal contacts to secure the services to which Mary Ann was entitled. I applied for her participation in Minnesota's Title XIX Medicaid waiver program with the hope that Mary Ann could live in a "supported living arrangement" with two other women with mental retardation who had similar needs. I thought that she could use her inheritance to buy a house and protect her assets. My vision for her future was, in some ways, her very own small group home purchased with her inheritance, yet controlled by the service system.

Fortunately, this dream never became a reality. She did not get a "waiver slot." Instead, Mary Ann moved into an apartment with a woman her own age who does not have a disability and she began to teach us what it truly means to support someone in the community. From an advocate's perspective, I wanted Mary Ann to get everything that she was entitled to receive. As a friend, I learned to support Mary Ann as she discovered what it is that she really wants.

Challenging the System

Early on in my involvement with Mary Ann's "service life," I became increasingly dissatisfied with her day program. I had a thorough knowledge of the requirements of the state rule on case management and I knew that one way to advocate for changes in her day program was to refuse to sign the individualized service plan, which authorized services. I returned the service plan to the case manager unsigned with a detailed letter that demonstrated my knowledge of the rule requirements. As an advocate, I had been taught that writing letters and quoting state rules were supposed to bring results.

However, by refusing to sign the service plan, I jeopardized a very good working relationship with the case manager who was responsible for bringing us together initially. Using the formal methods to express my dissatisfaction, I put at risk an important personal relationship. Fortunately, the case manager and I were able to come to an agreement without much difficulty, but I soon began to question my advocacy methods. Getting along with people so that we could work together to get things done became more important than being right. I began to understand that my relationship with Mary Ann would need to change from advocating for her rights from a safe distance to walking with her day by day to face the ordinary challenges of living.

A Different Place To Live—A Different Way of Life

Several months after I was appointed Mary Ann's conservator, I received the check from her inheritance. Within a month she was no longer eligible for Medical Assistance and she began paying the cost of her care at the ICF/MR group home. After several months of writing large checks to the facility in which she lived, I knew that it was time to do something. It was not going to be enough to keep telling people in the service system that Mary Ann had the right to live in "the least restrictive environment"; I was going to have to do what was necessary for her to begin to live her own life. I remembered the words of Tom Kohler, the director of the Savannah-Chatham Citizen Advocacy Office: "There are people out there waiting to be asked to do something important."

While considering how to handle Mary Ann's living arrangements, I thought of my friend, Sue. Sue and I were best friends and had known each other for nearly 15 years. She was at a time and a place in her life that a change in her living arrangement was welcomed. After many long and serious conversations about the implications of my proposal, Sue agreed to share an apartment with Mary Ann and provide support and supervision in exchange for rent.

What had started as an advocate's efforts to "get the most out of the system" had become a way for Mary Ann to simply get out of the service system, at least to a far greater degree than would have been thought possible. On June 1, 1988, just a week before her 40th birthday, Mary Ann moved from the group home into the apartment she would share with Sue for the next 4 years. Now that she was living "outside" of a publicly funded human services program, our relationship changed at a much more rapid pace.

Complicated Feelings

During the first year and a half that Mary Ann and Sue shared an apartment, problems occurred on a regular basis. Mary Ann would become angry and frustrated, and on occasion she struck Sue or threatened to hurt her. Many of these incidents were a result of miscommunication; some were a reaction to what Mary Ann understood to be unwelcome and unnecessary control. Sometimes Mary Ann would react to disappointment by becoming angry and blaming us for things over which we had no control. She would sometimes react strongly to correction or criticism, and would refuse to cooperate with reasonable requests, such as those that involved her personal well-being and safety. For example, once she took a package of frozen fish patties out of the freezer and put them in her room in her dresser so that no one else would eat them. When we tried to explain to her that the fish needed to stay in the freezer and that eating food that was spoiled would make her very sick, she became very angry and upset and began throwing things.

As Mary Ann's advocate and legal representative, I wanted to make sure that her rights were being protected. Was Sue making unreasonable requests? Did she have unrealistic expectations for what Mary Ann might understand or be able to accomplish? Yet, I was also Sue's friend and I certainly did not want her to get hurt. I had asked her to be a part of Mary Ann's life without really knowing what to expect. On several occasions, I found myself in the role of mediator, listening to both sides of the story, helping to sort out the facts and feelings, and suggesting ways to move ahead. I learned to "change hats" frequently and to listen with an understanding of both perspectives.

As I began to think of myself more as Mary Ann's friend than simply her conservator, I could acknowledge honest feelings of anger, impatience, and frustration. When there were difficulties and I was unsure if Sue would be willing to continue living with her, I wanted to say to Mary Ann, "How could you do this? Why do you keep risking what I have struggled so hard to make happen for you?" As a legal representative, it is easier to be objective, fact-based, and analytical. As a friend, it was possible to be impatient, hurt, and angry. Complex relationships, those that go beyond defined roles or job descriptions, require an investment in the full range of human emotions. It was not until I was able to get angry that I knew I could care deeply.

Defining Moments

In some ways, I can measure the changes in our relationship by the nature of our phone calls. When Mary Ann was living in the group home, our telephone conversations consisted of a quick hello and then, "When are you coming to get me?" Conversations were short and we would exhaust the possible topics of conversation quickly—"How is work? How are things at the group home? What did you do last night?" I did all of the questioning and she did her best to answer.

After she and Sue moved into the apartment, Mary Ann's life became more interesting and we had much more to talk about. Our shared experiences provided many opportunities for "Do you remember when we . . .?" But over time a more significant change occurred: Mary Ann started to ask me questions, "How was your day? How did your meeting go? Did you have a nice business trip?" During one conversation we were talking about her coming to my house for part of the weekend. Mary Ann asked me, "Is your house a mess?" I told her yes because it was. Her response: "I guess I better vacuum it tomorrow." As she began to show interest and concern about me, our relationship matured from the "advocate who can help the less able person" to "people who care about each other."

The "talking" in our relationship has certainly gone through metamorphoses, but far more important than our talk is our laughter. Sue and I discovered early on that Mary Ann did not seem to have a very good sense of humor. She reprimanded our casual joking and silliness with "you better behave," "that's not nice," or, simply, "stop that." We can only imagine the ways in which institutionalization stifles laughter and stunts the growth of one's sense of humor. From the beginning we made a conscious effort to "explain the jokes," to help Mary Ann understand that laughing is not only allowed, but encouraged. In a way, the changes in our relationship are reflected by modes of communication. As an advocate, it seemed to be important to "get it in writing." As acquaintances, I knew that we could build our relationship by talking to each other and by listening. And as friends, I am grateful for the laughter.

MARY ANN: FROM CLIENT TO FRIEND

Life as a Client

As a "client" of human services, lifestyle options are not only limited, but actually defined. Life as a client means that you are someone's "work." It means that you are supposed to do what others tell you because they know more than you do. It means a distance between people that is created by the role of "client," and fortified by the devaluation of those we have come to know as "different." Mary Ann had experience in the roles of client, patient, Medical Assistance recipient, group home resident, and person with mental retardation, cerebral palsy, behavior problems, and a seizure disorder. She had a Medical Assistance number, a social security number, a county case file number, a state ward identification number, and a number that was sewn into all of her clothes when she lived at the institution. When she first started living with Sue, she had no experience in the role of "loved one," and despite the dozens of people in her life, she had no real friends.

There is no way that I can truly understand Mary Ann's life experiences. She was placed in an institution before she was 10 years old and had no contact with her family after that time. I talk to my parents weekly and cannot imagine a Christmas when we will not all be together. Mary Ann does not remember going to school, although she can write her name and read simple words. I went to high school, college, and graduate school. When I met Mary Ann, her understanding of money was simply that quarters were for pop machines. I have a mortgage, a car loan, credit cards, and overdraft protection. As far as I know, when I first met Mary Ann, she had never traveled by plane, taken a vacation, or made a long distance telephone call. I have accumulated several free trips through my frequent flyer program, my current car has more than 100,000 miles on it, and my long distance phone bill includes calls to family in California and friends in Georgia. No matter how I try, there is really no way in which I can fully comprehend life as she has experienced it.

Roommates

We tried to prepare Mary Ann for the many changes that would take place once she moved from the group home into the apartment. The idea of having a roommate may have been familiar to her because she almost certainly shared a bedroom in the institution. However, living with just one other person who was not going to be "staff" but was going to be a "roommate" seemed to be exciting and new to her. The three of us went out to dinner on "moving day." As the hostess showed us to our table, Mary Ann announced that "she's my roommate." Moving into an apartment seemed to be secondary to this new kind of relationship—a person who did not have a disability and was connected to Mary Ann in a novel way.

Initially, Mary Ann seemed to interpret the idea of a roommate as someone who is a constant companion. She was jealous of any time that Sue and I spent together and resented not being included in everything. Because she did not *have* a friend, she did not know how to *be* a friend. It took nearly a year for her to understand that Sue could be her roommate and my friend at the same time. For Mary Ann, the first steps in changing roles from client to friend were simply to experience friendship—to have people in her life who cared about her, who wanted to spend time with her, and who enjoyed her company. In time, those people would also come to accept and appreciate her gifts and contributions.

Feelings and Friendship

I recently asked Mary Ann to tell me what it means to be Sue's friend. She said, "Well, I *want* to get along with Sue." For perhaps the first time in her life, she understands and is willing to make an investment in a relationship. She *wants* to get along, whereas previously in her life she was told that she *had* to get along. Staff come and go; generally if you wait long enough, the staff that you do not like will leave. Unfortunately, so will the staff that you like.

As we were first getting to know Mary Ann, the only way she seemed to be able to express emotions was through anger. She had frequent and troubling episodes of yelling, throwing things, and hitting Sue. During these episodes, it sometimes seemed as if she became a different person; her mood swings were sudden and perplexing. We tried to help her talk about her feelings before she became uncontrollably angry, but during the first year these "problems" (as we came to call them) were a weekly, if not more often, occurrence. During those first few difficult months, when Mary Ann was angry she would tell Sue, "I don't want you to be my roommate anymore. Go away. I hate you." However, Sue did not go away. Once Mary Ann began to understand that we were not going to leave and that we would have to find a way to get along with each other, the significant changes began to happen.

By the end of the second year of living together, Mary Ann was better able to get angry and then get over it without totally losing her composure. We made conscious efforts to help her identify different feelings—disappointment at not being able to do something she wanted to do, worry about an upcoming change in her routine, confusion about the schedule of events, and resentment at being corrected or confronted. We reassured her that it was alright if she was angry and that she should be angry if people were bothering her, but that when people are angry, it is not alright to hurt each other.

Eventually she would tell Sue after "problems" that "something is wrong in my head." She began to accept responsibility for her actions and to understand that what she did might hurt other people. It does not seem unreasonable that a person with Mary Ann's life experiences would have difficulty expressing feelings in ways that are generally accepted in society. It was as if Mary Ann was using her anger to guard and protect herself from people getting too close. She used "violence" not as a weapon, but as a shield.

Mary Ann consistently would maintain that she was strong and that everything was fine: "I'm not sad," "I didn't hurt myself," "I'm not lonely," or "that doesn't bother me." Surviving the institutional life of 30 years ago obviously builds character in a unique way—build a wall around your emotions to keep yourself strong; it may keep others out, but it is the only way to survive. After she started living with Sue, she learned that she was not alone in the center of her universe, but a part of a fragile web of people who were learning to care about each other. Once she was able to let down her guard, it was as if she was more willing to let people into her life.

On Being a Friend

When asked about friendship, Mary Ann explains it in terms of what one does not do: "When you don't holler at them," "No yelling or screaming," "Shouldn't hit nobody," or "Leave her alone and don't bother her when she's working." When asked what friends are supposed to do for each other, she said, "Well, you got to stick up for them and be nice to her and be good to her." She gave as another example, "Like we were running out of soap and she let me use hers." Mary Ann also talks about friendship in terms of concrete actions: "Like you ask them if they want coffee," and "Tell her that she looks nice."

For Mary Ann, friendship happens in moments of everyday life. It means that someone is there to help you and to compliment you. It means that you can get angry at each other and say mean things and then be able to apologize and forgive. Friendship means that you share the conviction that the household cats are the cutest and funniest cats in the world. Friends stick up for each other and pray for each other and care for each other. Friends can say, "I love you," and not get embarrassed. Friends are there for you, even when you cannot be there for them.

SUE: FROM STRANGER TO FRIEND

Sue and Mary Ann were basically strangers when they started sharing an apartment. Before the move, the three of us went out to dinner and a movie, spent time looking for a place to live, and did a lot of shopping for the apartment. Once the day finally arrived, none of us really knew what to expect. Sue and Mary Ann signed a 6-month lease; Sue and I agreed to evaluate the arrangement on a month-to-month basis. None of us knew when we started how long the arrangement would last or how it would develop. Given the typical pattern of staff turnover in residential services, anything over a year could be considered a long-term arrangement.

One of the first obstacles was being able to understand what Mary Ann was trying to say. Although her vocabulary was adequate in some ways, her conversations were filled with "you know, that thing," "remember when that happened last week," or "you know, what you said." When she was excited and spoke quickly, it was often difficult to understand what she was saying; words blended together and syllables disappeared from crucial places in key words. Deciphering her speech was often a time-consuming task. Sue recalls that the relationship had a chance to develop once it was "less work just to converse." Both Sue and I took time to explain the meanings of words to her and started to expect more of her when she talked to us about what was going on in her life. Because she was starting to have more interesting things to talk about, we wanted others to be able to understand her.

Once actually understanding each other was less of an issue, the challenge for Sue was to support Mary Ann as she discovered her emotions. Mary Ann was very unpredictable; her immaturity in dealing with the ups and downs of everyday life made living with her not unlike a roller coaster ride. Expressing her anger was not difficult, but sharing other feelings was more of a challenge.

On a Friday afternoon 5 months after Sue and Mary Ann moved into the apartment, Sue's father had a heart attack and was hospitalized in intensive care. Mary Ann spent a lot of time with me over the weekend while Sue joined her family at the hospital. We talked about how Sue was worried that he would not get better, that he might die, and that Sue was very sad and needed us to be her friends. A week later, Sue's father passed away. Mary Ann and I attended the funeral and did our best to support Sue and her family during this difficult time.

Mary Ann was able to relate in her own way to Sue's loss because both of her parents had passed away. Being able to share in this sadness seemed to "soften" the rough edges of her interactions with Sue. Mary Ann will still recall the time when "we were sad." Mary Ann rarely cries, but when she does, she is likely to say it is because she is "sad because her mother died." On the next Father's Day, Sue and Mary Ann decided to send a card to my father. Sharing in someone's sadness and grief was an important part of Mary Ann's learning to give of herself to others. She still reacts strongly when Sue or I tell her that we are sad, and she will say, "Please don't be sad; I don't like it when you're sad."

Sadness is not the only emotion with which Mary Ann has struggled. Before she could be comfortable with humor, Mary Ann needed to know that the laughter was not directed at her. I am sure that she has experienced ridicule at an intense and painful level sometimes in her life, and that her defense had been to respond with "that's not funny" or "stop laughing." The changes happened over several years, but now she knows when something is funny. Sue's two cats have made a significant contribution to the process. Mary Ann tells this story about Shadow, one of the two cats: "Sue was making her bed and Shadow was under her sheet. Sue said, 'Mary Ann, come here. I've got something to show you.' In her room Shadow was under her sheets. Shadow is so funny." Cat antics provided a safe and nonthreatening way for Mary Ann to learn to laugh. She has even learned to laugh at herself. Due to her mild cerebral palsy, Mary Ann occasionally falls when she loses her balance. On one occasion recently, she lost her balance and fell down for no apparent reason. Whereas in the past she might have said, "Look what you made me do" or "Why did you make me fall down," this time Sue reported that Mary Ann just started laughing so hard that they both found it hard to stop.

Until the communication issues and the roller coaster mood swings started to diminish, Sue found it difficult to think of Mary Ann as a friend. She noticed that her feelings toward Mary Ann began to change when Mary Ann started being able to apologize after she lost her temper. Also, once Mary Ann started to express appreciation for things that Sue did for her, she found it easier to enjoy being with Mary Ann. A barrier was removed with the mastery of simple lessons of childhood—learning to say, "I'm sorry" and "thank you."

Watching the relationship between Sue and Mary Ann develop, I was intrigued with the social maturation that Mary Ann was experiencing. At first, she reminded me of children at the summer camps where I worked while in college. Almost every session of the summer, a camper would develop a "crush" on one of the counselors; we called it the "neatest, coolest counselor syndrome." The camper would try to sit next to the "neatest, coolest counselor" at every meal, and would become extremely jealous if another camper got extra attention from that staff person. Children will create the heroes that they need; during the early stages of their relationship, Sue was Mary Ann's hero. Over time, as Mary Ann and Sue got to know each other, I could see that they were relating to each other much more as equals. Mary Ann no longer idolizes Sue; she will "stick up for her," but as she has become more mature, she is able to share in a more adult relationship.

Sue talks about her relationship with Mary Ann as follows:

> At first my role was undefined. The aim was to aid Mary Ann in her transition from an institutional setting to noninstitutional living. For a while she put me in the role of staff because that was what she was used to.
>
> One role I played was to open her eyes to the world around her. She was totally self-involved at first. I have seen her learn to not think only of herself, but to think of other people and show her concern. Now she volunteers for community events with me and takes delight in the stars and sunsets.

WIDENING THE NETWORKS

Although Mary Ann lives in what many would consider an ideal situation, she still has relatively few friends. Over the past 4 years, Sue and I have made conscious efforts to include Mary Ann in as much of our lives as possible. We may not be able to make people be her friend, but we have certainly created and supported as many opportunities as possible.

Nancy and Mary Ann

For the past 10 years, Sue and I have gotten together on a regular basis with two other friends, Nancy and Leslie, to play cards; we usually meet sometime during a holiday weekend and rotate the hostess duties. When Mary Ann and Sue first started living together, Mary Ann attended the card parties, but her role was basically a "tag along." We tried to include her, but the four of us had a "history" of get-togethers that formed the basis of much of our story-telling, conversation, and laughter.

After a while, Mary Ann became more comfortable as a part of the group. She was willing to sit at the table when we played cards or board games, even though she did not want to play along. She had lots more to say and as she became a part of the group's "history," she was able to join in the "remember the time when" sessions with the rest of us. Nancy and Leslie welcomed Mary Ann into their homes and over time they became genuinely interested in her life.

As time went on, Nancy and Mary Ann discovered that they have several things in common. Both believe that the Minnesota State Fair is above all an "eating event" and they both enjoy the rides on the midway. In 1990, 2 years after Mary Ann and Sue moved into the apartment, we planned a day at the State Fair. The year before I had gone with Nancy and disappointed her by refusing to go on the double Ferris wheel. But this time she had a friend who was willing to risk the ride. (I stayed on the ground and took pictures.) As we retold the story at a later card party, Nancy said, "None of my other friends would go on the double Ferris wheel with me, but Mary Ann would."

The next weekend the five of us took a trip to Chicago to visit my family and see a few baseball games. In the van on the way back home to Minnesota, Nancy was having difficulty opening a cooler. From my "back-seat driver" position, I kept telling her what she was doing wrong and repeatedly giving her directions on how to do it right. In the midst of all the commotion, Mary Ann turned around to me and exclaimed, "She's trying her best!" Nancy's response: "That's right. I am!" In that one moment, I understood reciprocity as I had never before. As Mary Ann has told me, friends "stick up for each other." She defended Nancy with the best defense anyone had ever used for her. At that moment, Nancy needed a friend and Mary Ann was the one who was there for her.

Extended Families

When Sue moved into the apartment with Mary Ann, Sue's friends at work were understandably curious: "Who was this person?," "Why would Sue want to live with a retarded woman?," "What was she like?," "How much was Sue getting paid?" Explaining the relationship was difficult, especially during the first year when there were ongoing problems. Sue's friends at work were introduced to Mary Ann gradually. One of Mary Ann's goals at her day program had been to learn to take the bus downtown and to find Sue's office in the department store. Some of Sue's co-workers first met Mary Ann, not in a social situation as Sue's roommate, but as part of a group of adults with mental retardation taking a rather unusual field trip to the general accounting office of a department store.

During the 4 years in which they have lived together, Mary Ann has been included in a number of social gatherings of Sue's friends from work, including a wedding. Now, when Mary Ann and I stop in to visit Sue at work, Mary Ann knows more of Sue's co-workers than I do. Sue reports that they regularly ask about her, and have shared in Mary Ann's excitement over a recent new job. I am not sure that they would consider Mary Ann a close friend, but I am sure that at least a few of them would be willing to help in a time of need.

We have also tried to support Mary Ann in building connections by helping her to send Christmas cards and other greeting cards on special occasions. The first year that I helped her with her Christmas cards, we struggled a bit to come up with even a dozen names. Instead of sending one card to Sue's sister, brother-in-law, and their daughters, each member of the family received their own card proudly signed, "Mary Ann Dowswell." Three years later, I helped Mary Ann send out 34 Christmas cards. As I was making the list, Mary Ann just kept rattling off names. We mailed cards to Sue's family members here in Minnesota, my family in Illinois, both current and past staff, and many people from Sue's work.

T-Shirts and Mugs

Sue works for a major department store company that is known for its corporate citizenship. Through work, Sue has numerous opportunities to volunteer for a variety of community events. Sometime during the first year that Sue and Mary Ann were roommates, Sue began to include Mary Ann in her volunteer work. Because Sue was willing to include her, Mary Ann has volunteered twice at the Twin Cities' Marathon, helped with spring cleaning at a state park, and served lunches at a Mothers' Day event at the arboretum. Every summer a variety of local groups and organizations sponsor a "paint-a-thon" at which volunteers paint homes for senior citizens or other individuals who request assistance. The first year that Mary Ann volunteered at the paint-a-thon with Sue, her job was to "supervise" from a lawn chair and help keep track of the other volunteers' wallets and keys. Two years later I asked Sue if Mary Ann was still "supervising." Her response was "No, this year I handed her a scraper and told her to get busy."

The three of us did volunteer work for the U.S. Olympic Festival in 1990, and also volunteered as skyway guides when the Super Bowl was held in Minneapolis in January 1992. On one level, Mary Ann enjoys participating because she usually gets a t-shirt or a mug and a free lunch. But on another level, she knows that she is making a contribution. When television ads mention volunteer work, she will point to the TV and say, "I did that. I volunteered."

WHAT WE HAVE LEARNED

Being a part of Mary Ann's life has enriched my life immeasurably. I have learned important lessons about the nature of relationships and have come to appreciate more fully the gift of friendship. Both Sue and I have also learned some things about supporting persons with disabilities in real-life situations and what it takes to be a friend.

Friendship takes a great deal of time. It is not something that you can accomplish by taking a person on a community outing every Thursday from 4:00 P.M. to 6:00 P.M. It happens when people find themselves on the same journey. It deepens when the travelers come to depend on each other—to read the map, to know where the next gas station is, to take pictures to capture the memory. An important part of friendship is just wasting time together—remembering shared experiences, being tired from a hard day's work, watching the sunset, or listening to the evening traffic.

It is the little things that matter the most—being able to laugh at something silly the cat did, enjoying the same television program, bringing a cup of coffee to help a friend wake up in the morning, remembering her favorite song, or offering a hug at just the right moment. It is the hundreds of little moments over time, like the hundreds of threads in a woven tapestry.

Most of us have friends that we see infrequently; yet, when reunited, it is as if no time has passed. In most of those instances, the relationship was built on a strong foundation of time spent together. Being a part of Mary Ann's life has taught me that we need to include people with disabilities in the whole fabric of our lives if we are serious about supporting relationships over time. Until, as a society, we abandon stereotypical responses to people who are seen as different, the stigma of devaluation will too frequently create a barrier to friendships among people with and without developmental disabilities. It is not enough to provide "community integration activities" as a part of a habilitation program. It's not enough to provide supported employment in fast food restaurants. We must truly include people in our day-to-day lives, every day, one day at a time, for as long as it takes.

EPILOGUE

Four years and one week after Sue and Mary Ann moved into the apartment, they moved out; they moved to a duplex that they purchased together. Sue lives upstairs and Mary Ann lives downstairs. They are no longer roommates, but they are neighbors. When we started our journey 4 years ago, no one in her life would have thought that Mary Ann would be able to live by herself. As much as I was dedicated to challenging old ideas about persons with developmental disabilities, I could never have predicted what I have seen happen. Mary Ann is living in her own home by herself, but she is not alone.

Looking Ahead

Last weekend, I went with Mary Ann to the church that is down the street from her new house. It is an older congregation that is struggling somewhat since many of its members moved from the city to the suburbs years ago. We were instantly recognized as newcomers and welcomed enthusiastically. The pastor asked Mary Ann her name, and during the coffee time after the service several women, including Mary Ann, started a conversation. As we left to walk back to her house, they said, "See you next week!" Stay tuned.

REFERENCES

Lutfiyya, Z. (1990). *Affectionate bonds: What we can learn by listening to friends.* Syracuse, NY: Center on Human Policy, Syracuse University.
Strully, J., & Strully, C. (1985). Friendship and our children. *Journal of The Association for Persons with Severe Handicaps, 10*(4), 13–16.
Taylor, S.J., Bogdan, R., & Racino, J.A. (1991). Introduction. In Taylor, S.J., Bogdan, R., & Racino, J.A. (Eds.), *Life in the community: Case studies of organizations supporting people with disabilities* (pp. 1–13). Baltimore: Paul H. Brookes Publishing Co.
Tyne, A. (Ed.). (1988). *Ties and connections.* London: King's Fund Centre.

13

That Which Binds Us
Friendship as a Safe Harbor in a Storm
Jeffrey L. Strully and Cindy Strully

During the 1980s, we worked hard to facilitate friendships for our daughter. We came to understand that it is friendship, not skills or competencies, or even quality services, that is most important in her life. We have come to realize that friendships are neither easy to achieve nor guided by an exact path to follow on one's journey toward inclusiveness.

However, it is friendships that make life worth living. Facilitating friendships for our daughter requires intentionality. Friendships are not going to be achieved unless people purposefully work on forming these relationships. This issue raises many questions for which there are no easy answers. However, unless we take the time to start asking these questions and attempt to determine why friendships happen and what we can learn from them, we will never learn how to be better at facilitating friendships for people with developmental disabilities.

Friendships require hard work. They force families, integration facilitators, focal people (persons with labels), and their friends to live with tension. Friendship for our daughter has been a series of peaks and valleys. When friends do not want to go out with her or they want to change their plans, she must live with these disappointments. Asking friends to do things places a potential strain on the friendship. It may move from being freely given to fulfilling an obligation. These are often very delicate situations that need to be addressed.

Friendships come and go. They are difficult to maintain and even more difficult to describe to people. However, one knows what friendship is really about when it is happening, which makes it worth all of the work that was required to develop it. Working on friendships

---

This chapter is dedicated to Leslie New, without whose assistance our daughter would still be a "stranger"! Thank you with all our love!

places us under the constant strain of attempting to reach for something that cannot be guaranteed. However, it is friendship, more than skills, money, power, and control, that makes life worth living.

Shawntell, our daughter, can live without many things in her life (e.g., learning to feed herself, learning to use the bathroom independently), but she cannot live without friendships. For years, we spent our time teaching Shawntell and working on her physical, occupational, and speech therapy goals. Although this learning was important to each of us, there was a subtle implication that Shawntell was a broken person who had to be fixed. If she learned the things we were teaching her, then we assumed that somehow her quality of life would be improved. What we learned over time was that Shawntell was not broken, therefore, she did not require fixing.

In all of the recent discussions and writing about relationships, what has not been discussed often enough is the pain and frustation that exists when people start working on friendship. Although friendships are important, even critical to our daughter's life, we would be living in a dream to say that there has not been pain and frustration in facilitating Shawntell's friendships over the years.

Although there has been and continues to be frustration and pain, it is well worth the effort because there are no other real options. It is friendship that will ultimately mean life or death for our daughter. It is her and our only hope for a desirable future and protection from victimization. Families and the human services system (including the educational system) have spent all of their time training, teaching, working with, and habilitating people with developmental disabilities. When one spends time with adults with the label of developmental disability, it is easy to see that their lives generally lack true quality. Being a client in a system, even a good system, is nothing to brag about. People still live in poverty; have limited control over their lives; and have few, if any, relationships. Staff come and go in their lives and life is a series of programs and learning sessions geared to enable people to function better to become valued individuals in our society.

This chapter is about what we have learned during 12 years of working on friendship—beauty and excitement, as well as pain and anguish. It is about learning from doing and then learning some more. It is about working on something that is well worth working for. It is all about friendship.

A NEW BEGINNING

The journey of our daughter's life took a new direction as she began college as an incoming freshman in the fall of 1991. Starting college is

an exciting time in the life of an 18-year-old. It is the beginning of a
new set of challenges and experiences. There are new people to meet
and friendships to form. Leaving home is difficult for any young person; it is frightening and exciting. Yet, no matter what happens in the
future, those of us who care about and love Shawntell are going to
continue to dream about her desirable future and work together to
make her dreams come true.

The journey toward inclusiveness begins when people recognize
what is worth working on and what will lead in the wrong direction.
For us, getting Shawntell just to be a regular student who is learning
all she can, having fun, hanging out, and being with people who care
about her because they are her friends, was and still is what we believe is at the heart of the matter. The journey is about being welcome
and invited in, as well as hospitality and circles of friends. It is about
not being the "stranger" on the outside, but being a "regular."

As Shawntell's high school days have come to a close, it is time to
reflect on what her educational experience has taught us. Shawntell
moved with us to Littleton, Colorado, from Louisville, Kentucky, in
1986. In her first year in Colorado she was in middle school and even
though she was in regular education classes in her neighborhood
school, things were far from perfect. However, we knew what the
"gold ring" looked like and we were not going to give up until we
achieved it! Knowing what is worth working on and devoting time to
is critical. You need to determine which of all the things that you can
spend your time on is the one that will really matter. For our family,
the answer is friendship for Shawntell—the single most important
thing in her life.

During the late 1980s and early 1990s, Shawntell traveled the road
in high school, finally attaining the status of a graduating senior. The
classes that she enjoyed the most were French, American literature,
music appreciation, economics, science fiction, and adult issues. She
enjoyed the drama club, Amnesty International, working on the year-
book staff, and being involved with the Wild Warrior Women—an exclusive club with the exclusive membership of female seniors.

Shawntell has enjoyed spending weekends in Steamboat Springs (a
nearby Colorado resort) and traveling to Mexico, California, Chicago,
and Florida with her friends! As long as she is with Joyce, Denise,
Brandi, Cyndi, and Ruth, she is happy. They plan things to do together
(e.g., going to the movies, a concert, or shopping; cooking dinner together; choosing a video; and talking late into the night). These
young women have come to recognize that Shawntell is the social
glue that binds them—she is the reason they came together and the
reason, in part, that they stay together. This group of friends is not
just for Shawntell; they rely on each other in order to "make it" at

school. In their daily lives, all of Shawntell's friends care about her
and have learned to care about each other.

For all teenagers, the desire to belong and fit in is paramount. The
young women speak openly about feelings of alienation and being
lonely among many types of people. They search for connectiveness.
Although academic achievement is important, it is the feeling of belonging to a group that is critical to make it not only in high school,
but in society today.

Being on the Right Path

Knowing where you are going is important. For many years we jour-
neyed down a road that we believed was the right one. It was supposed
to be the one that would help Shawntell the most by increasing her
skills. For years, she worked on physical therapy exercises to achieve
new milestones. We listened to every professional; we read every
book; and we attended every conference, seminar, and parent meeting. But one day we realized that all of this work was focused on
Shawntell's labels, which caused everyone to see her only as a litany
of deficiences. As parents, we did not see her "deficiencies"; few
other people saw her as the gifted person we knew. Although helping
Shawntell learn new skills will always be important, this path of deficiency labels was leading us toward a future filled with human services, paid caregivers, segregation, and isolation.

The dream Shawntell and we have is to live a life of rich experiences, all the while having friends with whom to share them. We envision a series of different futures. Among the ones we see are:
Shawntell living in her own place with people she wants to live with;
learning things that are important and useful, but also fun; doing new
things with new people; and having close and meaningful friendships
and relationships. These visions encompass what quality is all about
for Shawntell. For those among us who see only her deficiencies,
these dreams are undeniably what they consider part of a good quality of life for themselves. We do not see a future of congregate care,
residentially or vocationally, for ourselves. Rather, we continue to explore different possibilities and take new paths while being committed to enjoying a meaningful life now.

Shawntell started college last fall as did millions of 18 year olds
across the nation. This was the beginning of her journey to adulthood. College is where many people are practicing independence,
emancipation, and self-reliance. College is a place where Shawntell
can take several years to determine what she wants to do with her
life. Shawntell does not need transitional living—she needs to become her own person.

We do not know where this journey will lead Shawntell. There are no longer any annual goals and measurable objectives for a good life. Life is a mystery worth living. As long as she has love, friends, caring, opportunities, choices, control, and power in her life, the journey will be a good one. Without these variables, life would look very bleak.

CAN THE SYSTEM HELP US?

Shawntell does not need a service coordinator, nor does she need to be a client in the system; however, she does require support and assistance to live a good life and to develop relationships with others. Being part of life does not mean that she should be part of the human services system. We have worked hard to keep Shawntell out of the system; whether this will continue to be possible over time remains unknown. It is in Shawntell's best interest to have control of her money and the decisions that affect her life, rather than being thought of as a client who generates revenue and expenses for a vendor providing services.

We currently have a real dilemma because Shawntell definitely requires support; she needs to have people around her who are paid to introduce and connect her to her neighbors, classmates, and others. She needs other people to provide day-to-day support that her friends cannot be expected to assume on a daily basis.

For Shawntell to receive the various supports she requires, she needs financial control, the power to make decisions, and a genuine say in where she goes on her journey. This causes a dilemma between the system and Shawntell, with the system demanding that she alter her journey to conform to the system's needs and requirements and Shawntell demanding that her unique journey be respected and assisted. If real control is provided to Shawntell, then the system will be required to rethink and refocus where and how people spend their time. What will be discovered is that the system will need to spend time connecting people rather than teaching tricks. The system can help people become part of the community rather than be separated from the community. It has potential when the power is given to the person with disabilities and/or his or her family.

WHAT HAVE WE LEARNED SO FAR?

During Shawntell's 18-year journey, we have learned that:

The journey starts with a dream.
Desirable futures are possible.

Friendships are at the heart of any desirable future.

Friendships can and should be nurtured and supported.

Circles of friends benefit everyone involved.

Needs do not require a formalized system response.

Control and power over one's own life is critical.

Opportunities to explore new paths on one's journey are paramount.

New paradigms need to be considered for people; the old paradigms do not help bring people into the community.

The journey toward inclusiveness is not like a road map—it is an adventure to be lived.

Shawntell's journey is not the journey others should follow—each journey is unique to the traveler.

There is a need for paid and unpaid relationships to facilitate the journey.

There are times on the journey that will cause a need to rethink, change, or modify the path.

Intentionality is required for some people if they are going to be connected to a group of friends.

From School to Adulthood

The experiences children and young adults have in the school system will bring very different expectations to adult services than what has been provided so far.

Young adults and their families expect the adult services system to rethink how it spends its time and energy. The system will be expected to help foster and maintain relationships and friendships that were developed in high school as well as support and foster new relationships.

For some people, learning what has been successful with the school-age population and applying it to adult services are difficult. This difficulty may be due to the fact that all children have a common place—school—but adults do not. Rather, adults spend time in many different shared areas, such as the work place, community college, figure and fitness salon, ballfield, and local restaurants.

A lesson to be learned from the successes in facilitating friendship for children is that assistance is required. The failure of some of us to learn that lesson has led to the mistaken belief that adults do not need to have someone assist with connections. The assumptions that "I can do it by myself" or "it should happen naturally" or "you can't force people to be friends" have caused many adults with labels to continue to be disconnected in their communities. Adults with and without disabilities need people to help introduce them to others, and sometimes to help them stay connected.

Throughout life there are a variety of excuses that people hold on to about why friendships cannot happen. Often, we hear that adults without disabilities have careers, family, and social networks that will not allow them time to meet and spend time with adults with developmental disabilities. However, there are many people in our communities who want to know people, with or without disabilities. If people without labels really have the opportunity to meet and be introduced to people with developmental disabilities, they could discover some valuable friendships and become more connected in their own lives.

Adult support workers should spend time introducing people in their community and helping them to connect with one another. These connections require intentionality. Without intentionality, relationships for Shawntell would never have become a reality. It is difficult for some people to accept that the facilitation of relationships requires purposeful involvement in people's lives. It requires a third party, at least in Shawntell's life, to help to introduce her to others, invite other people to get to know her, find places that people can link with her, and fulfill other strategies to help build bonds of friendships.

Before relationships can develop, people need to be in the community together. A person has to be present in other people's lives before people will become familiar with him or her. Facilitation is required with both adults and school-age children.

The Integration Facilitator

A third person may be required for people to become acquainted with other people in the community. The integration facilitator, as this third person, introduces people and tells a person's story to others (see Forest & Snow, 1986; Strully & Strully, 1989). Additional activities of the facilitator are to interpret to others, make introductions, find opportunities for people to get to know each other, and represent the person as if he or she were that person.

When we began to think about friendships for Shawntell in secondary school, it became obvious that parental involvement was different between elementary and secondary school. In elementary school it is acceptable and even advisable for a parent to be actively involved; however, in middle school, this level of involvement changes as children learn to become more independent.

In middle school, it was obvious that Shawntell needed someone from the outside to devote attention and efforts to facilitate her friendships. When Shawntell began attending high school, a "teacher" was assigned to facilitate friendships for her. The teacher was also responsible for other students with complex needs. Shawntell had several relationships but these relationships were not of the quality and intensity that we felt she needed. The relationships were fairly superficial and basically at a caregiving level; they were not friendships based on mutuality and reciprocity. Although this teacher assisted with the facilitation of these relationships, she was unable to devote the attention that was needed to take these relationships to a plane beyond just caregiving.

When the next school year began, we decided to hire an integration facilitator who would be responsible solely for Shawntell. After we hired this facilitator, Leslie, the Colorado Department of Education and our local school district decided to become more involved in this effort.

Leslie fulfilled the role of facilitator for a little over 2 years. She was the ingredient that had been missing in trying to build friendships in Shawntell's life since she had started secondary education. Leslie's love for Shawntell made her an excellent facilitator. She is committed to Shawntell and is able to understand and experience what life is like through her eyes. Living in a society where people only see a person's disability is lonely; Leslie felt the pain of isolation that Shawntell had experienced.

Leslie's role was to bring people together around Shawntell and form a circle of friends. When searching for friendship, it is necessary to meet many people before friends are found. Many people have approached and become involved with Shawntell only to move on after a short time when the newness or uniqueness wore off. Others stayed past the initial stages of friendship. They learned that being a true friend to Shawntell requires being committed through "thick and thin." Those people who are really committed are not many in numbers, but they do exist. They are true friends.

Sometimes commitment is not enough, sometimes personal circumstances have an impact on people's ability to remain involved. College, parental issues, moving, and work are some of the variables that are often beyond a person's control. Some people who truly cared about Shawntell and became her friend left the friendship. These departures are also a part of understanding friendships, relationships, and the difficulty of being part of another person's life.

The summer after Shawntell graduated from high school, a new integration facilitator was hired. Angie was the same age as Shawntell and was new in Shawntell's life. It took some time for them to get to know each other; however, in the short time Angie was involved with Shawntell, her social life improved as her social calendar filled up. Shawntell became involved in different types of young adult activities than she had previously experienced. She developed new friendships while maintaining and enhancing her old relationships.

Angie was faced with many challenges, including forsaking a certain amount of individuality to see things from Shawntell's perspective. Yet, Angie has the same need as Shawntell: to be connected to a group of friends. Both young women were searching for a sense of belonging and acceptance in their lives.

Although Angie and Shawntell have experienced many positive interactions at Colorado State University, there is still much to do. There is perhaps an unreasonable expectation that anyone who assumes the role of integration facilitator will be able to fill the void that exists within Shawntell's life. To be unable to fill the loneliness that exists for Shawntell causes pain and disappointment to those who care about her.

After 6 months, it was decided that Angie was at a point in her own life that she was unable to make the personal commitments that Shawntell needed. Just before Christmas 1991, Angie resigned as Shawntell's facilitator. She was replaced by Cheryl, who has started to develop a strong circle of friends for Shawntell at Colorado State University.

As a result of Cheryl's work, Shawntell moved into her own house with three other college students in August 1992. It is an exciting time in Shawntell's life to move away from home and be with other young people who are also attending college. New adventures wait for Shawntell and new opportunities to meet the friends of her roommates are on the horizon. Terri, Janna, and Natalie are very excited to be living with Shawntell and it is our firm belief that this move has the potential of increasing Shawntell's circle.

Without an integration facilitator in Shawntell's life, many positive developments would never have happened. Without intentionality, Shawntell's experiences would be far less than they are. This raises many questions: Can and should everyone have a facilitator? Who should be a facilitator? What happens if there is not a facilitator available? If one is not available, what can be done and by whom?

Pain and Frustration

Pain, frustration, and anger are emotions that we have experienced as Shawntell's parents. Being involved with the facilitation of friendship for Shawntell is not always one glorious celebration after another. There are times when it hurts. There is pain when we see that friendships are not happening for Shawntell or when people are either not aware of what they are doing or do not understand their negative view of disability. Being disabled in America still places people on the lowest rung of the ladder. People's views of those who have been labeled are conditioned by what they see and grow up listening to, as well as their lack of daily interactions with people with disabilities.

People do not recognize the extent to which disability has an impact on our schools, neighborhoods, and communities. People's lack of awareness, knowledge, and, at times, understanding, is profound. With all of the positive relationships that Shawntell has had over the years, she remains a lonely person. Shawntell is patient with people who are trying to get to know her, her communication system, her dreams and fears, and her desires and wishes. Many people come into Shawntell's life not realizing how difficult her life is. Most of these people are not able to remain involved with her because it is hard "being in her shoes."

As Shawntell's parents, we recognize the ingrained nature of prejudice that she faces on a daily basis in her struggle to be free. At every bend, there are professionals and human services organizations wanting to implement some sort of activity, program, or service that will distance Shawntell even more from the community. Or, someone enters her life and then looks for a way to escape so that he or she does not have to think or feel what it must be like to be Shawntell on a daily basis.

It is because of this loneliness that we have worked so hard to build relationships and friendships for our daughter. When things are going well, we feel hope this work will provide some sort of safeguard for her. It is our firm belief that friendships can provide one primary safeguard in Shawntell's life. We know that the friends in her network care about her very much. However, even they do not really understand the sense of urgency that we feel as we search for people who will stay around for a while.

It is a profound realization that Shawntell's life, because of her friends, is far richer than the lives of the vast majority of people with disabilities in our country. Knowing Shawntell's life is richer makes us feel good that we are working in the right direction; however, knowing how fragile her friendships are makes us constantly anxious as we wait for something to happen.

If our feelings are even close to being accurate reflections of the feelings of other parents, then it is easy to understand the sense of urgency that families with adult sons and daughters must feel as they know that there are few, if any, people who just want to be around their children because they care about them. Therefore, parents often place all their eggs in the human services basket, hoping that at a minimum their adult children will at least not be harmed. When all families can hope for is that their adult children are not being harmed, then it is time to rethink what we are doing and how we are doing it.

The pain and anguish of seeking friendships are not always as blatant as described here. Sometimes, it is felt in little things, such as

Shawntell being left out of a party or a concert or waiting around for someone who knows that she will always be there, even at the last minute, to call her. This part of Shawntell's life is difficult for us. We want so much for her to be active and engaged all of the time. That she gets out to be with friends three or four times a week is both wonderful and disappointing. We want so much more for Shawntell, but accept with appreciation what she has.

Since Shawntell was a young child, we have done everything in our power to try to increase the opportunities for her to get to know people, for people to feel welcome at our home, and to do the little things that will provide Shawntell the chance to be with others. These efforts have paid off, but at the same time we have had to bite our tongues and accept less than what we envisioned for our daughter. Knowing when to ask, how often to ask, when to let things slide by and how frequently, fighting quality versus quantity arguments, and other issues continue to be faced on a daily basis.

It is important to recognize that, in her own way, Shawntell senses what is happening to her. She knows what she would like to do (i.e., go out every night and be with people who care about her), but it seems that she knows this will not happen; therefore, she accepts the opportunities that do come by and enjoys them. She does not understand why people do not come by as often as she would like, even though they may have a good excuse.

Despite the many difficulties, Shawntell's life is good. Yet, it can be better, and we will work to make it better. With all of the fanfare on friendships and relationships these days, it seems that there needs to be at least an understanding of what the "other side" feels like. Why is it that we work so hard on friendship at the cost of everything else (e.g., helping Shawntell learn a specific skill or competency)? The reason is simple—without friendships in Shawntell's life, gaining additional skills and competencies is useless. Shawntell will be at increased risk of abuse, neglect, and exploitation without friends and relationships in her life. She will never have a chance to go for the "gold ring" if we do not work to facilitate friendships and relationships for her. At least we know that our efforts are leading us in the right direction.

THE IMPORTANCE OF FRIENDSHIP

As this chapter was written, a situation occurred that clearly frames the issue on why friendship is so critical in Shawntell's life as well as in all of our lives.

Shawntell was eating dinner at a restaurant with three of her friends. We received a call from Cyndi informing us that Shawntell was choking and that the paramedics had been called. We rushed over to the restaurant to learn that not only had Shawntell choked, but that she had gone into a grand mal seizure. As Shawntell was coming out of the seizure and was being transferred to the hospital, her friends forgot about needing to be home by a certain time. All they could focus on was getting to the hospital to be with Shawntell. Two of the young women (Denise and Cyndi) went to the hospital together and the third, Joyce, came with us. Joyce never left Shawntell's side. She talked with her and made sure that Shawntell knew that she was right there. She defended her when the nurse was asking foolish questions about Shawntell's functioning level.

On their way to the hospital, Denise and Cyndi were in an automobile accident (fortunately, they were not hurt). We received the call about the accident as the three of us were with Shawntell in the emergency room. They were lucky that their impatience with red lights and the speed of other cars did not result in a more serious accident. It was their concern for their friend, Shawntell, that caused them to hurry to the hospital.

That evening and the following few days were difficult for all of us. However, if we ever become depressed again about Shawntell's life, and we may, we will never forget the way her friends rallied around her that evening. Their care and concern for their friend in a time of need clearly answers the question of why friendship is so important in our lives. No one should ever experience a time of need without the presence of people who truly want to help because of their care and love for the person.

CONCLUSION

We asked Shawntell's friends to have the last word. The following are their thoughts:

Brandy: "I have always had friends in school, but I never really did anything with them outside of school and now we are starting to do things together and now my life is richer."

Ruth: "Shawntell made it through high school. She will do OK at CSU. It won't be easy, but we will help her."

Joyce: "Times are changing, why aren't you?"

Denise: "Shawn has helped me to look deeper into myself. Before I met Shawn I was a physically handicapped person striving to be a 'normal' person. Because of my friendship with Shawn I am able to accept myself for who I am."

Cyndi: "Shawn's friendship is a wonderful addition to my life. Shawn accepts me as I am and I do the same with her."

As Shawntell's parents, we are excited about our daughter's journey toward inclusiveness. It is her friendships that will provide her a safe harbor in her journey. It is our belief that together we will work to make our communities more caring and accepting for all people. There are two reasons why this is important—*because it is time and because it is right!* We hope that your journey will be as exciting as ours has been. As long as you keep your eye on the prize and keep dreaming, you cannot go wrong! Good luck in your search for inclusiveness for yourself as well as for the people whom you love!

REFERENCES

Forest, M., & Snow, J. (1986). *Support circles: Building a vision.* Downsview, Ontario: G. Allan Roeher Institute.

Strully, J.L., & Strully, C.F. (1989). Friendship as an educational goal. In S. Stainback, W. Stainback, & M. Forest (Eds.), *Educating all students in the mainstream of regular education* (pp. 59–68). Baltimore: Paul H. Brookes Publishing Co.

14

Opening Pandora's Box

A Parent's Perspective on Friendship and Sexuality

Betty Pendler

Parents of individuals with developmental disabilities, professionals working in the field, and the general public often believe that discussing the topic of sex is like opening Pandora's box and letting loose the floodgates with no notion of how the rushing waters can be controlled. In today's society, those gates are already open. Learning to talk about sex when a person would prefer not to has become an unavoidable necessity for everyone who has a genuine desire to see that people with developmental disabilities receive their full social and sexual rights.

Much of what is expressed in this chapter is applicable to parents, professionals, staff working directly with people with developmental disabilities, and the general public because all of these groups have similar fears, doubts, misgivings, and discomforts. Also, all of these groups are affected by societal attitudes, so it is often difficult to separate and clearly delineate the role each group plays in the full sexual expression of people with developmental disabilities.

Furthermore, although this chapter primarily elaborates on sexuality issues for persons living in group homes, the same general issues apply to persons who live independently, in a supported apartment, or at home with their parents. The message is the same, that is, for friendship to be fully developed in the community, there is a need to recognize all persons as sexual human beings, to impart knowledge, and to teach social awareness skills.

Some professionals and agencies indulge in the tempting proposition of reducing the needs of persons with developmental disabilities to only biological urges and of reducing sex to a simple behavior that can be programmed away. However, the truth is that we do not view our personal loving relationships only from a genital perspective. We have caring and loving relationships, including the desires to touch, caress, and hold hands, and we have to recognize that people with developmental disabilities also have the capacity to love and care for others. This recognition should, perhaps, be the first step for parents, professionals, and society at large. It is impossible to talk about human relationships for people with disabilities without looking at one's beliefs in the ability of these individuals to love, develop a healthy self-concept, and have caring relationships similar to the rest of society. Encouraging friendships has long been a goal for parents and staff within the human services system; therefore, it is necessary to recognize that one of the aspects of friendship must be the subject of sexuality.

It is important for a person with developmental disabilities to feel comfortable with people of the opposite sex. One way to achieve this comfort is to be involved in a variety of activities, such as belonging to a community center, recreation club, church organization, or YMCA, or going to movies, local pizza parlors, or parks. It is heartening to see two young people who may be living in a group home go to the movies together, hold hands, share popcorn, and experience a feeling of being connected. Yet, there may be some parents who would not permit even the beginning of such a friendship for fear of what may ensue.

Parents must be convinced that the professionals working with their children can adequately teach proper social skills. There are many standard techniques that are effective in enhancing friendships (Griffiths, Quinsey, & Hingsburger, 1989). Those parents who fear that talking about sexuality will open up Pandora's box must realize that exposing their son or daughter to sex education does not create sexual feelings—those feelings are already there. Rather, it is the responsibility of parents and professionals to help young people deal with these feelings. The fear that prevails is that if we teach people about sex and protection, we may be encouraging them; the truth is that experts agree that the knowledge of the subject encourages appropriate behavior. For example, the increased publicity on the subject of AIDS will hopefully reduce the incidence of that disease.

In general, the subject of sexuality is often very difficult for parents of all children to discuss openly in any context; however, because society is filled with even more ambivalent feelings on the topic of sexuality as it relates to people with developmental disabilities, that subject seems to be fraught with even more emotion and controversy. The question of whether or not a person with developmental disabilities should be involved in sexual activity or sex education often reflects common myths about the sexual nature of such individuals. Typical myths include the perceptions that they are either asexual or oversexed.

It is encouraging to see an increase in professional training and the number of articles in professional journals on the subject of sexuality (e.g., Ames, 1982; Ames & Boyle, 1980); hopefully, these increases will generate more public discussion and more dialogue within the human services system. As soon as professionals and parents deal with their discomfort in discussing this subject more openly, it is hoped that their candor will also affect the general public and its ability to be more at ease with the subject. It should not be implied that sexuality is more important for someone with disabilities than a typical person, but it is certainly no *less* important. With the advent of community residences, supported employment, and the push for inclusion in the community, this issue must be faced and all of the myths about this population must be dispelled.

IT IS OKAY TO FEEL UNCOMFORTABLE

Few people are free of discomfort in approaching the issue of sexuality with young people with disabilities. Often, professionals approach teaching about sexuality with great reluctance because it is such a sensitive and personal topic. David Hingsburger (1990), a well-known expert in this field, suggests that people allow themselves "the freedom to feel uncomfortable" (p. 89). When professionals are working with parents on this subject, it is very important for them to recognize parental discomfort and validate it, as well as to recognize their own discomfort when it is present.

It is also important for both professionals and parents to consider whether the hesitation in freely talking about the subject reflects an unconscious feeling that perhaps people with developmental disabilities should not have the same sexual rights and feelings as everyone else. Although everyone might agree that all people are entitled to sexual expression, people might react differently when they see, for example, a couple in a sheltered workshop affectionately embracing (on break time, of course) behind the lockers. It must be realized, however, that these two people do not have the same opportunities as nondisabled couples; they do not have a private home, the opportunity to go to a motel, or other privacies that are taken for granted by nondisabled people. Is it any wonder that they seize every chance they can? They should be given credit for their ingenuity. Rather than trying to "eliminate inappropriate behavior," it is hoped that the workshop staff would help such a couple to have some privacy and confer with either the parents, group home supervisor, or other personnel about the provision of private space and time.

Helping Parents Deal with Their Feelings

If both parents and professionals deal with normal sexual activities in a wholesome way, this style will determine to a great extent how much sexual freedom the person with developmental disabilities is going to enjoy. Therefore, it is important for parents and staff to envision sexuality and sexual expression as normal, to view both without anxiety, and to accept this part of a person with developmental disabilities with dignity. These attitudes will certainly enhance friendship in the community by fostering good feelings on the part of the individuals with developmental disabilities and creating the understanding that the term *sexual* is more than physical contact—that it is a warm, friendly feeling.

It is vital, therefore, that when staff attempt to help parents deal with their fears and anxieties, that their parental concerns be treated as valid. Parents need to know that professionals respect their concerns as a reflection of a legitimate value system, that they sincerely believe in the parents' love and care for their children, and that they understand that these concerns are reflections of this love and care. There are, indeed, many very real and understandable concerns regarding sexual behavior of an adult with developmental disabilities, and establishing a respectful tone when dealing with parents will convey appreciation of the difficulty of the issue.

One technique to deal with the discomfort of parents is to use group discussions. Such groups give parents an opportunity to talk about sensitive issues in a supportive environment. To make life in the community successful, parents often need nurturing and extensive group sessions to point out the needs to "let go" and not overprotect under the pretext of parental love. Parents must encourage their sons and daughters to participate in sex education courses, and staff must encourage parental discussions. These discussions can include pointing out that restricting sons or daughters only adds to their children's differences. Unless parents accept their sons or daughters as full sexual beings, they are doing them an injustice and making an unconscious statement that their children are not full human beings.

Parents have legitimate concerns and it is important that these concerns be discussed openly. The group process can be very helpful for this purpose. Because validating concerns is so important, the first group session could be one of sharing and honoring these anxieties. The concerns would most likely include: "Will my son or daughter be able to control his impulses? What does he or she have to learn to avoid being exploited? Will he or she learn social skills to manage in the community?" A good facilitator can divide the concerns into two categories: 1) parental feelings and 2) concerns for the child's safety, such as fear of exploitation, unwanted pregnancy, and sexually transmitted diseases. It is not easy to explore one's feelings on this subject; very often parental concerns may reflect unconscious attitudes they have about their own sexuality, which hopefully will emerge in a good group session. An effective facilitator can start such a session by asking: "What two things did your parents teach you about sex?" The answers will generate much discussion, and no doubt laughter, as people share stories about their youth.

Unconscious Attitudes

The advent of the principle of "normalization" (Wolfensberger, 1974) brought the perspective that persons who have developmental disabilities are fully human. However, that perspective presents a dilemma: if they are human, that means they are also sexual. Most of us can handle the human part, but are we prepared to deal with the sexual?

The unconscious public attitude about sexuality and people with disabilities was reflected in a conversation I had with my beautician. She knows my daughter Lisa, who has Down syndrome, because Lisa used to accompany me to the beauty parlor. When I mentioned to the beautician that I was going to make a presentation on the subject of sexuality for persons with developmental disabilities, she asked me very sincerely and kindly if I really thought that Lisa had sexual feelings like "other people." I proceeded to tell her that whenever I teased Lisa about her workshop supervisor, on whom she had a terrific crush, she would blush. I submit, therefore, whether I like it or not, something is happening inside her to bring that flush to her face.

It is rare that parents or staff ask, "What is this person thinking or feeling?" Often we are so overwhelmed by our own fears and anxieties that we are not even aware of the impact that our attitudes have on the person with disabilities. Therefore, unfortunately, persons who have developmental disabilities are often the victims of both parental and societal attitudes. People must overcome the myth that individuals with disabilities are either asexual or uncontrollable, and, therefore, their sexual feelings should be ignored or confined.

It is true that parents have an excuse when accused of overlooking the sexuality of a person with developmental disabilities. Unlike his or her typical brothers and sisters, this person is already somewhat dependent, has limited peer relationships, and might be facing physical restrictions and a lack of privacy that limit his or her experimentation with both social and sexual relationships. Indeed, many parents and professionals, as well as the public, never acknowledge the potential for adulthood and independence on the part of persons with disabilities; therefore, it is not hard to understand their reluctance to perceive sexual needs. Parents tend to vacillate from one extreme to another—they point out their children's deviations, their lack of judgment, and their disabilities, and then they ask that society accept their children just like everyone else. They see sex "for them" as dangerous because it adds to the parents' already anxious lives; therefore, they adhere to the proverb that sex is private and decide not to talk about it. Because of their consuming anxiety, parents often prefer to continue to believe the myths and misinformation.

PROFESSIONAL AND AGENCY RESPONSIBILITIES

It is easy for many people to espouse the belief that every person, even one with the most severe disabilities, has a right to be a social, sexual person; however, it is quite another matter to take an active role in proposing specific goals that will secure that right. A provider has ethical and professional responsibilities to persons with developmental disabilities regarding sexual development, and to staff charged with the responsibilities pertaining to health, teaching, and day-to-day welfare. This provider role applies to all ability levels and program settings of persons with developmental disabilities, including those who are living in residential settings with 24-hour supervision and those who are living in the community under minimum supervision. These five-fold provider responsibilities are:

1. To develop a broad encompassing philosophy of habilitation and resulting policies and procedures that foster the underlying personhood and affirm the sexual needs and rights of the person with developmental disabilities.
2. To hire staff ready, willing, and able to commit themselves to the agency's positive philosophy and policies on sexuality; to hire program supervisors trained and experienced in overseeing effective sexuality training, education, and counseling. (All program staff will probably not be qualified to provide sexuality education and counseling, but no one should be on staff or in contact with individuals with developmental disabilities who is not prepared to give "permission" to an individual working on sexual development issues.)
3. To provide ongoing inservice teaching that maintains staff perspectives and skill levels, and compensates for the frequent turnover of staff working in programs; to provide regular case man-

agement supervision and clinical supervision that facilitate and enhance both learning and opportunities for optimal functioning of staff.

4. To affirm and support the supervisory and direct-care staff over-seeing residential living and providing sexuality education and counseling, and to set clear guidelines and procedures protecting against sexual abuse.

5. To actively promote positive attitudes and approaches toward sex-uality within the agency's programs, among parents and families, in the local community, and in the professions represented in the agency; to disavow such terms as *perversion* and *sexual inade-quacy*; to confront the lack of understanding that is distortive and demeaning to the person with developmental disabilities.

It is hoped that professionals do not fall into the "yes, but" trap described by David Hingsburger (1990). The moment one says "yes, but," what he or she is really saying is "no" to whether persons with developmental disabilities are sexual beings. Some typical "yes, buts" include: "yes, but" can this person fulfill the duties and respon-sibilities of marriage; "yes, but" what if they have a baby; "yes, but" do they really know what they are doing? Although they appear to be legitimate, in reality these questions place a set of obstacles in the way of persons with developmental disabilities and prevent, or at least discourage, their actualization as social-sexual persons. Why should we assume that just because some people may not be able to control their own finances, or perform certain tasks for which they may need support, that they are not capable of having warm relation-ships, loving, hugging, and flourishing with a healthy self-concept?

SELF-STIMULATION

The subject of masturbation, one form of self-stimulation, must be discussed when talking about sexuality. Today, many parents are be-ginning to ask that their son's or daughter's individualized education program (IEP) include information about body changes and social sex-ual development, and that information about these changes be intro-duced in health and other classes. Braver parents are asking that their sons or daughters are taught proper self-stimulation. Many people have to relearn that touching one's body can be pleasurable. It is much wiser to see masturbation as a necessary function instead of a punishable crime. Having come from a puritanical background, I re-call my discomfort the first time I noticed Lisa masturbating. I gulped, braced myself, and forced myself to say calmly to her that I knew it felt good. I did try to distract her, or at least direct her to a room other than the living room. I am convinced that my casual attitude did not increase her desire to do it more often, but rather took away any guilt feeling she might have had.

Scientists and educators have discovered that masturbation is good for everyone, young and old, as it helps relieve tension. Once good feelings are encouraged through self-discovery, it is easy to go on from there and encourage a good self-image. The body plays an important role in human development, including tactile stimulation and body movement; self-stimulation allows the child to have a feeling of self-sufficiency that contributes to a sense of physical and emotional well-being. It is the attitude that is the important factor, and it must be acknowledged that masturbation is a normal sexual expression; it becomes self-destructive largely as a result of feelings of guilt. James Maddock (1974) wrote that such self-stimulation can be viewed as an adaptive behavior, a coping mechanism, rather than a maladaptive behavior. Studies have shown that after persons with severe behavior difficulties were taught how to masturbate properly, their level of acting-out behavior decreased considerably.

HOMOSEXUALITY

The subject of sexuality is not complete without mentioning homosexuality. It must be acknowledged that some people choose this option and that they should not be deprived of their choice of physical contact with the same sex. It may be difficult to determine if homosexuality is truly a matter of preference for people with disabilities and not representative of exploitation or the lack of choice in a supervised setting in which units are of the same sex. In terms of friendship, we must acknowledge that this form of human expression is a matter of choice. We should be able to accept the fact that homosexuality is a perfectly appropriate and acceptable style of life for some people, including people with developmental disabilities.

IMPARTING INFORMATION AND TEACHING SOCIAL SEXUAL EDUCATION

In order to prepare children with disabilities for friendship and life in the community, it is important to be able to impart information. Experts agree that a basic knowledge of sexual matters will prevent experimentation rather than stimulate it. Research on cases of sexual abuse has shown that often such abuse is due to a lack of knowledge, and that more information produces more responsible behavior (Gordon, 1974). There is a role for human services professionals in this area: to provide sex education and to do so in a comfortable and relaxing manner and environment for persons with developmental disabilities. It is important to realize that teaching sexuality must be approached with the same determination and positive attitude as applied to the teaching of toileting, grooming, or other adaptive skills. Leading sex educators claim that in their years of providing sexuality education and counseling to persons with developmental disabilities, they have yet to meet a nonsexual person (Ames, Hepner, Kaiser, & Pendler, 1988). Professional sex educators have found that even among persons with severe disabilities, their sexual needs and capacities are essentially the same as nondisabled people; they can learn functional and appropriate ways of expressing their sexuality and they can become as responsible in this area as they can for their own adaptive skills.

The types of education to provide and the types of skills to be learned are varied. Social interaction skills, such as learning how to make conversation, are necessary for people living in the community. Protective skills that can be accomplished through role play help identify responsible behavior. Sexuality refers to the whole identity of a person, the total way an individual interacts with his or her world as a male or female; therefore, teaching should address not just methods of sexual activity, but also skills to express feelings and emotions. Through such methods, individuals can learn that social behavior has causes and consequences.

As stated earlier, it is easy to use the "yes, but" excuse that persons with disabilities may not understand, but in my personal experience, I am convinced that people with disabilities *do* understand. I recall speaking to my daughter when she was very young about boys who might want to hug and kiss her. As she began to travel by herself, I tried to tell her about not letting anyone touch her vagina; I used as nonthreatening a manner as I could. Even though she has an IQ of 49, I learned that she did, indeed, absorb what I was telling her. Before she moved into a community residence, I used to take her to visit various group homes run by our local Arc. She knew many of the young men residing there because they worked in the same workshop. On one of our visits, I noticed a young man sitting next to her, sliding his hands slowly up her knees. While I tried to be unobtrusive, I did overhear her say, as she removed his hand, "That's a no-no." In this and many other instances, Lisa has proved to me that she is well aware of her actions.

Professionals can help young people learn about their bodies, assist them to see themselves like others, and teach them to avoid situations in which they could be sexually exploited. Sex education should help young people communicate about their sexuality with others without guilt or embarrassment.

PHILOSOPHICAL ISSUES AND MORAL VALUES

Each individual with developmental disabilities has the right to achieve his or her highest reasonable potential in the continuum of human sexual development. Because there is no such thing as perfection in sexual matters, all people have the right to develop and accept themselves. Certain people with developmental disabilities, as well as typical people, may never develop beyond an infatuation with their own bodies; others may progress farther along the continuum to creative emotional relationships. Hazards and risks are inherent in growing up, and to use the excuse that "they don't understand" is usually an excuse on the part of parents and/or staff to justify restrictions.

Often, parental over-protection arises from fear of pregnancy, which is a consuming and unconditional fear. However, this fear does not address the fact that there are many cases in which people with developmental disabilities, when learning what is involved after having been given enough information necessary to make an informed choice, elect not to have children. Having the type of information necessary to make an informed choice underscores the importance of family life education at an early age.

With the changing social mores in our society and the significant movement into group homes and other community settings, one has to look at the attitudes toward the entire subject of premarital relationships. If such relationships are acceptable for the nondisabled population, then they should be acceptable for people with developmental disabilities as well. As I faced this issue, I had to tell myself that if I truly believe that Lisa is as fully human as her brother, and if I accept this behavior on his part, even though it is counter to my own moral values, then I have to agree that it is acceptable for Lisa. In not doing so, I am subtly saying that she is less of a person than her brother.

Jennifer Hamilton (1977) has reported on her wrestling with her conflicting morals on this subject. She wrote that although she was desperately anxious that her son be spared the isolation that so often accompanies retardation, she had to face the fact that he may never get married. She admits her dilemma with the morality of family values that says sex belongs in marriage, but recognizes that for the sake of the happiness of the individual with disabilities, the standard of the moral code might have to be adjusted to allow for these special circumstances.

ISSUES AND CONCERNS IN RESIDENTIAL SERVICES

There is no doubt that the current lifestyle in most group homes, as well as that of other community-living arrangements, allows for much greater exposure to male–female relationships than institutional care. This community exposure brings up such issues as the right to privacy, developing relationships, avoiding exploitation, and other issues that were not examined to the same degree before the advent of inclusion in the community.

With regard to the right to privacy in a group home, I have an amusing personal experience to relate about my daughter and her first few months living in a community residence. She happened to be the only person in the house with Down syndrome; her roommate was a young woman who was quite "high functioning" and already had a sexual relationship with a young man who did not live in the residence. I was informed by the director of the residence that while the staff do not necessarily encourage sexual relationships, for those persons who can handle it and know about birth control, they do not discourage it. He was quite relieved to see that I was not shocked by this attitude, and we were to discuss the subject more fully at a subsequent time. Lisa's roommate introduced me to her boyfriend and referred to him as "Loverboy," which became the name Lisa used for him. I was quite pleased to see how nicely they all got along. One night Lisa telephoned me and happened to mention that the previous evening the residence showed two movies, one about grooming and one about sex education.

Shortly thereafter I was preparing to visit Lisa, but there was a severe snowstorm and I had to call her at noon to cancel my visit. She cheerfully responded, "That's okay because we have company anyhow—Loverboy is here." I inquired as to what he was doing there so early as he did not live at the residence, and she explained that he had spent the night. Once again in my life I blundered and gulped, and foolishly asked her if she remembered what she had seen on the film on sex education a few nights earlier. Then I gingerly asked her if "Loverboy" had touched her, and her immediate innocent response was, "Of course not, he is M's boyfriend."

The setup in that residence was that two people shared a small apartment; Lisa slept in the living room and her roommate had a small bedroom off the living room. Naturally I was quite upset, and called the director the next morning. He, too, was quite upset, as they do have rules that no one can spend the night; apparently "Loverboy" had snuck in. However, the real issue was one of privacy—the couple's privacy as well as Lisa's. The director explained that they usually dealt with this issue on an individual basis and generally arranged for privacy.

I do not mean to create fear about residential programs because many of them do have excellent programs on sex education as well as set policies. Typically, the issue of each resident's sexuality is dealt with adequately, and the issues of privacy and responsibility are fully discussed. Rather than being unique to group homes, this incident represents an issue that is probably not much different from college when a roommate wants to invite a friend in.

In addition to the broad areas of responsibility for all human services described above, I believe that people who run community residences should consider the following issues:

1. How to teach a person who is developmentally disabled to be selective and not promiscuous
2. How to allow for privacy without imposing on the rights of roommates
3. How staff should encourage natural contact and relationships with the opposite sex
4. How to reach a balance between the parents' and resident's points of view
5. How to maintain consistency of attitudes among the staff so that the residents are not at the mercy of a variety of individual attitudes
6. How to prevent sexual exploitation disguised as tenderness and affection

All of these issues reflect genuine parental concerns, as well as the concerns of those who run the residences.

I confess that I count on the good judgment of staff because at this time they are closer to my daughter than I am. There are other questions that I have as a parent, including: does the residence have a qualified sex educator to teach both staff and residents? More and more, agencies are hiring professional sex educators. Usually their teaching includes the ability to interpret the behavior of people with developmental disabilities, how to determine consent with residents who are verbally limited, and counseling for people such as my daughter about how to understand the consequences of their actions and accept responsibility for their behavior.

CONCLUSION

The task of encouraging positive attitudes of parents is not an impossible one. The first messages that professionals give parents should not be negative. They should point out that parents actually have a moral responsibility to their son or daughter to help them achieve an appropriate sexual identity, and point out that it is unethical to deny persons with developmental disabilities access to information that will make them aware of their options.

Sex education is seen as necessary for the person with developmental disabilities, but it is equally necessary for staff and parents. Sex education programs can help with what staff and parents must remember: that persons with developmental disabilities have a right to choose, a right to disagree, and a right to self-determination. Honoring these rights is a big task because over time sons and daughters are taught to comply with powerful people in their environments. The power of staff and parents to set restrictive rules and the traditional acceptance of the status quo usually result in the young man or woman seeking approval rather than expressing their real needs and wants. However, personal power can be taught through individual or group sessions to help individuals with developmental disabilities take responsibility for their actions.

What is usually completely lost in the picture of sex education and programs is the perspective of the young man or woman with developmental disabilities. In accordance with the exciting new thrust of self-advocacy, it is important for us to find ways to encourage real choices and responsible decision making by these young men and women, and to find ways to help parents and professionals listen to them. We have to learn to be directed by them instead of directing them.

When people with developmental disabilities are treated with dignity and provided with privacy, when they receive age-appropriate and situation-appropriate expressions of affection, and when they are taught to say "no" to advances they do not want, they can begin to take responsibility for their own sexuality. Like anyone, they can love and be loved. As more and more young people with disabilities are moving into the community, making new kinds of friendships, and seeking social-sexual satisfaction, they are creating new paths in our society. We no longer have to fear Pandora's box, but can welcome this new social revolution.

REFERENCES

Ames, T. (1982). Some considerations for effective sex education and counseling with the developmentally disabled. In J.J. Levy, P.H. Levy, N. Liebman, T.A. Dern, R. Rae, & T.R. Ames (Eds.), *From the 60s into the 80s: An international assessment of attitudes and services for the developmentally disabled.* New York: JAI Press.

Ames, T., & Boyle, P. (1980). The rehabilitation counselor's role in the sexual adjustment of the handicapped client: The need for trained professionals. *Journal of Applied Rehabilitation Counselor, 11*(4), 173–178.

Ames, T., Hepner, P.R.H., Kaiser, F., & Pendler, B. (1988, June). *The sexual rights of persons with developmental disabilities: Guidelines for programming with severely impaired persons.* New York: Coalition on Sexuality and Disability, Inc.

Gordon, S. (1974). *Sexual rights for the people who happen to be handicapped.* Syracuse, NY: Center on Human Policy Press.

Griffiths, D.M., Quinsey, V.L., & Hingsburger, D. (1989). *Changing inappropriate sexual behavior: A community-based approach for persons with developmental disabilities.* Baltimore: Paul H. Brookes Publishing Co.

Hamilton, J. (1977, December). Another view. *Exceptional Parent, 7*(6), Y26–Y28.

Hingsburger, D. (1990). *I contact: Sexuality and people with developmental disabilities.* Mountville, PA: Vida Publishing.

Maddock, J. (1974, January). Sex education for the exceptional person: A rationale. *Exceptional Children, 40*(4), 273–278.

Wolfensberger, W. (1974). *The principle of normalization in human services.* Toronto, Ontario, Canada: National Institute on Mental Retardation.

15

Held in Each Other's Hearts

*Members of Speaking For Ourselves
as told to Karl Williams*

Speaking For Ourselves is a self-help and self-advocacy group founded in the early 1980s in Philadelphia. Its speakers have traveled across the United States and to other countries, and they have talked with legislators and made depositions in court cases. The organization publishes a newsletter, is involved in a national project to ascertain the best practices among self advocacy groups and a project to interview employees of sheltered workshops, and planned the celebration of its 10th anniversary in 1992.

In 1988 Speaking For Ourselves was asked to contribute a chapter for a book on quality assurance. For the last few years the group's annual leadership retreat has been held in the fall at Fellowship Farm. One Saturday evening in 1988, after the planning work of the day was done, those members who were interested gathered in a circle in a large open room, set a tape recorder on the floor in the middle of the circle, and began to talk. The session lasted about an hour, but many of those who participated were up all night. The questions that framed the discussion seemed innocent enough: Are you satisfied with where you live? How do the people there treat you? But the answers that these questions drew out—answers that told of physical and psychological, and, much later in the evening, sexual abuse—hit nerves in the organization that had never been struck before. From airing their personal troubles in a more open way than they had ever been able to do and from admitting for the first time to the level of constant fear in which they lived, the members came to realize just how difficult—and for some of them untenable—their living situations were. Even those with no pressing problems felt tied by the very disabilities that had landed them in a community-living arrangement; their disabilities made them feel vulnerable with the people who were hired to assist them.

The advisors to the group found themselves tied too—by their un-official (and, thus, powerless) standing within what is called the ser-vice community. They had tried advocating for the members of the group many times before with no results. They despaired now at the thought of trying to go to the state for help with improving the condi-tions in which the members lived. In addition, many of the advisors were reeling from having heard the net results of their approximately 20 years of hard work to promote community living. The Pennhurst State School was closed, but people seemed hardly any better off now than they were before. But most importantly, despite the difficulties they saw before them, the advisors felt compelled not to let this hour of truthfulness slip by unaddressed, this hour of truthfulness that had come about, they felt, only because of a kind of hard-earned trust built up over the years by the mutual support and respect among the members and the advisors within the organization. What was crucial was that no one deny what had been said and what was being felt. This had always happened before—people's voices were ignored be-cause of their disabilities. The commitment was not to let that hap-pen again.

Over the next week or so the situation became so tense that several of the advisors went to talk with Carol Cobb-Nettleton, a woman with a Ph.D. in clinical social work who agreed to help the group sort through its troubles. Two meetings were scheduled. At the first meet-ing the advisors put their view of things on the table; the members who attended this first session did so only as observers. On the sec-ond day, the entire original group assembled. It was at this second meeting that Carol began to implement the idea of partnership.

What happened on the retreat was called a flood by some—a flood of truth that had been hidden and a flood of emotion, unleashed and disturbing, in response to the sudden revelations of that evening. What Carol Cobb-Nettleton saw was an organization that was being torn apart, that was tearing itself apart under the strain of dealing with all that had been revealed. Her analogy of the situation was to the work in a hospital emergency room—first and foremost, the bleeding must be stopped and the breathing must be started. What she suggested was a way for individuals to do what the organization was finding impossible. The bleeding to be stopped was the burden of phone calls and meetings with members who were most at risk, which had fallen on the shoulders of several of the key advisors who were quickly losing their capacity to deal with the situation. The breathing would be started with the idea of partnerships to create a two-way relationship between member and advisor; the advisor could give expression to his or her own troubles just as the mem-ber did.

A second meeting time was set aside for the mechanics of the plan, and, following Carol's suggestions, people asked each other to be their partners and a list of names, addresses, and phone numbers was put together. No one in the organization knew what would happen next.

The partnership project—as it is sometimes called because there is no funding involved—has been in existence since 1988. Each fall at the annual retreat the idea of new partnerships is promoted. Planning is currently underway to offer the idea of partnership to other members of the group and to other groups. Many of the partnerships are between a member of Speaking For Ourselves and an advisor; some partnerships are between two members; others between two advisors. Many of the people involved started off with more than one partner. Some of the original partners began communicating with each other immediately; some took a year or more to begin; some never caught on.

Part of the groundwork for this chapter was done at a day-long discussion about partnerships held early in the fall of 1991 at the organization's office. But most of the work consisted of interviews conducted at the 1991 retreat at Fellowship Farm. The interviews took place throughout the day and evening on a Saturday and Sunday in October in a first-floor bedroom. When it was possible, both of the partners were interviewed together. These were some of the questions asked:

How did you become partners?
How do you communicate?
What do you talk about?
What problems have you faced?
What do your friends, your family, and the people you live with think of your partnership?
Have you been disappointed at any time?
What was your best time together? Your hardest?
What are your hopes and plans for the future?
What part has Speaking For Ourselves played in your partnership?
What advice would you give to other people?

Perhaps partnership is just another name for friendship. Perhaps friendship needs another name these days. Or, perhaps partnership is a kind of stamp of approval given by this organization to friendship. Perhaps what the organization has done, by giving friendship another name and by adopting a simple ritual in which an agreement is entered into willingly by two parties, is to open many pairs of eyes to the importance of other people in one's life. Perhaps partnership is the next step that needed to be taken, the next step of approach. Perhaps this next step, which puts the power of friendship finally within the reach of people who have never known that power before, is the one that breaks through the barriers that disability sets up between human beings.

KAREN AND BEA

Karen has a brisk cheerful personality and an animated way of telling her story. Bea's manner is markedly unguarded and genuine but at the same time she is one to keep her private life to herself.

Karen: My name is Karen H. and I live in West Chester. I work at the (restaurant). And I do like it very much there. They're all real nice; they're a bunch of kidders. I'm actually a dishwasher. But when I'm not busy I help the cooks. I've been working there since July, about 3 months. Before that I worked at West Chester University. My job coach got me my new job. She had somebody in there, but he didn't work out. And one day I was off, and she said, "Karen, do you think you'd want to go over to (the restaurant)?"

I said, "Do I have a choice?"

She said, "No." (Karen laughs.)

And I said, "Oh, really?"

And she says, "Yeah, well I need somebody really bad."

So I went over there and I was helping the other guy out. His name was Ricky, but he wasn't doing too good. It was like taking forever to do the bus pans. They needed somebody faster—somebody to do the work, not just play around. And he was like daydreaming in nowhere, you know? And I started helping him and Jeff says, "I'm going to hire her."

So I was basically right on the spot. I go, "Thank you, thank you."

So ever since, I really get the work done. I don't play around.

Bea: And I'm Bea R. and I live in Soudertown, Pennsylvania, which is about 2 hours away from Karen. I've just actually moved a half of an hour farther away. We had been about an hour and 15 minutes apart. I'm the mother of four children who are just grown; they're college-age children. I'm a person that's very involved with people in my life —who likes people.

I think I would have to say that Karen and I do have a real friendship. I mean, we enjoy each other's company. We got started when Carol Nettleton told us to choose partners and I guess Karen and I had already sort of hit it off. Each time we'd gotten together, we seemed to wind up talking together. So it was a natural thing. I have to give credit to Karen for being the one that really called the first couple of times. I'm a hard person to catch up with.

Karen: Yeah, she is. She's definitely a hard person to catch up with.

Bea: But I found that each time Karen called I really enjoyed our conversations and we always wound up trying to set something up at that time to get together at a later date. It was something I looked forward to.

Karen: No, it's not that big a problem—I don't make that much telephone calls to people anyway. I can always work something out. I mean, I can try and maybe like take the bus down to meet her or something. And she'll make sure I get the right connections. I don't have a problem with buses. As long as I can get connections I'm alright.

Bea: And it depends on where we're going or what we're doing, I mean, as to how we get together. We're going to have to rearrange it now that I've moved. But before, we talked about you coming in on the city bus and meeting me at work. And other times we've connected it with Speaking For Ourselves and we've done something from there. But it's also involved a third person from time to time—when we've gotten together with Sally Ann.

Karen: Sally Ann, yeah. So we've been really trying to keep in touch, trying to do things together.

Bea: But we are with different chapters of Speaking For Ourselves: I'm with Montgomery County chapter.

Karen: And I'm with Chester.

Bea: But we went to Longwood Gardens together. We've gone out to dinner together several times. Karen's come out and spent the night.

Karen: Yeah, I spent a night with her one week.

Bea: And you met my son and my family.

Karen: Very nice family. I got to meet all of her animals and stuff. She has two.

Bea: I've been out to your apartment.

Karen: Right.

Bea: And I've met your cat and your roommate. And a friend of yours. And I guess it's just been whatever we're thinking of, you know. I think our greatest thing has been to be able to talk with each other.

Karen: Yeah. When I feel down, she's always there for me, you know, so I don't feel that I need somebody to talk to; she's always there. I have a lot of problems with—remember I was telling you at a Speaking For Ourselves picnic?—I was telling you about how can I deal with my boyfriend? And she was giving me some advice, what I should do, you know, how I should go about it.

Bea: I guess it's woman-to-woman talk.

Karen: Yeah, woman-to-woman talk, you can say that. She gives good advice when you need it.

Bea: And I guess there was that time when you were getting ready to have an operation. And you were kind of afraid of that and we were able to talk about it.

Karen: Yes, something like that. But she's there for me when you need her.

Bea: But likewise, it's been very good with different things that have happened in my life that I wanted to tell Karen. When my daughter was expecting a child, and then had the baby. And now there's another wedding coming up. And my new home. We're both looking forward to her coming out and visiting my new home.

One of the things that was very important to me in purchasing my new home was to have a place that I could have people visit because I wanted Karen to come out.

As far as other people are concerned, we haven't really told too many people that we're partners. I haven't told too many people. So people don't really know what Speaking For Ourselves and what partners really are. On the other hand I have to say that my family all knows who Karen is. Because you've met my oldest son. Did you ever meet Ann-Marie when she was home? Or was she just there when we were talking on the phone?

Karen: No, I never really met your daughter.

Bea: So, OK. But my family does know who Karen is. And as I said, there's another young lady that I've introduced Karen to and we've had a chance to talk. She looks forward to seeing Karen every now and then, too.

Karen: Sally Ann?

Bea: Sally Ann, yeah.

Karen: I like to share some things with Bea once in a while. I was telling Bea that my parents invited me to Florida this year for Christmas. For the very first time. My ma, she called and she said, "Well, Karen, we decided this year that we should all get together for the whole month of January."

So I told Bea the news and she was really happy that I got a chance to go to Florida this year. I never have. Bea's there for me when I want to talk. My mother or father, because she lives so far away, I don't call much. But Bea's there. Anytime I'm feeling that way, I'll call Bea or something like that. She tells me her stuff that goes on in her family, and I tell her stuff, you know, that goes on with me. Which is nice. I like having Bea for a partner because she's very understandful.

Bea: And I enjoy having Karen for a partner. I mean I think it's been a real mutual enjoyment for both of us. I guess I've enjoyed having Karen for a friend as much as I've enjoyed any other woman as a friend. Karen is a friend that I really enjoy being with. It came about through Speaking For Ourselves, but I do enjoy planning things and being with Karen. I have children that are away and I have really looked forward to the times that we get together. It makes my life fuller for me.

Karen: I feel the same way.

Bea: No, I guess the only disappointment here is that we were really looking forward to the Flower Show. But then we were able to schedule Longwood Gardens to sort of make up for that.

If I had to talk about high points, I'd just say that I've enjoyed laughing with you. I think it's just that we both seem to have somewhat of the same type of a sense of humor and I've enjoyed laughing. And acting silly sometimes.

Karen: On the future, I hope that I'll be able to spend more time with Bea. Like get over there and start taking buses and stuff like that. Planning to see each other a lot more.

Bea: I would—and I really haven't said anything to Karen about this because it hasn't been something that was possible this year—but I would actually like to go on a mini-vacation with Karen. It's something that I would hope to do at some point. Because last year, with so many things happening in my life, I didn't take a vacation. We were hoping to go to Massachusetts—remember about the project on state advocacy? And it's different now that you have both Saturday and Sunday off. That's going to be a benefit because before Karen used to work every Saturday and the only thing we could do was to get together on Sunday. That was another thing that we did together. You came to my church and you were part of the service with me in church.

Karen: That was the day we went to Longwood Gardens.

Bea: Yeah, I guess that was the same day. And I think we've had good discussions about that, about spiritual life.

Karen: Well, Speaking For Yourselves got me in a partnership. I just thought to myself that Bea would be a good partner for someone. And that's when I asked her, when they first started partnerships. I went up to Bea and asked her: "Bea, would you be my partner?"

She said, "Sure."

And so she did. So that's how I really got to know Bea really well.

Bea: And then we got together when we went over those stones. That stone I picked is still on my desk at work. We were asked to pick a stone out to describe ourselves and we talked about it with our partners as to why we picked a specific stone and what it meant. And to me it was so revealing because I hadn't really opened up and talked about myself that much before. But I felt very comfortable telling Karen at that time why I picked that stone. It was a stone with many cracks and crevices and dimensions to it. And I guess that night what I was talking about was very meaningful to me.

Karen: I know there's a lot of people out there right now who are in Speaking For Yourselves and they don't have partners. And what we could do is maybe we could, me and Bea and I could 'courage them on what partners are all about.

Bea: I think that partners are a very good thing. I know that initially people were told that they had to ask each other and had to agree to be partners. I do think that the make-up of people and the compatibility is important. There's a person I'm thinking of who chose me as a partner who is no longer a part of Speaking For Ourselves. This is the person that we've referred to; that we've sometimes been a trio with. This Sally Ann. And I am still pretty much a friend of hers equally and aside from Karen. But again, although I myself would like to be partners to anyone that asked me, it's been very easy for me because Karen and I just fit. And it's been equally as easy for me with the other person. But I think there has to be some meshing. Now, whether people can develop themselves, I guess is another question. I mean you've got to try it, work on it. I think it's more than just a phone call and saying you're partners. I guess that's what I'm trying to say. Karen and I have both worked on this relationship.

Karen: I feel that I have other partners, but I keep more contact with you than I do with the others. Jim S. doesn't keep in touch at all. So basically two or three others. But I have always keep more up to date with Bea.

Bea: This word *partners* and the whole thing from when we first talked, at one of the sessions with Carol Nettleton, and the importance of being a part of that other person's life—there was a solemness, a commitment that we weren't doing this lightly. Which is different than meeting someone, becoming acquainted, and going to the same church Sunday after Sunday. Or being part of the same tennis team. In other words, this was something that we made a commitment to. And out of that a very good relationship has grown.

I guess one of the hardest times for me has been when Karen was very open to me about some of her dreams and my knowing there's nothing I can do to change things or help her. That's been very hard for me. Because there are times I would want to suggest to her to do something—something I would say normally to anybody—and yet I know that there are barriers for Karen. And I would like to just take those barriers and break them down so that I could see her dreams come true, the way she'd like to have them. That's been a very hard thing for me. I think you (Karen) know what I'm talking about.

RICHARD AND THOM

Richard is a stocky man with neatly parted hair, strong vocal chords, and a straight-ahead look. Thom has an easy smile and a beard turning grey some years earlier than it might have been expected to.

Richard: I do the lobby mainly; I clean the lobby at McDonald's— sweeping, mopping, tables—what's called the lobby. The dining room, actually. And I live in Morrisville. I live with my parents and I have four sisters and four brother-in-laws and one niece and two nephews. I've been working at McDonald's for about 4 years. Yes, I've seen everybody come and go. I guess I'm one of the long-term employees. I remember at last year's retreat, I talked to Carol Nettleton. She asked me why would I want to become a partner. And I asked for a simple reason: I feel that partners can talk together. And then last year Carol asked me, "Who do you think would be a good partner?" And Thom Cramer's been my partner since last year at the retreat.

Thom: I think I remember that, because Carol also came up to me later and she said, "I think you're going to have a good partner in that Richard H." But the other part of that is, you know, that you came and asked me. I was really honored by that. It's nice to be asked.

Richard: I was the chapter president at that time and I felt I needed a little more support and partners do give you support.

Thom: I think more of our partnership has been about chapter stuff than anything outside of that. I don't get out Richard's way too often. But when I do, I try to stop and have a burger at McDonald's.

Richard: We talk together about different things.

Thom: Mostly I've been calling him. He doesn't do a whole lot of the calling back yet. We've been working on that together.

Richard: We're working on that together.

Thom: We both have such crazy lives.

Richard: When I'm at work, he's home. And when I'm home, he's . . .

Thom: I'm at work. Also Richard has his own kind of circle of some friends. I'm talking about the men in your church.

Richard: Yes, yes, I do.

Thom: That's not really a part of the partnership.

Richard: No.

Thom: But I think it's a big thing about what goes on in your community.

Richard: Yeah.

Thom: I'll just mention it and you can tell more about it. Richard's in a men's breakfast club, a church breakfast club that gets together . . . how often?

Richard: Once a week, every Wednesday morning.

Thom: And how many people are in that club?

Richard: Well, it's about, maybe it ranges about 15.

Thom: And you bring them to McDonald's, right?

Richard: (laughing) No, no, no, no.

Thom: That would work in business. But this is the male members of the congregation. There's a lot of them?

Richard: Yes.

Thom: And it has nothing to do with disabilities.

Richard: No, no.

Thom: It's just an interest group of men who get together. And then in the summer what did you do? What was your vacation this summer?

Richard: Well, in the summertime my vacation was I went up to Maine. It was my church group. We did different projects like sheet-rocking and painting. We did 10 different projects in 1 week.

Thom: And they celebrated your birthday, didn't they?

Richard: Yes, they did. And it was a surprise to me. I didn't even know that they were going to make a cake at that point.

Thom: Anyway, so that's what Richard does for me is he tells me all these great stories about his adventures and things that he does. I'm trying to see if maybe sometime he'll invite me to breakfast and I can meet some of these guys that are your friends. Richard and I, we've known each other . . . Well, you came to some of the first Speaking For Ourselves meetings 9, 10 years ago. Bucks County was the first chapter that started. Back then it was all just called Speaking For Ourselves, until it got big enough and then the idea of chapters came up. And I was living in Doylestown at the time and we invited some folks that we knew to come and we started a chapter up there. And Richard you got involved in it shortly—I don't even remember when or where.

Richard: I don't even know either.

Thom: But I know you showed up at one of the meetings we had at a church. Then we went to the community college, but it's hard to find.

Richard: It's hard to find, but it's more central located, I think.

Thom: And then Richard was elected president.

Richard: Actually I was not elected, Thom.

Thom: What would you call it—more like appointed?

Richard: Yeah, more appointed.

Thom: Well, no, there was an election. I remember I was a lot more controlling at that time.

Richard: Yes.

Thom: But we had a real election and you were elected by the majority of the vote. That was after Louis; I guess you followed Louis?

Richard: About, yeah, about 4 years after.

Thom: So we've always had this working relationship. But the partnership seems to have kicked things into a different gear. It has a different quality to it now; it's more personal. You never told me those stories about your travels before. A partnership is a different kind of relationship. It's a conscious kind of a joining with a person rather than being together because of work. I think we could—we can—probably get together a little more and do more. But that's as much mine as it is yours. That's just life. Richard never comes over to take care of my kids for the weekend.

Richard: Oh yeah, right, Thom. And Thom never comes over . . .

Thom: I don't come over to flip hamburgers at McDonald's.

Richard: No. And Thom never comes to my house.

Thom: No, I usually just drop you off. Because by that time it's like 9:30, 10:00 at night and I want to go home.

Richard: But you never come for a weekend even.

Thom: Hey listen. (laughing). Don't make that offer.

Richard: I guess when we moved to Bucks County Community College, I guess it mainly was because we had that conference there.

Thom: Yeah we did, we had a real successful conference there. Although it was a lot of work. I guess Richard was the m.c. at that time.

Richard: Yes, I was. Boy, after that, my voice was kind of raw.

Thom: We had 100 people.

Richard: And our chapter there, when we first started it, we had about four or five people attending. Now we have, I don't know exactly how many people.

Thom: Like 28 people or something.

Richard: Yeah. We've grown.

Thom: Now with the new president, we'll probably have *good* meetings.

Richard: Yeah. (He registers what Thom has said.) I don't know about that. I don't know about that, Thom.

Thom: If there's one thing that Richard and I share it's a terrible sense of humor. But we're able to use it on each other.

Richard: But I kind of think with the new president, Charlie B.—
I think I can give him support that he needs.

Thom: So now you've moved on to bigger and better things. What
are you now?

Richard: Secretary of the board.

Thom: No, I probably wouldn't have known Richard without the
organization.

Richard: Oh, that's right. I probably wouldn't have known Thom
either without the organization.

Thom: And my association with people in Bucks County especially was usually through referral from the base service units. But
then it's usually because of problems and since you're such a
troublemaker. . . .

Richard: Oh, oh yeah, right.

Thom: Actually, I'm too serious. My personal relationship would
have been kind of therapist to client. But this way, I mean, with
Speaking For Ourselves, it's just a relationship. I don't even think they
know what I do. And it doesn't even matter.

Richard: No, I don't think people in Speaking For Ourselves
know what I do either. I don't think it really matters.

Thom: But you're learning a lot of skills. Richard has figured out
public transportation now; he can get from here back to Morrisville, I
think. Of course, he'd have to take the train into Trenton and then
cross the river, but he's got it down. I think you're also getting a lot
of confidence, too. I just watched you grow and I've really had fun
watching all of the things that you're doing. Also watching your parents. You do a whole lot more than you did 6, 7 years ago. But I think
it's almost essential to have some kind of sponsor, some kind of
framework to help these relationships either get started or, if they
were already there, get onto a new level. I mean, Richard and I would
always have a relationship. But not at this level. Partnership is a conscious reaching of the hand from one to the other, a kind of affirming
of one another, saying, "Yes, you are my partner." Which is different
than, "Yes, you're a fellow member," or, "Yes, you're my advisor."

It's a whole different flavor. If Speaking For Ourselves were to stop,
we'd still have a partnership. But it wouldn't have started if it hadn't
been for Speaking For Ourselves. I think in a broader sense the partnerships enriched the whole organization. It's nothing that you can
put your finger on. You get this feeling that people are much more
deeply involved in each other's lives. But this summer was crazy with
the new baby, so Richard and I really didn't get in touch.

Richard: Generally we don't have meetings in July and August.

Thom: And normally I wouldn't even think about that. It was like those were almost days off—I mean months off—from having meetings. But I thought about you. I thought, I need to give Richard a call. What I didn't do is do it.

Richard: You didn't do it to me.

Thom: Well, I have a crazy schedule in the summertime.

Richard: Well, yes, I think I did feel a little shaky about it. I thought we should do more.

Thom: Yeah, we were both thinking it, but neither one of us acted on it. But that's on another plane. I mean, at least we were thinking about it. The summer before that, there wasn't even a thought.

Richard: No.

Thom: It's the whole idea of what is freely given. There's a certain quality to it. It's not because of some other duty. Even though the work that I do with these guys is voluntary, it was still almost like a job kind of a thing. But everyone should have friends. That's really what partnership is about. And unfortunately people that are not part of the community are going to need some structure to help them make those ties. But once the ties are made, you know, they last.

Richard: I think that the partnership has supported me a lot. I do agree with that. And even my church group that I belong to (has) given me a lot of support. And then my parents have been giving me support too, I think. But my parents don't like the times that I take days off from work.

Thom: Your parents like hard workers.

Richard: Hard workers, yeah. But I like to work, too.

Thom: It seems like partnerships have given the go-ahead to people to deepen their relationships. You already had a relationship of long standing, but it stayed at a certain point.

Richard: I didn't know how to go about it until the retreat last year. Now I have a whole different structure in my life. And I would miss not having a partner (to go and talk to if I had a problem).

Thom: It's interesting that you say that because we really haven't had any problems that we've had to resolve.

Richard: No.

Thom: I've seen this from other people that I talk to about the partnership thing. There's just that knowledge that there is someone to go to outside of family or staff. Almost like knowing that you have your wife.

Richard: I felt that Thom was always a friend to me. Even when we met with our chapter, I felt you were my friend. But I didn't know how to go about being a partner.

Thom: You've done pretty well; you figured it out: You moved out to me. But if I had to say anything else I'd say that I would like you to call more.

Richard: Yeah.

Thom: And I'll call you more, too.

Richard: (He looks for something to say next.)

Thom: What should I call you?

Richard: Oh, oh, oh (laughing). (The time comes to close the interview.)

Thom: Say, "Salutos, amigos!"

Richard: Salutos, amigos!

Thom: Richard also speaks Spanish. And not too bad, either. Is it Mexico? Your sister married a Mexican prince or something?

Richard: A Mexican person. And now I have a 4-year-old niece. And you know, my niece stayed overnight last night.

Thom: Oh, great! You know, actually your niece and my son were born right around the same time.

KELVIN AND STEVE

Kelvin is a compact man, with brown skin, and a subdued twinkle in his eye. He gets from place to place in a wheelchair. He often leaves long spaces between his words when he speaks, but he is quite fluent—also very quick—when he stumbles on the notion that he's after. Steve has a pale complexion, black hair, and a captivating smile. He gets around by means of crutches into which his forearms fit. He speaks thoughtfully and quietly, but his voice rises when he wants to emphasize something humorous.

Kelvin: My name is Kelvin A. I go to (he names an agency that provides services during the day). And that's about it during the week.

Steve: My name is Steve D. and I live in Folcroft by the Philadelphia Airport. Mostly all my time is taken up by Speaking For Ourselves. If I have board meetings or something like that, that night, I usually go in early in the morning and stay. I help the office out. I just got back from Massachusetts. (Speaking For Ourselves has contracts to do surveys of self-advocacy groups in four nearby states.) And while I was in Massachusetts, we went to Gunnar Dybwad's house and had lunch with him. Him and his wife are 82 years old—both. He showed us the deck he has built on his house in the backyard. He asked about what Speaking For Ourself was doing these days. He told me how he also wants to write another book on it. So we can never tell what Speaking For Ourself is going to do from day to day.

Kelvin: Yeah, I live near—not near—in West Oak Lane.

Steve: We talk once in a while on the telephone. If he has problems, he usually calls. But we haven't got together. With schedules the way they are, we're getting to be so busy. My family thinks it's great. Because I've got Mark (Mark Friedman is a full-time advisor to Speaking For Ourselves), I've got Kelvin, and myself. We had to go ask each person if they would like to be our partner. And what we did is we went in the big hallway and we exchanged phone numbers and then what we did is each person had asked the other person if they want to be their partner. And luckily for mine, Mark said, yes. I mean, he could have said, no. But, you know, luckily he said, yes. That must be a thing in my favor. I spent a lot of time with Mark—going on trips, things like that—we spend a lot of time talking about what a partnership does for each other, how has it helped me, and how has it helped him to be a partner. When I have a problem, I can call the office. And if he doesn't get back to me right away, I understand that. Mark and Diana they both work in the office. When I come in, either one of them will take me to lunch. The last time I was there, we ate Chinese food. I think it also helps me too because they understand what our "handi-capable" people come from. You know Debby has problems (Reference to the physical challenges of Debby R. who is the current president of the organization. She uses crutches like Steve's.) We both understand what's going to happen to both of us. She has problems walking and it takes her a little longer to get around, but she gets around just like myself. And Kelvin—it takes him a little bit longer to get where he's going, but—pretty sure—you get there, where you have to go. You may have somebody push you and all that, but at least you get there. I think you have to understand if God would have made you the way Mark is, then you wouldn't have to use crutches, you wouldn't have to use a wheelchair or anything like that. I think you would feel better about that. But God, I think, has his own special people to go out and do his work for him, even though they do have handicaps. I feel every day of my life that I could have passed away a long time ago. But thank dear God that I'm around today to help other people understand what handicaps are. You know I commend Kelvin for doing what he's doing for this organization, going different places with different people. That's what it taught me: to go out and do these things with other people. I'm never home anymore. I usually don't see my room anymore unless it's on weekends or something. I'm on the road doing other things with other people. I feel good about that for myself. Kelvin, when you go out, I think you feel that way too. You feel probably that you help other people out to understand what your capabilities are and where you're coming from.

Kelvin: Yeah. Yes, I do. (He has a point he wants to make here, but he is unable to find the words for it. Finally, he tries another way.) But I don't quite hear from him as much as I would like. Some of the stuff that he's telling me now, he never really goes over with me. I would like to talk to him more. But I do like the partnership and my parents are, gosh, supportive. This sounds so mushy. But I still like this idea of partnership. And I do agree with a lot of the things that he said. I never really thought of my disability that much. I can do almost anything a quote—oh, I hate that word—"normal person" can do. The only problem I really think about is when some little kid comes up to me and says something like: "What's wrong with you?" or something. I have always myself found it difficult to answer a question like that. I mean I know they need to ask. It's good for them. But I just don't know how to tell them. Myself, I just have to find the way of answering that question. I do like the fact that I think I'm a little bit more open than I was.

Steve: Mark and I usually see Kelvin at board meetings and things like that. So we either brainstorm that night or the morning of the board meeting. It's not really my fault, it's not really Kelvin's, it's not really Mark's. But it's where I took on more responsibility that I know I can handle. I've got Kelvin, I've got Mark, and last year I took on an added responsibility, my pet project, to answer questions for the people in Mon Valley (the newest chapter of Speaking For Ourselves, near Pittsburgh).

Kelvin: Well, it's a bit more simplistic, but I think partnerships are just to be able to go over how you're feeling or how your day went or things that you are doing. Not necessarily connected to Speaking For Ourselves. It could be how in a sense your life is outside Speaking For Ourselves.

JEROME AND HEATHER

Jerome is an older man with the deep olive skin and the change in color running to black near his eyes that signal the Mediterranean origin of his family. He carries a cigar in his shirt pocket. Heather was unable to make the retreat.

Jerome: No, sir, I live in Coatesville, Pennsylvania, PA. And Heather is my partner. She live in Norristown, PA. I'm the vice president in charge of fund raiser and I get paid for my job and I got a-sponsibility. I did for a while without pay. But June the 25th of 1991 the board picked me for . . . July, August, September, October . . . about 4 months I'm working for Speaking For Ourselves.

Heather is working in Norristown. I can't answer for Heather, for my partner. I miss my partner when she not here. She give me a support. We go out and have dinner and then we start talkin' about different things. I give her my support and she give me her support.

Speaking For Ourself asked us couple of year ago do we want a partner. At the meeting they said that we could have one or two or three. So, I asked Bill first and then I asked Heather. But it take a while with Heather because I still had Bill. He teached me how be a partner and he teached me how, anything happen to him, I could help my other partner. I don't want to get into detail. I still miss Bill, because Bill was a part of Speaking For Ourselves and plus he was a partner. I don't want to get down into detail and tell other people what happened. I'm going to keep that private.

But Heather and I, we keep in touch with each other. I call her, then she call me, then we ask could we go out and have dinner. If we don't have too private things to talk, then we 'vite couple other friends. And we got something 'portant it would just be Heather and I. Well, both times we went over Heather 'partment; she just moved in in Norristown. She got on Market Street, a nice 'partment. And other times we go out and had dinner. Sometime we go out in the country. Heather will always say it will be up to me and her where we want to go. We just make a plan and then we go from there.

Heather ain't too far from Speaking For Ourself office; she right in Norristown. I can take the transportation, I can take 98 bus from Plym' Meeting Mall and take me right to her office.

Trans-a-tation is hard all around Pennsylvania. My partner live in Norristown; I live in Coatesville. But I travel all time. The other one could do it, but the staff won't let them go because the staff say, "That's not our part to take you anywhere; we don't get paid for it."

Same as when you're married, you can't do it. You got to be home wit your wife. And sometime you say, "Why did I get married for? I'm sorry to get married now."

Yes, sir, I always did live by myself. Sometimes you get bored, but I have something I can do. No, sir. I don't have no contact with my family member. I'm still hurt what happened my first partner. And what I say, I don't want to talk about it. Because my other partner not around; Bill D. is not around. And I just can't talk about it right now because I'm hurt when he did suicide. It just hurt my . . . It just hurt me, the hard time that I had when I lost Bill. I didn't want any more partner. But Heather did prove herself. She gave me more support and it feel like that's what I need and that's what a partner all about. You got to give your other partner support. After Bill died, I didn't talk to Heather for a while. I was in shot (shock) for a couple of month; I didn't talk to anybody.

But Heather, when we first start, we didn't try to be a partner. You know, it's hard to be a partner. But she did prove herself and I'm proving myself. Her and I working like a partner. We can show other partner how to be a partner and then would be up to them how they feel.

But as far as the good times, oh man, we're having a good time right now; we having a ball. In the future I don't know what Heather and I are going to come up yet. We got some plan that I don't want to get into it because my partner ain't here. So far, we might go out on a trip. We talking about go down the shore for a couple of days. And I asked Heather if she like to go down the horse race.

But I got a hope in the future: hope we could do more and help other partner in Speaking For Ourself. I think I'm going to talk to Heather —could we have a meeting somewhere, show the other partners in how to be good partners, how could you help each other out if they just watch Heather and I do it.

I can tell you this—without Speaking For Ourself I don't know how to do anything. I wouldn't know how be the president in the Chester County, Philadelphia. I wouldn't know how to be the vice president. But most important how I can do the vice president job is John F. Kennedy. Kennedy say not what the country could do for you, but what you could do for your country. And that's how I learned to be the vice president.

Did we have the pro'lems? I don't know, I can't say; I can't remember. I did tell Heather I got permoted, that I'm the vice president in charge of fund raiser and I'm getting paid. And she said congratulation to me. She make me feel good. But sometime I feel down in the dump when I call her and I just tell her, "Can you keep something in private?"

And she said, "Whatever we talk about, if we want to keep in private, I will."

And I don't have any other body over there sometimes, just her and I.

BOB AND GEORGE

Bob is a big man with a small t-shirt. He holds his sides in excitement over being interviewed and laughs, revealing the missing tips of the two teeth at the top of his smile. George is tall and wiry. He has an intense air about him, but it is crossed with an almost perpetual smile, at least throughout this weekend, evidently brought on by his standing within this organization.

Bob: I'm Bob C. I live on Second Street. Bridgepor'. I work on Marsha'. On Concha'? (At Marshall's in Conshohocken.) I clean all the stores. Vac' the rugs.

George: My name's George W. I live in Drexel Hill in an SLA situation. I go to (he names a rehabilitation center) during the day. I clean; I'm a custodian. I do the same thing Bob does.

Bob: Up here . . .

George: . . . last year. I talked to Diana about getting a partner and she hooked me up with Bob. (Diana is the office manager for Speaking For Ourselves.) Yes, we do live far apart. But we started calling each other right away. And we kept making plans, but we never got around to getting together. We want to go to the mall or something like that for the day. Hang out, you know? Go to the movies.

Bob: You check the newspaper. We never got to it.

George: Something kept coming up. Yes, we both take public transportation. Maybe he come over my place for a long weekend.

Bob: Come to my house.

George: If your mom lets me come over your place for the weekend, you know.

Bob: Yeah.

George: Uh-huh, I'm allowed. Only thing I got to do is tell Michael. Call my coordinator, my counselor, a week in advance and that's it. That's no problem.

Bob: I like raps. You know—raps?

George: Oldies. (This in answer to a question about their common interests.)

Bob: You used to work at Hardee's, remember?

George: Yeah, I used to have a job at Hardee's and that didn't work out. That was just recently. They . . .

Bob: . . . fire you.

George: No, they didn't fire me; I quit. They wanted me to work too many hours and they wouldn't give me a break. Yeah, it did help me to talk. See, where I lived at before, it was a restrictive CLA. That means you don't have all the freedom you want. And I refused to live in that kind of situation. So that's why I pushed, pushed, pushed my way out of that place. And the way I feel—if those people, those counselors that I don't get along with, if they do see the article, I don't care. It don't bother me. You know what I'm saying? Cause I'm just telling the truth. And if they don't like it, you know where they can go. That's the way I feel.

Bob: I live with my mom. I'll gi' you my alldre' (address). Yeah, Michael, Jennie. Michael's is my stepbrothers in the group home. And Jennie's in a group home, too. Ray's is my father. And my mom is...mom. The one girl in there had the jumpsuit? She send the letter home (Diana).

George: My mom thinks it's good for me. She likes me to keep myself occupied. She likes me being involved with this organization.

Because I used to have a problem before—just sitting around and all. I would hear all these voices. And, you know, I don't want to. I don't want to get talking about this, because this is something that's passed. You know what I mean? I'm moving on to the future, not the past.

Bob: I miss George. No, I'm with the libri' chap'er (the Montgomery County Chapter meets at the Norristown library).

George: I'm Delaware County. Israel's my boss, 'cause I'm the vice president of Delaware County now. (Israel is the president and George's recent election to the vice presidency is apparently one of the reasons he's happy.)

Bob: When did you call me, Geor?

George: A week before . . .

Bob: . . . you get the jo', workin' at Hardee's.

George: Yeah, that was a hard time, when I was in that other program. I was only allowed 15-minute calls at a time.

Bob: He got out. Move out.

George: Someone got me involved working with the county. My county case manager. And my therapist from (he names an agency that provides services . . .). And my therapist's boss and my therapist and the county must have got together and got me this help. 'Cause they knew I was fed up with it. That's the only thing I can think of.

Bob: Listen. Yeah.

George: You have to listen.

Bob: Talking to people, yeah. That's what. Talking to people and no talking back.

George: That's what partners are.

DEWEESE AND SHARON

DeWeese's control of the world around him seems to extend far beyond the bounds of the wheelchair he sits in. He has a winning smile and can talk, apparently, for hours at a time—maybe for days—with only the most imperceptible of nudges to get him started. Sharon was forced to reschedule for the next day.

DeWeese: You don't have any of this on tape? I'm just trying to make sure that it's working this time. I've already done this a couple of times and I got everybody down.

I don't know how Sharon came to Speaking For Ourself. You'll have to ask her yourself. All I know is she met me and she hasn't regretted it a day since.

I was trying to be the brave soldier, okay? Nothing was gonna get through to me. I tried to hide the fact that I was hurting. I didn't fit anywhere. I was trying to be a superman. I was struggling with my own identity. People said, "You don't let nobody in unless it's absolutely necessary."

I met Sharon at this retreat and we started talking and the next thing you know, we started really becoming close. I guess one of the ways I think that me and Sharon kind of hit it off is because she's so warm, caring, and sensitive. Now that doesn't mean to say that she doesn't have a temper, okay? Like when I got all the bad news all in one year about my family, I just wanted to get out of here, Okay? I wanted to go somewhere where nobody knew me and I wanted to start over again. Which I'm still going to do eventually. But where Sharon got fed up at this point in our relationship, she said that, "Alright, DeWeese! Look, enough is enough! okay? I've had it! I don't want to hear it. You're not going to move to Texas." You know? And it's like I got mad at her. Because she thought that I was talking about leaving at that moment. My dream is still to own a ranch, but you got to do it step by step. I guess what I was trying to get her to do was to get prepared for when I *do* move to Texas. Because eventually I want to get out of Pennsylvania.

But I was running away and my running away wouldn't have solved nothing. My grandmother always used to tell me that. Running away from something doesn't solve it. It doesn't make it go away. It's still there when you get right back to where you are. So running away from something didn't make it any easier for me.

Sharon and I have arguments and disagreements. Like if you're married, I'm sure you have arguments with your wife. But because you're married, you all got to come through them. And that's the way me and Sharon's relationship work out. It worked out because God saw that we were two special people.

Now there's a lot about Sharon and me. We're friends because we're both honest. And we're both older now. So I don't have as much time to say, "Well, I want to move to Texas." Even though that's in the back of my mind.

I'm planning to start my own woodworking business now. And when I get it going good, I won't be at the workshop anymore. One of the things that I find about starting your own business is that it's rough. If I don't like the way a piece of wood is, I have to draw up another whole set of plans. And one of the things I've found by hanging in there with Sharon is that she will do anything for anyone. She got $100 from her church and I put $20 to it so that made it $120. And we bought an electric saw and a leveler and gloves and a T square. And I have the wood. I made my pastor a birdhouse and I have different prices for different things. I'm making hope chests. I'm making spice racks. I'm working on two spice racks now as a matter of fact. So Sharon's helped me realize that there's a lot of good and there's a lot of bad. But there's more good-hearted people than there are bad. Sharon's helped me realize that as long as we work together, everything will be fine. She's helped me to realize this. Stuff that I wouldn't have even thought of. I wouldn't have thought of going to the board in the church and asking them for $100. Thanks to her 'cause she's helped me see that maybe it isn't bad that I start my own business. And I told Sharon that Jack G. said that I could start my own business in our group home. He's the director of (he names a local agency); he's the big boss. I was happy. I called Sharon first. I was just like a kid. Going on and on. I was just real happy that he said yes. But he told me, "I don't want you to quit your job—OK?—until you get set up."

So, I got to turn my room into an office. I haven't done it yet. I have to first get all set up with tools and stuff and different kind of stain.

She went with me after I came from Philadelphia one time I had to go to court. The judge sent me home, 'cause she said, "Well, I don't need anybody today." (Apparently the court proceedings didn't go according to plan and they weren't able to get to DeWeese that day.) And so I was kind of upset. But I was kind of glad too. Because that day she sent everybody home, Sharon said, "You want to go do some shopping?"

On the day that I finally did have to go to court to deal with this case from 5 years ago—and this case was about a man who raped me; the owner raped me who owned this home where I lived. It was real hard for me because after all the case was 5 years ago and I thought they had the guy and he only did 30 days probation. So I had to dredge up the old memories of what he did. I couldn't say, "You raped me." I had to just stick to the facts that my lawyer wanted me to stick to: Was the food any good; what kind of clothes did you wear? You know, stuff like that. And Sharon was really supportive. She got mad when she first heard. But I was like, "Will you calm down? I'm the one that's got to testify."

And she knew how hard it was for me 'cause I wasn't sleeping.

Well, to wrap this up. (He takes a deep breath.) Okay, that Sharon is the warmest person that I've ever known. She's open, she's honest, she's fair, and she's straightforward. If she feels like somebody is going to hurt somebody that she cares about, she'll speak on it. 'Cause she's just that kind of person. Partnership to me means that we hold each other in our hearts. My final thought in closing is this:

Sharon is one of the most caring people that I know and I'm glad we're partners because it just proves that we can go through the good, the bad, and the not so good, and still remain friends. That's it.

DeWeese and Sharon (continued the next day with Sharon)

Because she does not come to Speaking For Ourselves through her work (she is not employed by an agency that provides services, nor is she a therapist), Sharon has a somewhat unique air about her. She is neither a "newcomer" nor an "insider."

Sharon: When I moved to Pennsylvania I didn't know anybody and so I asked my friend Carol Nettleton how I could meet people and she suggested that I try Speaking For Ourselves. She said that this group was outstanding. It was like being drawn into a network of folks who are really talented and creative—it gives you a lot of energy. But I still didn't know how to join in. Everyone seemed to be so close to each other and I still felt like an outsider. The partnership idea gave me a way to deepen a relationship. DeWeese and I are in the same chapter and we met there. But it was here at Fellowship Farm 2 years ago when DeWeese was going through a time of grief. He'd had some losses in his family and he had parked his wheelchair out here on the lot. He was by himself and I just went over and started talking to him. I think because of some of the experiences that I've had in my life with a loss, we just really connected with each other on that level. And it was that same year that Carol was here and that's when we committed to be partners. DeWeese asked me to be his partner.

And then immediately after that, when we came back home, his birthday was the next week and I had him at my house for his birthday. Because his family didn't do anything for him. And I began to see how important his family was to him, but how disappointing. And that he needed my family. And so since then we've celebrated all the holidays together. And we go to church together—eventually he joined my church—and we talk on the phone every day. Those kind of things.

My husband gets along really well with DeWeese. At church on Sunday we have two levels in the building and we have to get DeWeese onto a lift and then up and down the steps. So Dan helps me with that. And my youngest daughter, Janette, loves DeWeese. She likes to help push the wheelchair and just kind of hang out with him. My oldest son doesn't want DeWeese around. I think he's kind of threatened by anybody who's different. Also, his friends make fun of people a lot and I think he's kind of torn. His loyalties are torn between his friends and how he relates to DeWeese as a person. So I'm really hoping that he'll grow in that way, to accept people as they are. My middle son is cordial when asked to be, but he has his own agenda.

Perhaps I have been disappointed in the partnership now and again. But it's because of me: I'm a person who's so oriented to caring and fixing things and, you know, making things good for people, that I don't always see my own needs. And so I think one way that I'm disappointed—but it's my own fault—is I'm just not vulnerable enough. And DeWeese is really teaching me that, just as he can call me and talk to me about anything, he would like me to be able to do that too with him. I tend to do that more with my husband and maybe one or two other friends. But I'm learning. And I think it's very important in a partnership to have that. I've also learned a lot about what I would call caring and not curing. When you're talking to someone, not trying to give advice or fix everything up but just to listen and be someone who's there. And DeWeese appreciates that. A year ago in August my brother was killed in an accident and DeWeese was very supportive during that time. Because of the losses that he'd had, he could really understand. He let me be angry and he let me be hurt and that was really good. And sometimes DeWeese is just like me, you know? He tries to fix me up and he wants everything to just be wonderful in my life. And I have to remind him that I just need him to listen, too. So I think we've both grown in that way.

One of the best times we've had together came right back to back with a very hard time this past week. DeWeese had to be in court 2 days to testify in a trial and it was a painful thing emotionally to go through because it brought up a lot of memories. But our church gave him some money to help him with his woodworking business. So we planned to go out to lunch and go shopping right after this trial. It was really fun to do that together.

I think our partnership works well because we live so close to each other. We're just 10 minutes away and I know that if DeWeese really needed me, I could be there very quickly. I just have a very strong sense of DeWeese as part of my life. And part of my family.

But living in a group home makes the relationship harder sometimes because the person does not have total say over what happens in their life. Everything has to be filtered through that experience. And I find that very frustrating sometimes.

Speaking For Ourselves has helped in the partnership because it brought us together. But also I watch people in this organization and they model relationships that are really positive and caring. That's an important role that the organization plays.

I think if other people wanted to have partners, they'd need to consider the time commitment, because it's major. It has been for me. Or you could decide as partners how much time you're willing to give. But make sure the other person understands that and be clear with what you're able to do, to avoid some disappointment.

DeWeese has gotten started on his business. I went to his house to see what he was up to, expecting this little bird house. The bird house was this tall and this wide. (She indicates with her hands a birdhouse an eagle might feel comfortable in.) If a baby bird was ever hatched in the bottom, he would die there. There's no way he could get out. Unless he learned to fly in the box, I guess that's a possibility. But you know, DeWeese did his level best on it and he only had hand saws. He actually did a very good job making the corners neat and making it actually a square box. But he's going to work on some spice racks now and I just can't wait to see them. He's so sincere and he really wants to make this work. It's hard for me not to be the voice of caution and discouragement. I just set my lips. And yet, on the other hand, I'm working with him to explore some training possibilities. The workshop doesn't seem to want to get him out of there. I think they're dependent on those people for their funding and so they don't work very hard on getting them real jobs. But I've been trying to build a relationship with his job coach, just to let her know that I'm someone who cares for DeWeese, that I will advocate for him, and that I really think he's capable of being out there. He was before. And he really wants to get out. That's the bottom line: he wants to get out of there. So I feel it's important for me to honor that and try to guide him or encourage him any way I can. So the college partners idea is very intriguing. (This is a new program Speaking For Ourselves has been asked to get involved in.) I'm going to graduate school starting in February. But if I can work in somehow to get him 1 day a week in the classroom, that would be really neat. It's just so great to hear him talk the way he talks about what he wants, about what he envisions in his life. He always has had dreams. For a long time he wanted to go to Texas and be a cowboy. And—I'm sorry, I just could not help it, you know?—I just let him know that I didn't think that was going to be possible. He says, "Well I'm not talking about leaving tomorrow. This is my 5 year plan."

I said, "I can learn something from this man."

Some days I can't cope with today—you know? And he's got a 5 year plan. He really did help me. And so he's taught me that you do have to have dreams. Because I'm not a dreamer. I'm a real practical person. I can think of a million reasons why you shouldn't do something. So he's affected my life, too. And I'm just really thankful for the chance to be a part of it.

The other thing I really like about DeWeese is that he's black and I'm white. And I think not too many people get a chance to have friendships across race in our culture without doing it very intentionally. But it seems just very natural for us. Definitely a person-to-person relationship. No, the issue doesn't come up so much between us, but in the ways in which race affects DeWeese's life and how his family has rejected him, saying that he's gone over into the white world and white values and ways of doing things. I can't imagine what kind of conflict that would create in a person. But it's a very alive issue for him. We talk about it. It's tough (she laughs). It's a tough one.

DOMENIC AND BETH

Domenic is slight and swarthy with a slightly nasal quality to his voice. Beth is several years younger than Domenic with the look of a person who believes that the world—or at least the part of it she inhabits—can be set right.

Domenic: I live in Norristown and I worked for Jessup Company 7 years and I get tired of it. I want somewheres to work somewheres else in Montgomery County. And every time I try to talk to people they say they don't want people with handicap. Where I'm working at now is terrible. They mistreat me. Stuff like that. It was better when I was there the first 2 years. Then after, it went downhill. They blame everything on you. If something goes wrong with the machine, they blame it on you. I got tired of it. Yeah, the boss changed a lot during that time. No, there's nobody working on another job for me. You know how the 'conomy is.

Beth: But something too, Dom, that we were just talking about today was using your contacts. That's something of what I do is support people in finding jobs over in Bucks County. So what we were thinking of doing is doing it together. But with not just me, with Dom's other contacts. You know, Terry. He's a contact. Dom met Terry through myself. Terry's down at the Sixers (Philadelphia Seventy-Sixers basketball).

Domenic: I love the Sixers. I keep an eye on the college and I tell them who's good guys for the Sixers for next year. I didn't contact him yet.

Beth: Well, no, but that's part of networking. You're looking to build like a circle around you.

Domenic: Right. Yeah, I do so good for the other people, right?

Beth: Uh-huh.

Domenic: But nobody supports me.

Beth: Oh, am I chopped liver? (She responds to a question.) Yeah, it's easy for me because I have a car. I'm living in Montgomery County now, but I work in Bucks. I'm hoping to eventually get back to Bucks County. I guess we're about 20, 30 minutes away from each other.

Domenic: Right. That's why I'd like to learn how to drive. That's another thing I wanted my partner to help me with: learn how to drive. I know I don't have a car. I just wanted to learn in case of emergency. And let's see, Hope and Bea lives in Montgomery County. Sharon lives in Montgomery County. And later on I'm gonna build more people onto it. Right now is the people here (the people attending the retreat weekend). I'm difficult trying to pick out a good day to pick.

Beth: But have you got commitments from anybody?

Domenic: Not yet. I know Beth would do it. I was thinking putting Joe on it.

Beth: Joe?

Domenic: H. (a local politician). (He stops to consider his plans.) Beth is like a sister to me.

Beth: I guess it's just taken a lot of hard work to get there.

Domenic: It didn't click, me with her, with Beth, until right after the, what?, the ninth conference?

Beth: Is that what you think? I kind of thought it was before. I always liked you. You always made me laugh.

Domenic: 'Cause I know how to make her—make people— laugh. And when she's depressed, I know how to get her out of it.

Beth: It's been a true give-and-take. There's some people who wonder how that can be. But I think I can truly say it's been a really hard year for me and Dom's been there. My grandmother was in the hospital. We were going to get together, but this stuff came up. So Dom came over with me instead and was able to . . .

Domenic: Help her out . . .

Beth: . . . share that.

Domenic: Share. Help her with her problem. Because I went through it. I just went through it. In '75 my mom died. And in January 8 years ago my grandmother died. And Aileen was born 2 weeks after that.

Beth: Oh, that's, that's something else that we clicked on, too. Aileen is Dom's niece who was born to his sister who's a single mom. And in my family I have a nephew who was born to my sister who's a single mom. And so there were . . . commonalities and things. Shared experiences, I guess. And we found that we enjoyed it. It just kind of grows. Dom always worries that I won't call him back. He worries about establishing trust and everything.

Domenic: I'm a-scared of people leaving. People leave who was with me for around 6, 7 years. They just up and left and dint tell me why. When I was living in Ken-Crest, a friend—a good friend of mines—left. And I felt hurt. They dints explain it why. I leave so many messages on her machine and she never calls me back.

Beth: But haven't you had other people move into your life, too?

Domenic: Yeah, I got two friends of mines, Teresa and Lucy. I used to work with them. Teresa got laid off. And Lucy—I can't say anything about it. I told her. I can't say anything about it. And I'm trying to find a girlfriend who lives near me. Like around Norristown or Conshohocken.

Beth: Can I tell what we were talking about this morning?

Domenic: Yeah.

Beth: There's this male/female stuff, too. We were saying it would be easier if we were both guys or we were both women. That male/female barrier sometimes is there. And it's hard to sort the feelings. But we talk it through, I guess. It's been pretty important. Different, I guess. Different friends for different needs.

Domenic: And sometimes I call Mary. She came to the second conference when we had it at Plymouth Meeting Mall (Speaking For Ourselves holds an annual conference). She's not with Speaking For Ourselves, but she calls me "buddy." She calls me "bud." And that made me feel good. That's what Beth doesn't call me. You call me "pal," but no "buddy."

Beth: I do call you "pal." Is that something you want me to call you—"buddy?"

Domenic: Yeah. It makes me feel better.

Beth: Okay. I never knew that.

Domenic: Now you know.

Beth: Now I know. Okay. How is that different from pal?

Domenic: Pals is just like guys. And between a woman and a guy. . . .

Beth: So buddy is okay. I never thought of that.

Domenic: That's why sometimes I don't call you. I call her and see how she's doing or I call Teresa. She calls me back and I tell her I love her and she says she loves me. Not even my sister don't say it. And to this day nobody says it until she says it. Teresa says it. When I say I love her.

Beth: There's two different loves now. What are they again?

Domenic: Well, you mean like the love between family members or friends? Friend love. That's what I show Beth, friend love. I can't think of that word. It starts with a P.

Beth: Platonic?

Domenic: Yeah. And the other love's between your girlfriend. I can't even pronounce it.

Beth: Amorous?

Domenic: Like a girlfriend-boyfriend. I can't think of it. To this day, I don't know how to say it.

Beth: Sexual?

Domenic: I don't know. I really don't know what it is. I'm trying to figure out what it is.

Beth: Passion?

Domenic: I don't know what it is. I got to look it up.

Beth: Okay.

Domenic: I don't know how to spell it though. (Another question is asked.)

Domenic: It's hard to go see people. The only time I see Beth is on retreat and conferences.

Beth: I don't agree. I'll pull out my date book. See, I disagree. We see each other about twice a month or so. We go back and forth. You've come to my house for dinner. We had that barbecue. Or we meet at the mall.

Domenic: Right. See and now I'm looking around for a good computer. A guy I was talking to said I got parts of computer. I got a TV, and I got a disc drive, and I got a keyboard. And it's not working. I'm going crazy.

Beth: What the staff said at Dom's IVP is that you have to save enough money before you even investigate anything.

Domenic: And I don't have that much money.

Beth: Yeah, but it doesn't cost money, Dom. I know somebody who will come and look at it without it costing anything. So you don't have to sit and wait and save and all that stuff. You can move on it now.

Domenic: Right. I don't know what to do. I'm going crazy with it. No, I don't play with, I don't use it no more 'til I figure out what's wrong. I want to put my baseball cards on there, but I got so many of them. I got over 5,000 and nobody helps me write them down. I have to do it all by myself and it takes time.

Beth: Well, you want Brian's number?

Domenic: Yeah, but then he'll might be busy doing something, you know?

Beth: Might be, but you never know 'til you ask.

(There is talk now of the computer demonstration later in the day and Dom's work sending out postcards for chapter meetings from a mailing list. Then another question is asked.)

Domenic: Well, I know when Beth had difficults with her family, I know to leave her alone.

Beth: That was a hard time—this summer and then this fall.

Domenic: And I told her I like women with long hair.

Beth: Yeah, and what are my thoughts on that?

Domenic: I don't know what you said.

Beth: I think it's a sexist comment.

Domenic: I'm just telling you what I thought. I really do—I don't know why.

Beth: What I tell Domenic is: "Dom, you got to talk to Terry about that." 'Cause these are things that he's not going to get any empathy from me on because I just can't relate. Women with long hair . . . .

Domenic: Not that long.

Beth: You know what I mean. Terry would understand that and say, "Oh yeah, Dom." There's different bonds between guys, I guess.

Domenic: One thing, I never argue with her. I never argue with a woman.

Beth: I totally disagree with you. I think we argue all the time.

Domenic: It's not arguing.

Beth: Okay, maybe it's not arguing. But we talk and we disagree.

Domenic: Disagree. What I like is when we meet at the mall and go out to get something to eat, or we're just driving back from somewhere, and we stop. It seems like when we go out and get something to eat that there's more of a chance to talk. She treats me like a human being. Other people don't, but she treats me like a human being. Sometimes I'm always upset after work. This guy bothers me. He bothers me all day at work and then I come home and I get upset and I don't know who to call. And I look through my phonebook, and I call Beth. She's never home, right? 'Cause you work at night.

Beth: Dom, what you said about me treating you like a human being—that's never something that Dom's ever shared with me before.

Domenic: They treat me like dirt. Dirt! An object. You could pick up a chair and throw it. But you can't throw people's feelings.

(Domenic returns to his urgency about getting the people and the date and the location nailed down for his circle of friends meeting, because he will soon be leaving for Maryland for a conference.)

Beth: Yeah, we have to figure out a day. I got an appointment

book with me. I want to do it too before the winter starts.(Nancy No-
well comes in. It was her idea that Domenic have a circle of friends.
She wants to make sure that he and Beth are making plans for it and
that they will let her know what is decided.)

Nancy: You need to find a date far enough in advance that most
people can come. I don't know where; it could be at my place. What
the trick is: you just pick a day far enough in advance and people
write it down. Domenic, people care about you and they love you.
They will show up; they will show up. (After a short discussion she
goes out.)

(Domenic contemplates where to have the meeting.)

Domenic: If I have somebody at my house this guy will say,
"What are these people doing here?"

And I have to say, "Don't worry about it. It's not for you; it's for
me."

Beth: Smitty would say that?

Domenic: He'll say that: "It's not your house."

He'll say, "Did you tell Jim? Did you tell Keith?"

I don't have to tell them. The way he told me, he doesn't like me
because my attitude. And I'm thinking that nobody likes me. And
it hurt. It really hurt me when he said that. And I say to myself,
"Wait a minute! I do got friends. I do got friends who like me. In the
organization."

Beth: Having friends is different from being a part of Speaking For
Ourselves, from being part of any organization. Friends is different.

Domenic: This is the only organization I'm belong to. I don't
want to go to church. They say the same thing over and over and over.
And you get boring, saying over and over.

(The talk turns to birthdays. Last year Domenic gave Beth a neck-
lace for her birthday. This year they want to plan to go to dinner for
his birthday. He will be 39 years old.)

Domenic: No, not 29. *Thirty*-nine. When I say I'm 40, okay?—
everything hurts on me. When I say I'm 39, nothing hurts. Like I have
a bad knee now and if I fall down the steps, I get real hurt. How the
heck I'm going to come to these retreats. I know Beth would be concerned—right?—if I got really hurt. I know my knee's starting to
hurt. I don't know why. I do my exercise and after I do exercise, it
hurts. And I got a woman doctor. She's real nice to me, real, real nice. I
had all men since K. I never had a woman doctor. And I have to go to
dentist next month. I got so many things to do. Then the conference
comes up, planning things for the conference. The brochure, I got to
figure out how to put up the brochure. Lucy told me that we got to get

together and talk about it. For the 10th year anniversary. I can't believe it—10 years! Make me feel old. I can't believe it. We started in June; it was '82, June 18th.

(The time has come to close the interview.)

Domenic: I like Beth being my partner. I know she's there. She's like a sister. My other two sisters never there for me. They're always working or they're busy with Amy, busy with Aileen. And Margy's going to have a baby. I hope it's born this time. Last time they lost it. The baby was born without a brain. Her son was born with no brain. How could that happen, you know? And my friend Melissa's baby was born blind. Everything's going haywire for me now.

I got two people who called me. I put an ad in the paper for a ride from the library to H. Avenue. Yeah, I put ads in the paper before—that's how we got Diana. I don't know which should I do because two people called. One said for free and the other one said he's on scale, that he's getting $10 towards gas. Should I give him $10 after the chapter meeting or after the board meeting?

Beth: Not 10 bucks each way? Ten bucks a month, right?

Domenic: Ten bucks a month.

Beth: For two rides a month. My gut reaction is it sounds like a lot.

Domenic: My sisters won't do it. And my father told me to get out of this racket.

Beth: He told me that, too. I couldn't believe it! I wanted to meet Dom's dad so I could straighten him out. Yeah, he called this a racket.

Domenic: And a taxi's like $7, $8 a ride.

Beth: So you would be saving money? Are they reliable, the taxis?

Domenic: No, they're not reliable.

Beth: Well, as long as you trust these guys. Did you ask them would they be reliable?

Domenic: Yeah, I'm going to ask them.

Beth: Let me know what happens.

JOCELYN AND HOPE

Jocelyn is a young woman with rich brown skin and a shy but engaging smile. She chose not to use her real name. Hope's smile betrays her decidedly optimistic outlook on life. She is of medium height with dark hair and glasses.

Jocelyn: I'm Jocelyn W. and I live in Philadelphia. I'm just sitting home. Getting tutored. And going to meetings for the Speaking For Ourself.

Hope: And my name's Hope S. and I live in Bridgeport and I work for Weight Watchers.

Jocelyn: I think we had a meeting and we sat around and they figure out who wanted to be partners and so me and Hope say we could be partners. I guess it took a little while because I had a letter and I wasn't too sure when I should of called and everything. So it was a little later and we got together and called each other.

Hope: That's true. It was probably about actually a year from the time that we agreed to be partners. I was afraid, really, to call Jocelyn. Mainly because I really didn't know how to start it. I found it more comforting when I found Jocelyn was feeling the same way. We just needed to make that first move. Somebody needed to make the first move.

Jocelyn: 'Cause I thought, you know, she probably wouldn't want to, you know, be a partner or whatever. So I guess that's what happened. Then we started talking. That's when we really got to know each other—by telephone and over my house. Hope came over for my birthday.

Hope: I really enjoyed that—celebrating Jocelyn's birthday— because I really got a chance to see a different side of Jocelyn. I felt like I got closer because of that experience. First celebrating her birthday with her and then just, you know, being able to act goofy and have fun—talk about guys. Right?

Jocelyn: My mother really likes it because she says, "Well, you do need a partner to talk your problems . . . " and everything. She have no problems with it. She's really happy, you know, because it's just me and my mom and my sister, but she doesn't live there. So my mom doesn't have no problem being a partner.

Hope: I have four sisters and I told two of my sisters about Jocelyn. They thought it was really neat to be able to have some kind of relationship like that. I think the main thing that I said to my sisters was that Jocelyn and I have a lot of common interests. Like we like to go out dancing. We like to stay active.

Jocelyn: Well, no we haven't—not yet. It will probably take a little while to go out and things. Sometimes you really can't plan it. But talking on the phone is nice, you know.

Hope: We did try one weekend. I think you were busy. And then one weekend I was busy. So it's really kind of hard to connect with each other, but I think it'll be interesting to see where it goes from now. I think I'm definitely getting closer to Jocelyn. The different things that Jocelyn is facing, I faced. Or I'm still feeling, which is just really interesting. Like when she says different things, I'm like,

"Wow! That's . . . " We can just really connect with each other. Some of the things that Jocelyn has been struggling with, I struggled with. We kind of experienced the same thing. I was more disappointed in myself that I couldn't reach out to Jocelyn, in the sense of starting it. But when we finally did talk on the phone, Jocelyn was like, "Well, I could have called you."

And I was like, "Oh, I didn't even think of that."

Jocelyn: Well, I have a difficult calling people and talking on the phone. I mean to be a first person to start the conversation, pick up the telephone—usually I don't do it. I talk about it, but I really don't do it. And sometimes, you know, I figure, "Well, maybe she didn't want to be bothered."

Whatever. And I supposed to write to her, but I didn't do that. But, you know, when she called me, I was really surprised. It was a very nice conversation and I felt kind of happy, you know, 'cause I have somebody that I could talk to sometimes.

Taking the buses? Well, sort of and not really. I mean, no. Not really go out on my own to catch the buses and everything without my mom taking me. 'Cause I've been really retective. Over-retective. And so usually she'll do more for me 'cause I'll just sit back and let her do that, 'cause—like I say—she's used to doing that. So I have to say, "Mom, I have to take charge of my life and go on transportation and everything on my own."

And try a little bit more about doing that.

Hope: Which is one thing that I shared with Jocelyn. I just couldn't believe it. Jocelyn was saying that she's been very over-protected by her mother and I experienced the same thing when I was living at home. I grew up in a very protective environment where I had no—let me see—experiences. Because everything was done for me. So taking transportation when I didn't have a car was traumatic: Oh my gosh! Am I going to get off the right stop?

And we were talking about that and it was like, well, we could go on a bus and go on down Atlantic City with each other—supporting each other.

And it would be fun instead of being forced. For me, I think I would like to see if we could do more things with each other. I think talking on the phone and building that trust is good, but I think in the future I'd like to see if we could do more things together. 'Cause you had mentioned yesterday that you wanted to start doing things more like on your own and more with people your own age. Remember you were saying that? Which is kind of the same with me, too. It's easy to stay at home. But actually going out—doing some dancing or whatever—that's one thing that I would like to be able to see in our partnership.

Jocelyn: A partner's like a friend to talk to and go out with. And talk about your problems with. That's all.

Hope: The partnership for me is to be with my partner no matter what. Sticking by. When there's tough times, to stay with it. When it's fun, to go along with it. And when it gets scary, to stick with it, too. I think that that's kind of neat—to be able to have a partner like that, to be able to build up that trust and go with it. That's the main thing: making the commitment with each other. For me, partnership is just for both of us to be able to feel free to be ourselves and not have to put on any airs.

Jocelyn: Well, I would say it's nice to have a partnership, you know, because you can share your problems with them and perhaps go out. Maybe you should try it.

CONCLUSION

Although it is very obvious to those in Speaking For Ourselves who make decisions about the future that the partnership project has benefited those members and advisors who are involved in it, there is still no desire to formalize it. In fact, it is barely viewed within the organization as a project at all, except by way of its initiation. That is, the organization only records the names and addresses and phone numbers of those people who have approached each other to become partners. After that, what happens or does not happen and when it starts to happen or how long it takes to start happening is nobody's business but that of the two people involved. The only desire is that as many people as possible should find out about partnerships and that they, too, should get partners. Even the question about how to refer to the concept has changed within Speaking For Ourselves since the initial meetings with Carol Cobb-Nettleton. Why does it have to be called anything at all—a program or project—if it does not require money? Perhaps this need to name is worrisome because in some ways it creates the possibility that the "system" will get involved. These partnerships have worked too well on their own for Speaking For Ourselves not to be justifiably concerned at any mention of becoming programmed.

Partnership is not a program; it is a bond between two individuals. For this, it seems, the organization has been necessary. Without Speaking For Ourselves the members of the organization would still be what the outside world has always condemned them to be: less-than-human beings, with one or more disabling conditions, whose primary role in life is to receive services. Speaking For Ourselves has brought people together as *individuals*. Through these partnerships, it has given the impetus and its blessing to the possibility of true friendship. Now, it stands back out of the way and lets what might happen simply happen between the two people involved.

These partnerships are not a project or a program. If they are anything, they are simply a part of the struggle to be as fully human as possible. Programs and projects are set up by one group of people to cure, correct, or channel another group of people. A partnership means only that two individuals have somehow managed to get through all of the obstacles that the world puts between them. These include many of the same obstacles that exist between two "typical" people and then the added obstacles that occur because of the perceived disability of one of the individuals. But the partnership is not to be conceived of as the end of anything or as a solution to any problem or collection of problems. Rather, a partnership might be seen as simply a new door, a door we have not been able to locate before, a door that swings open to allow *any* person entrance into the world to which we all have a birthright, but to which some of us have been denied entrance. A partnership is *only* that, only the door. What happens on the other side of that door will be no more perfect for the newcomer than it has been for those of us who have lived here for a while. So jobs and marriages may fall through or fall apart. There are no answers in life; there is only the living of it. A partnership is simply the opening of the door that leads to true living in the world.

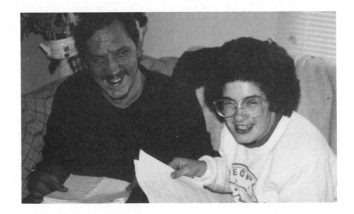

III

STRATEGIES FOR
BUILDING FRIENDSHIPS

A home-made friend wears longer than one you buy in the market.

Austin O'Malley

Many people working with individuals who have disabilities are aware of the isolation and loneliness that these individuals experience and the importance of supporting real friendships. However, many of these same people are stopped by not knowing how to initiate that support or how to be effective. One of the intentions of this book is to provide useful and concrete information about how to actually support community connections and friendships. That information is presented in this last section of this book.

A great deal has been written about supporting relationships in school settings; however, the content addressed in this section concerns the remainder of human services, especially programs and services for adults with developmental disabilities. Some of the approaches discussed here, however, have also been used to support friendships for children, especially when their schools are not doing much to promote integration. "Circles of support" and "circles of friends" have been extensively presented elsewhere (e.g., Perske, 1988), and will not be discussed in detail here.

Chapter 16 presents nine different reasons why working to support friendships is important. Different categories of approaches to support friendship, community participation, and community connections are also described. Using the analysis presented in that chapter, the information in the next three chapters is primarily about bridge-building (pp. 292–293). The methods discussed are predominantly initiated and intentional efforts (p. 293), and are particularly intended to assist human services agencies, families, community organizations, and others who care about persons with disabilities to engage in concrete efforts to support friendships.

Chapters 17, 18, and 19 present these concrete strategies and methods for intentional bridge-building with a different focus in each chapter. Chapter 17 summarizes the information from several different approaches and projects and presents a sequence incorporating various methods that have been used to plan community-building efforts, identify possible community connections, and introduce people to others. This information has been used successfully by many residential services agencies as well as day programs, advocacy agencies, families, and others. In Chapter 18, Wilson and Coverdale discuss the Friendship Project of The Association for Persons with Severe Handicaps (TASH), which was particularly aimed at supporting workers with severe disabilities; issues of friendship through employment and day programs are also addressed. In Chapter 19, Reidy presents specific strategies and information on how to assist individuals with disabilities become members of community groups and associations. Final thoughts on the issues considered throughout this volume and the future of friendship building are presented in the Afterword.

Of course these chapters do not present all that could be provided regarding strategies and methods, but they are not intended to duplicate specific information that is already available in other forms. Rather, more summary information is presented here and references to other resources and manuals are provided when appropriate. However, the intention of this section *is* to provide sufficient discussion of techniques and methods so that people who are attempting their own community-connecting for individuals with disabilities can use this information to be successful in their efforts.

It is important to remember, however, that no one approach provides all the answers (Roeher Institute, 1990). Each method has its place and its own strengths and weaknesses. Supporting friendship is not a linear process that involves following any set of steps or specific strategies. Many ways, methods, and models may need to be tried. Each person is unique and each relationship is different. The path to friendship and to community is not a straight, fast interstate highway, but rather a circuitous, winding country backroad—perhaps slower, but immensely more pleasurable.

REFERENCES

Perske, R. (1988). *Circles of friends: People with disabilities and their friends enrich the lives of one author.* Nashville: Abingdon Press.

G. Allan Roeher Institute. (1990). *Making friends: Developing relationships between people with a disability and other members of the community.* Downsview, Ontario, Canada: York University.

=====16=====

Working on Friendships

Angela Novak Amado

There's something wonderfully rewarding in being part of an effort
that does make a difference. And there's something sparkling about
being among other people when they're at their best too. When any
of us take inventory of the meaning of our lives, these special experiences have to be among the high points. Happiness is, in the end, a
simple thing. Despite how complicated we try to make it or the en-
trapments we substitute for it, happiness is really caring and being
able to do something about the caring. . . . In the course of these
efforts there is at work a silent cycle of cause and effect which I call
the "genius of fulfillment," meaning that the harder people work for
others and for the fulfillment of important social goals, the more
fulfilled they are themselves.

Brian O'Connell (1983, p. 407)

Building community relationships and friendships means contributing to moving the world from an "us and them" mode of operation to
an "all of us" togetherness. Supporting friendships in the community for persons with developmental disabilities extends beyond
many current practices of "community integration." Although there
has been tremendous progress made in the last 20 years in the number of people with disabilities living in small community homes and
working in offices and businesses (Amado, Lakin, & Menke, 1990),
most of these people are still lonely. Although many people with developmental disabilities are at least more physically integrated and
have the opportunity for activities in their neighborhoods and towns,

Information contained in this chapter pertaining to the Friends Project is in the
public domain.

The development of some of the information in this chapter was funded through
Grant No. 17673 to the Human Services Research and Development Center from the
Minnesota Governor's Planning Council on Developmental Disabilities under provisions of the Developmental Disabilities Act of 1987 (PL 100-146). This content does not
necessarily reflect the position or policy of the Minnesota Governor's Planning Council on Developmental Disabilities or the Minnesota State Planning Agency.

most are still not really part of their communities. The majority of these people have very few, if any, friends (Lakin, Burwell, Hayden, & Jackson, 1992). Support for friendships with community members extends the concept of "community integration" to a broader societal context: that persons with and without disabilities have active opportunities to be in meaningful relationships with each other.

The understanding of friendships between persons with and without developmental disabilities has evolved significantly throughout the course of history. Perhaps the entire history of services and of attitudes toward persons with disabilities can be seen as the evolution of relationships between the two groups of people. In Wolfensberger's (1976) formulations of the various roles that "deviant" people have held throughout history, such as object of menace, object of pity, or object of charity, all of the roles denote the attitudes of persons without disabilities toward persons with disabilities. Yet, that same history can be examined for instances and themes of contribution, friendship, and belonging. Some classic literary stories, for instance, have embodied the themes of both separation and of contribution. The beautiful La Esmerelda is initially repulsed by the deaf, one-eyed, disfigured Hunchback of Notre Dame (Hugo, 1831), but she becomes touched and moved by his deep feelings for her and his attempts to save her life. Benjy, the narrator of Faulkner's *The Sound and the Fury* (1929), although retarded, is both an integral member of his Southern community and critical to the unfolding of his family's drama. Lenny and George in Steinbeck's *Of Mice and Men* (1937) clearly have an interdependent relationship in which both are contributed to and contribute. If art can be seen to both reflect and shape the popular attitudes and values of the day, then the mirror is one of complex community attitudes—disability as both an opportunity for deeply personal and close interconnectedness and as a source of tragedy.

How caregivers and professionals perceive community attitudes toward persons with disabilities has also clearly evolved over time and throughout the latter half of this century. Medieval monasteries provided opportunities to early forms of "volunteers" for getting closer to God as they cared for the less fortunate. The 18th and 19th centuries saw the professional role as protecting the community from these "poor and evil wretches," as well as treating and curing them so they could return to regular society (Wolfensberger, 1976). Jean Vanier (1971) and (the) l'Arche movement initiated intimate communities in which persons with and without disabilities share lives together, belonging and contributing with and for each other. From the 1970s to the 1990s, educational models for encouraging friendships and relationships between students have evolved from total separation, to peer tutors, to mainstreaming, to fully inclusive classrooms. Models for adult day services and work have evolved from adult day programs as segregated versions of kindergarten, to industrial contract work, to segregated enclaves within community businesses, to supporting employers and co-workers in their own hiring, training, and supervision of workers with disabilities. None of these changes have occurred solely because of changes in professional attitudes; rather, the attitudes of community members have shifted in accompaniment with professional perspectives, both influencing and being influenced by professional practices.

Currently, large, multidimensional shifts are occurring in the general public's knowledge of and attitudes toward persons with disabilities, with numerous factors both contributing to and reflecting these shifts. More children with severe disabilities are living longer and remaining at home. Persons with disabilities share integrated classrooms from preschool through postsecondary education, and share workplaces in both supported and competitive employment sites throughout the country. The number of persons with developmental disabilities living in institutions has been more than cut in half in the last 20 years, and the number of individuals living in the very smallest community-based settings (from one to six persons) quadrupled from 20,000 to 80,000 in just 11 years (1977–1988) (Amado et al., 1990b). Many more people are living with severe physical injuries (i.e., postwar or postaccident) who previously would have died, and buildings and city streets are now accessible even in the smallest towns. The Americans with Disabilities Act (1990) is increasing awareness for every business and employer in the country. All these factors and others contribute to community members having more knowledge and daily experience with individuals with disabilities.

In 1991, Louis Harris and Associates conducted a major poll called *Public Attitudes toward People with Disabilities*. This poll demonstrated that a majority of Americans support increased participation of citizens with disabilities in community life. The poll addressed all types of disabilities, not just mental retardation or developmental disabilities. Harris (1991) described this study as "one of the most interesting and most important surveys our firm has ever conducted." Of those Americans surveyed, 98% believed that everyone, including people with disabilities, should have equal opportunity to participate in American society. Nine out of ten said that society would benefit from having persons with disabilities become more productive and contribute to the economy. Ninety-six percent supported public places becoming accessible. One of the most intriguing factors in terms of public awareness and knowledge is that almost half of those polled said they knew people with disabilities as friends, relatives, neighbors, or workers, and almost a third of those polled reported having a close friend or relative with a disability.

The enhanced visibility of persons with disabilities in the media has also contributed to this increased awareness. The people who were polled reported that movies and television programs have had a powerful and positive impact on their attitudes. Individuals cited films such as *Rainman, My Left Foot, Born on the Fourth of July*, and *Children of a Lesser God*, as well as the television programs *L.A. Law* and *Life Goes On*, as influencing their attitudes. For 3 years in a row (1988–1990), one of the persons winning an Academy Award as best actor or actress was either a person with a disability or someone who portrayed such a character. Not only is there currently a television series with an actor who has Down syndrome (*Life Goes On*), but the television show, *L.A. Law*, with its subplots about characters with mental retardation, was one of the highest-rated television shows in the country for several years. Millions of people have been exposed to these television characters week after week, seen these films, and read stories in newspapers and national magazines concerning individuals with disabilities.

Yet, even though many people surveyed in the Harris poll reported personally knowing people with disabilities, most reported continuing to feel somewhat awkward or embarrassed around such individuals. Seventy-seven percent said they feel pity toward people with disabilities. Interestingly, in another recent survey, Levy, Jessop, Rimmerman, and Levy (1992) documented that personal knowledge and experience may contribute to more comfort and acceptance on the part of community members. In a survey of *Fortune 500* businesses, the employers who were the most positive and accepting of workers with disabilities, even those with severe conditions, were those who experienced positive contact with such workers in the past. In addition, other research has documented that it is the quality of contact that is important in affecting attitudes in integrated situations (Allport, 1954; Jeffries & Ransford, 1969). Children growing up in integrated schools and inclusive classrooms today will bring those values into a much different adult culture in the next 10–20 years, forcing human services systems to adapt or be left behind.

The receptiveness of community members to meeting persons with disabilities and getting to know them has been documented in several efforts and projects that were focused on establishing community ties for persons with developmental disabilities (Amado, Conklin, & Wells, 1990; Arsenault, 1990; O'Connell, 1990; Tyne, 1988).

The attitude that the community is ready, willing, and able affected the success of these community-building efforts.

WHY WORK ON FRIENDSHIPS

There are several reasons why it is important to support more friendships and community connections for persons with disabilities.

1.   Relationships Are Important to All People

Relationships are probably the deepest and most satisfying facet of life. Sometimes relationships are so integrated into the fabric of day-to-day existence that their number, their nature, and their crucial role in moving all of life forward are taken for granted. The importance of friendship has been discussed in writing since at least the time of the Greeks and is an ancient issue for all humanity (see Gaventa, chap. 3, this volume).

Friends are important for several reasons. They provide intimacy and affection, help people feel important and valued, provide companionship, and encourage risk-taking (Roeher Institute, 1990). For most people, their sense of identity and what is possible in their lives has been gained through their experiences with other people. For individuals with disabilities, friends also help in having a life beyond human services, provide support and advocacy, and help a person have a greater chance for a "normal" life.

2.   People with Disabilities
Report the Importance of Friendships

People with disabilities report that friendships with nondisabled community members are extremely important to them. They indicate this importance both in direct statements and indirectly through their behavior. Self-advocates have stated that support for getting out in the community and meeting community citizens is one of the most important ways in which human services programs can help them (People First of Washington, 1985). For persons who have difficulty speaking or expressing themselves, the behavior changes they exhibit when they have a chance to be with and interact with regular community members is an extremely important communication (see R. S. Amado, chap. 4, this volume; Baker & Salon, 1986).

From 1989 to 1990, the "Friends Project" operated in Minnesota with six residential agencies (this project is more fully described in A.N. Amado, chap. 17, this volume). During that year, one of the participating agencies sponsored a one-day planning workshop with the executive director and 15 consumers served by the agency. An outside facilitator coordinated the workshop. One assumption made at the meeting was that staff could not help everybody with everything in life that they needed; therefore, if staff could not do everything, what was the consumer's perspective concerning the areas most critical to support? What are the most important things for staff to spend their time on? The group made a list of everything the staff could help them with (e.g., shopping, managing money, getting a job); then, they made choices between pairs of items—this one is more important than that one. A list of 15 items was narrowed to 7, then 7 was narrowed to 2. What the group determined to be the two most important areas for staff to help them with were: 1) to help them have more friends, and 2) to help them get along better with people. This group process was one method and instance of documentation that persons who receive services will, when given the opportunity to be heard, express in their own way how important relationships are to them.

Others often report this importance in more subtle ways. For example, when a stranger enters a program with a large number of people with disabilities (e.g., a group home or day activity center), almost invariably one or more of the people with disabilities will immediately approach the person, shake hands, say "hi," introduce him- or herself, ask the person's name, and/or touch the stranger. Contact with typical persons, other than staff and other people in the program, is directly sought and extremely significant. There are also numerous cases in every agency where the reports about people served say that the particular individual "prefers staff," or will relate better to staff than to their peers. Training programs and objectives abound for peer–peer interaction; however, given that in most cases there seems to be an already-existing importance to relationships with community members, perhaps a more productive path would be to support those relationships.

3.   Health and Well-Being

As more fully explicated in Chapter 4 of this volume, loneliness has a severe impact on one's overall health and longevity. Lynch (1977) documented that people who are alone are more likely to acquire illness than people who are married. House, Landis, and Umberson (1988), after reviewing 20 years' worth of medical studies, concluded that people who are isolated are twice as likely to die over the period of a decade or so as are others in the same health. They found that lack of social relationships constitutes a major risk factor for mortality and that social isolation was as great or greater a mortality risk than smoking.

There is tremendous attention in our society about the health risks and dangers of smoking. At the same time, there is tremendous attention in residential facilities and other programs on health needs of persons with disabilities; this attention is reflected in the number of nursing care plans, medication administration training for staff, documentation of medications, and other common features of the care system. Yet, no medical care plan addresses having friends as part of the overall health plan, even though it is just as, or even more, important a factor in overall well-being.

4. Recognizing the Fact that People Have Very Few Friends

Various research studies concerning deinstitutionalization and community integration over the years document the lack of friendships in people's lives. A question that recurs in studies of the quality of life of persons in community programs is: How many friends does this person have? Many of the results in these studies indicate that people only have one or two friends, a sufficiently alarming indicator of the limitations of the social network; however, the percentages of people for whom *no* friends are reported are even more startling.

In O'Connor's (1976) national study of community programs for persons with developmental disabilities, staff reported that 33% of community residents had no friends. Gollay, Freedman, Wyngaarden, and Kurtz (1978) studied deinstitutionalized persons who remained successfully in the community and those who were returned to an institution. They found that 99% of the persons who remained successfully in the community had at least one friend, whereas 31% of those who returned to an institution had no friends. Hill, Sather, Kudla, and Bruininks (1978) compared the friendships of persons in institutions with those in community-based private facilities. They found that 63% of those in institutional programs had no friends, compared to 42% in the private community facilities. For most of the people who had at least one friend, that friend was a peer (another person with disabilities), a staff person, or a former staff person. Only 16% of the persons in community facilities and 14% of institutionalized persons had a friend other than staff, former staff, or another person with disabilities. It should be noted that these studies of "community" facilities in the late 1970s included both small and large settings; even if a facility had 500 beds, it was called a "community" program if it was not a state institution.

In 1989, Hill, Lakin, Bruininks, Amado, Anderson, and Copher conducted a national survey of the smallest (six beds or less) community living facilities. The number of individuals living in these small settings had quadrupled from 1977 to 1988, rising from 20,000 to

80,000 people (Amado et al., 1990b). One of the major reasons for this study was to describe the quality of life in these smallest of residential programs. Three basic types of programs were studied: foster homes, group homes, and group homes that were funded as intermediate care facilities for persons with mental retardation (ICFs/MR) (under Title XIX of the Social Security Act, Medical Assistance). For these types of facilities, the percentages of residents who staff reported as having *no* friends are shown in Table 1.

These percentages are very similar, and in some cases even more extreme, than the percentages of people with no friends living in the larger community facilities reported in the earlier research studies cited above. From 1976 to 1989, social relationships have apparently not improved, even with more individuals living in the smallest community settings. Hill et al. (1989) also asked staff if the people with disabilities were satisfied with the number of friends they had. For those people who had *no* friends, Table 2 indicates the percentages of staff who reported that individuals were satisfied with the number of friends they had.

Many staff are perhaps unconscious of the issue of friendship, given that it has begun only recently to be reflected in program standards and regulations, or perhaps because of the ingrained tendency to think of "community integration" as activities rather than relationships. During workshops on supporting friendship, many staff have reported to this author, "Oh, I never even thought about this issue before." Other staff may recognize the issue, but may not consider it important.

Even persons living in the smallest, most physically integrated settings have yet to be fully socially integrated. A study conducted in 1991 of Minnesota's community programs that are funded by the Medicaid Home and Community-Based Services Waiver program examined many homes and apartments in which only one or two persons with disabilities lived (Lakin et al., 1992). The most residents in any of these programs was four. This survey found that only 5% of the program recipients regularly participated in community activities with friends who did not have disabilities.

Table 1.   Percentage of residents staff report as having no friends

	Foster home		Group home		ICF/MR	
Number of beds	1–4	5–6	1–4	5–6	1–4	5–6
Percentage with no friends	41	46	39	33	43	26

Adapted from Hill, Lakin, Bruininks, Amado, Anderson, & Copher (1989).
ICF/MR, intermediate care facility for persons with mental retardation.

Table 2.   For persons who have no friends, percentage of staff who report a person is satisfied with the number of friends he or she has

	Foster home		Group home		ICF/MR	
Number of beds	1–4	5–6	1–4	5–6	1–4	5–6
Percentage of staff	34	29	27	22	20	13

Adapted from Hill, Lakin, Bruininks, Amado, Anderson, & Copher (1989).
ICF/MR, intermediate care facility for persons with mental retardation.

Physical integration does not automatically mean social integration. If people are really to be part of their communities, moving them to small homes is not enough. More efforts and intentionality are needed to promote community relationships.

5.   Adjusting the Balance between Personal and Functional Relationships

George Durner (1986, June) has delineated at least two types of relationships, "personal" and "functional." Personal relationships are those that have no specific purpose and are freely chosen. In a personal relationship, the person is valued, the care and concern is about the person, and the person is more important than the program. "Functional" relationships have a specific purpose, which is often dictated. The person is not necessarily valued, the care and concern is with a particular attribute or characteristic of the person, and the program is more important than the person.

Everyone has both types of relationships. Personal relationships include those with our friends and sometimes family members; functional relationships can include those with employers, co-workers, doctors, and so forth. Most people who are dependent on the services system for a large majority of their life have an imbalance between functional and personal relationships, with most of their relationships being functional. For instance, individuals who live in a residential program and work at a day activity center or supported employment program are often subject to "active treatment" and "programming" from morning to night. Most communications or conversations they experience during the day may tend to be directive and goal-oriented. There is usually little time to spend with people who want to be with them just for the sake of being with them; and there are few relationships with people who like them for themselves, who freely choose the relationship, or who care about them rather than about their "program." Perhaps one of the most valuable ways caregivers can assist these people is to support a different balance between functional and personal relationships in their lives.

6. More Power and Control

Almost invariably, people who are dependent on the services system have fewer relationships than typical community members. Not only do they have fewer relationships, but these relationships are typically restricted to three areas: family, paid staff members, and other persons with disabilities with whom they live or work (Hill et al., 1978).

It has been documented that the number of persons in one's social network is directly correlated with the amount of power and control one has (Fischer, 1982). Chief executive officers and political figures typically have very large social networks. The President of the United States usually sends out about 100,000 Christmas cards. The most important source of getting a new job in any field is not employment agencies or advertisements, but "personal contact" (Bolles, 1990). An increase in the number of people in the typically restricted social networks of persons with disabilities helps increase the amount of control these individuals have over their own lives (Roeher Institute, 1990).

7. Reducing Personal Stress and Staff Burnout

When a high proportion of the total number of relationships in a person's social network is with paid staff, several results occur. First, staff turnover is reported as one of the major problems in operating human services (Hill, Bruininks, Lakin, Hauber, & McGuire, 1985). Staff come and go, receive promotions, and are reassigned. If a person with disabilities is dependent for a high proportion of their relationships on people they cannot trust to be with them over time, often a sense of personal uneasiness can result. People might question themselves; question if anyone really cares or if they are someone worth knowing; not fully develop a sense of identity; or "test" staff, especially new staff members.

Second, when a person is dependent on the services system, he or she might also be subject to a great deal of "coming and going"— being shifted around among programs, buildings, or groups, without much control over the situation. In particular, persons with challenging behavior who might be most in need of continuity in their relationships and building up trust over time are shifted most frequently. In communities with a variety of choices of provider agencies, a frequent solution to any type of problem is to "change providers," which only further contributes to discontinuity in relationships. One friend of this author was moved to 20 different programs in 7 years.

Third, if people are paid to be with a person, do they really care about that person? Are they there because they are being paid or because they really want to and like the person? When an individual with disabilities has a significant proportion of his or her relationships with paid staff, this confusion can also contribute to personal uneasiness, a diminished sense of one's self, and confusion about who is a "friend" (also see above discussion on personal versus functional relationships).

Fourth, a staff member may be an important person in the social network of a person with disabilities, but is the person with disabilities equally important in the social network of the staff member? There is often an imbalance or inequity in the relationship when one half of the relationship is a paid person.

Newton (1989) has listed seven functions that friends play in each other's lives, including: 1) information, 2) feedback, 3) assistance in making major life decisions, 4) emotional support, 5) material aid and services, 6) access to others, and 7) companionship. If there are fewer persons in the social network of a typical group home resident, and if staff represent a significant proportion of the total number of relationships for that resident, then a staff member has to provide a greater number of the functions than one single person has to provide in the network of a typical person. If an individual with disabilities has 10 people in their social network and a typical person has 100, then one staff member is "standing in for" 10 other people. The phenomenon of "staff burnout" (Edwards & Miltenberger, 1991) can then be appreciated in a different light—if one staff member is providing what 10 people provide for the typical person, perhaps that staff member's "burnout" is more than understandable.

If a staff person's job is altered to support people to have more variety and depth in their social network, then perhaps the impact in the overall network will not be so dramatic when staff move on. Perhaps one of the most important things staff can do with their time and role is to shift from "client"-staff exclusivity to connecting the person with disabilities to a much broader network.

8. People Change When There Is a Focus on What Is Important to Them

A number of studies have documented that when relationships are supported for individuals in services, the individuals begin to change. When people have others in their life who they know like them and they realize that these people will be there for them over time, other facets of their life also change (Amado, Conklin, & Wells, 1990a; R.S. Amado, chap. 4, this volume; Baker & Salon, 1986; Berkman & Meyer, 1988; O'Brien & O'Brien, 1992; Tyne, 1988; Wilson & Coverdale, chap. 18, this volume). This phenomenon has been documented primarily in stories about people, and more systematic understanding of these types of changes is warranted.

When community members become acquainted with and like individuals with disabilities, when they want to spend time with them, some people who previously had challenging behavior "improve." Others who have difficulty with assertiveness or motivation become more assertive or motivated when they start to have friends. Some individuals may have had "behavior programs" or "assertiveness programs" for years; however, when they have someone whom they value, someone to dress up for, places to go outside of their programs where they are appreciated, many times what were "programming issues" disappear. Once staff invest the time to find and support friendship, sometimes the staff's job actually becomes easier.

9. Providing Community Members the Opportunity To Receive Contribution

Human services practices have typically robbed community members of the opportunity to get to know individuals with disabilities. When community citizens do have these opportunities, they are often extraordinarily receptive. Several authors have noted that one of the most important reasons to support friendships with persons with disabilities is that these relationships help people who do not have disabilities learn about acceptance (Bogdan & Taylor, 1989; Forest, 1989; Perske, 1988). People with disabilities bring different or unusual gifts and contribute in very extraordinary and unique ways to others (Taylor & Bogdan, 1989). Wolfensberger (1988) describes 15 gifts and assets that people with mental retardation contribute that are not commonly recognized, such as "heart qualities," spontaneity, more ease providing unconditional love, trust, an unfettered enjoyment of life's pleasures, directness and honesty, and an ability to call forth gentleness and patience from others.

Many employers have noted the gifts that supported employment workers bring to their companies, including the opportunity to get to know these people as "people," a greater "family" atmosphere, and a real commitment to doing a good job (Levy et al., 1992). In more casual settings, community members also appreciate the chance to get to know people. When two staff brought one older gentleman to play pool in a local bar, the man got everyone in the place involved in their game, even though he has very limited speech. When they were leaving, the bartender asked the staff, "When are you bringing him back? Everyone had more fun tonight because he was here."

For all of the above reasons and others, working on relationships and friendships with community members is important. The next section describes various approaches that have been utilized.

APPROACHES TO COMMUNITY CONNECTING

Many different conceptualizations have been generated about both the importance of friendship for persons with disabilities and how to best support it. Several authors have used different analyses to summarize these approaches.

Roeher Institute Analysis

In 1990, the G. Allan Roeher Institute in Toronto published an analysis of different approaches and methods for supporting friendship with community members. They identified four main categories of approaches that have been utilized.

A. One-to-One or Matching   The one-to-one or matching approach is not new, but tends to be a formalized "volunteer" approach. The method was utilized in the Citizen Advocacy programs that originated in the 1970s; in "leisure buddy" programs in recreation departments; and in more current programs, such as "Best Buddies" and other matchings of university students with similar age peers, often for course credit or as a course requirement. Although formal relationships often overshadow the quality and informality of friendship, many long-lasting friendships emerge from these efforts. Other difficulties with formal "matching" approaches are incompatibility between the persons matched and overlap of friendship with other functions, such as providing advocacy. However, more recently, one-to-one introductions have been utilized successfully to encourage more natural forms of friendship (e.g., see R.S. Amado, chap. 4, and A. N. Amado, chap. 17, this volume).

B. Community Development with Self-Advocates   Self-advocacy groups engage in personal support networking and community development through organizing and consciousness raising. Individuals and self-help groups become involved with other community groups and voluntary associations with broadened opportunities to meet people who will eventually become friends (see Speaking For Ourselves, chap. 15, this volume).

C. Using Social Networks and "Circles" To Build Friends   In this approach, formal or informal methods and structures are used to strengthen the existing social network or establish a group or circle of friends around a person. One of these methods is to strengthen already-existing relationships and natural social networks around the person with disabilities and to use the existing friends to access new relationships for the person. For instance, part of the McGill Action Planning System (MAPS) approach (Vandercook, York, & Forest, 1989) is to examine the existing network of relationships for a person with disabilities and then determine how to use those relationships to connect with others.

For individuals who have few or no existing social networks, more formal efforts can be planned to build or strengthen friendships. One form of this planned approach is "circles of support" (Forest, 1987; Mount & Zwernik, 1989) or "circles of friends." A more formal "circle" can be established, with individuals who do or do not know the person invited to participate (Roeher Institute, 1990). One of the difficulties with these circles is that there is sometimes a collapse or confusion between whether the purpose of the group is friendship or whether the circle should operate more formally to improve services or obtain needed services. Many groups have found it important to sort out the difference between whether their purpose is for support or actual friendship. Some individuals with disabilities have used their support groups to obtain assistance with more formal systems while actually calling on others outside the circle for friendship. Sometimes circles lead to friendship, other times providing support can interfere with friendship.

D. Bridging to Community   Another recent approach is that of using bridgers or connectors who guide individuals with disabilities into the community and introduce them to people who will be their friends. The bridge-builder or community-connector introduces the person with disabilities to new places, guides them to new relationships, connects them with valued citizens in the community, and familiarizes the person with new opportunities. This approach is based on ensuring that a person is exposed to and in community environments, and also on a trust that communities have the capacity and willingness to become involved with people with disabilities as friends.

Some of the qualities that have been identified as important in a bridge-builder are an ability to focus on the gifts and capacities of a person with disabilities rather than their deficiencies, a capacity to work by trust rather than authority, a belief that the reason people with disabilities are not in the community is because no one has asked them to join, and a willingness to let go after they have guided someone into the community (McKnight, 1987; O'Connell, 1988). Since it was first developed and since the time of the Roeher Institute description, the role of bridge-builder has been structured by others in at least three different ways: 1) as a community member, 2) as a special job for a staff person, and 3) as part of the job for all staff.

1. Community Member   The original concept of bridge-builder was a person who is not formally connected with an agency that directly provides services to individuals with disabilities (O'Connell, 1988; Spierman, 1991). The bridge-builder might be someone connected with a community organization, such as a neighborhood association or a formal advocacy organization. In some efforts, community people who are locally known, active, and respected (e.g., the mayor's spouse) are asked to provide bridge-building for persons with disabilities to other community members.

2. Special Job for a Staff Person   Once human services agencies recognized the importance of relationships with community members, many began to structure more formal connecting efforts. One method is to designate one or more staff persons within the agency to have special jobs as bridge-builders. These staff have linked persons served by the agency to community life (see Wilson & Coverdale, chap. 18, this volume). Some agencies have identified community-building as their exclusive role, with all of the staff having this special job (see Bartholomew-Lorimer, chap. 10, this volume).

3. Part of the Job for All Staff   In some agencies, community-building is recognized as so important that it has been defined as a role or as part of the job for all staff. Job descriptions in residential, day program, and other agencies have been changed to include community-connecting as part of the job.

Different applications of the bridge-building approach are described in Chapters 17, 18, and 19 of this volume.

Other Analyses

Besides the four-part analysis by the Roeher Institute, other authors have also analyzed efforts to promote community participation and relationships. Lutfiyya and Reidy (1991) have reviewed different efforts and strategies to support community participation. They identified three varying dimensions in these efforts: 1) initiated versus spontaneous participation, 2) formal versus informal organizations, and 3) created versus existing settings.

*1. **Initiated versus Spontaneous Participation***   Initiated participation efforts utilize a formal facilitator who supports participation and interactions. Spontaneous facilitation is less planned—the person might be in an inclusive setting, but then any participation that occurs is on a spontaneous basis. Initiated efforts use more intentional forms of introduction and meetings with others (see Strully & Strully, chap. 13, this volume, for an example). Spontaneous efforts are aimed at getting individuals into integrated settings and then expecting or hoping that connections will occur.

2. *Formal versus Informal Organizations* Formal organizations have a history and operating existence independent of their current membership. Informal organizations or groups exist based only on the existing members or existing effort. Many community-building efforts have been aimed at identifying both types of organizations within a community for potential memberships (McKnight, 1987).

3. *Created versus Existing Settings* Created forms of community participation are activities or settings specifically established for persons with disabilities; therefore, they are often segregated. Other forms of support for community participation, and the ones most likely to promote connections with community citizens, use existing and ongoing activities, groups, and settings.

Different approaches evolve as more of what is possible and successful is understood, and as we deepen our understanding of both citizens with disabilities and other community members. For instance, ten years ago, children in regular education classrooms were encouraged to come into special education classrooms and volunteer or "buddy up" with special education students. Today, they are involved in circles of friends to support fellow students in fully inclusive classrooms throughout the entire day and outside of school hours. The limits of what is possible in relationships keep changing; professional attitudes need to be out ahead, defining new possibilities rather than lagging behind even the views of children.

Day Program and Employment Efforts

The variety of efforts in supporting relationships is reflected in almost every category or type of service that is provided to persons with developmental disabilities, including educational, residential, leisure and/or recreation programs, and advocacy and self-advocacy efforts. At least three different approaches for supporting relationships have evolved on the part of agencies responsible for the day program or employment of persons with disabilities: 1) support relationships on the job site, 2) seek places for community connection during the day, and 3) support the person in all of his or her social networks.

Support Relationships on the Job Site Many job coaches for supported employment workers have a specific role of assisting coworkers in understanding and becoming more involved with their fellow employees who have disabilities. One method of assisting employers in the hiring of workers with disabilities is to train company employees directly in the supervision of workers with disabilities, allowing for more immediate contact and more direct relationships (Karan & Knight, 1986).

Seek Places for Community Connection During the Day   Some day program agencies have specifically sought out daytime connections (see Bartholomew-Lorimer, chap. 10, this volume; Wade, 1991). For example, day program staff have assisted individuals with disabilities to become "regulars" in coffee shops and cafes, volunteers at the humane society and museums, and assistants in local daycare centers and businesses.

Support Persons in All of Their Social Networks   Some day program agencies have taken on the role of establishing connections and supporting friendships throughout a person's life. Once staff are familiar with the whole person (not just the vocational interests usually attributed to daytime hours), they use the person's interests and life priorities to link him or her to various aspects of community life. Staff in these agencies might support someone in the evenings or on weekends, not just during daytime programming hours. Wilson and Coverdale (chap. 18, this volume) extensively describe such an approach used by an agency in Indianapolis, Indiana.

CONCLUSION

The reasons for working on friendship make it clear that prioritizing this work is critical in the day-to-day lives of individuals with disabilities. In a society and era in which many people are lonely and need friends, supporting friendship and building community can recall and realign many hearts and souls to what is most important in life.

Perhaps the critical issue is that this area must become carved into professional practices. Other major initiatives, such as deinstitutionalization, community living, behavior modification, and independent skill training, have evolved significantly since they were first introduced. They all started somewhere and then expanded, developed, and changed. Supporting friendship and building community need to be started; they are awaiting the opportunity to further evolve.

Although not an exhaustive list, the different types of efforts that have been reviewed in this chapter provide useful ways to begin to understand different types of approaches that can be tried. The potential avenues are endless; perhaps the most critical factor is, as Confucius indicated, that the journey of a thousand miles begins with a single step. Failures and missteps will occur on that journey. However, through beginning the work of supporting friendships and relationships, and through examining what is successful and what is not, committed individuals will learn for themselves what is effective with particular people, situations, and communities.

With every true friendship we build more firmly the foundations on which the peace of the whole world rests. Thought by thought and act by act, with every breath we build the kingdom of non-violence that is the true home of the spirit of man.

Mahatma K. Gandhi

REFERENCES

Allport, G. (1954). *The nature of prejudice*. Reading, MA: Addison-Wesley.

Amado, A.N., Conklin, F., & Wells, J. (1990a). *Friends: A manual for connecting persons with disabilities and community members*. St. Paul: Human Services Research and Development Center.

Amado, A.N., Lakin, K.C., & Menke, J.M. (1990b). *1990 chartbook on services for people with developmental disabilities*. Minneapolis: University of Minnesota, Center for Residential and Community Services.

Americans with Disabilities Act of 1990, PL 101-336 (July 26, 1990). Title 42, U.S.C. 1400 et seq: *U.S. Statutes at Large, 105*, 587–608.

Arsenault, C.C. (1990). *Let's get together: A handbook in support of building relationships between individuals with developmental disabilities and their community*. Boulder, CO: Developmental Disabilities Center.

Baker, M.J., & Salon, R.S. (1986). Setting free the captives: The power of community integration in liberating institutionalized adults from the bonds of their past. *Journal of The Association for Persons with Severe Handicaps, 11*(3), 176–181.

Berkman, K.A., & Meyer, L.H. (1988). Alternative strategies and multiple outcomes in the remediation of severe self-injury: Going "all out" nonaversively. *Journal of The Association of Persons with Severe Handicaps, 13*(2), 76–86.

Bogdan, R., & Taylor, S.J. (1989). Relationships with severely disabled people: The social construction of humanness. *Social Problems, 36*(2), 135–146.

Bolles, R.N. (1990). *What color is your parachute?* Berkeley, CA: Ten Speed Press.

Durner, G. (1986, June). *Relationships of the heart—The essential ingredient*. Paper presented at the "Connections" conference of the Community Options Program, LaCrosse, WI.

Edwards, P., & Miltenberger, R. (1991). Burnout among staff members at community residential facilities for persons with mental retardation. *Mental Retardation, 29*(3), 125–128.

Faulkner, W.F. (1929). *The sound and the fury*. New York: Modern Library.

Fischer, C. (1982). *To dwell among friends: Personal networks in town and city*. Chicago: The University of Chicago Press.

Forest, M. (1987). *More education/integration*. Downsview, Ontario, Canada: G. Allan Roeher Institute.

Forest, M. (1989). *Action for inclusion: How to improve schools by welcom-

ing children with special needs into regular classrooms. Toronto: Frontier College Press.

Gollay, E., Freedman, R., Wyngaarden, M., & Kurtz, N.R. (1978). *Coming back*. Cambridge, MA: Abt Books.

Harris, L. (September 11, 1991). Press conference, National Press Club, Washington, DC.

Harris, L. and Associates. (1991, September/November). Public attitudes toward people with disabilities. *Word from Washington*, pp. 28–29.

Hill, B.K., Bruininks, R.H., Lakin, K.C., Hauber, F.A., & McGuire, S.P. (1985). Stability of residential facilities for people who are mentally retarded: 1977–1982. *Mental Retardation, 23*(3), 108–114.

Hill, B.K., Lakin, K.C., Bruininks, R.H., Amado, A.N., Anderson, D.J., & Copher, J.I. (1989). *Living in the community: A comparative study of foster homes and small group homes for people with mental retardation (Report No. 28)*. Minneapolis: University of Minnesota, Center for Residential and Community Services.

Hill, B.K., Sather, L.B., Kudla, M.J., & Bruininks, R.H. (1978). *A survey of the types of residential programs for mentally retarded people in the United States in 1978*. Unpublished report, Department of Psychoeducational Studies, University of Minnesota, Minneapolis.

House, J.S., Landis, K.R., & Umberson, D. (1988). Social relationships and health. *Science, 241*, 540–545.

Hugo, V. (1831). *The hunchback of Notre Dame*. New York: P.F. Collier & Son Co.

Jeffries, V., & Ransford, H.E. (1969). Interracial social contact and middle class white reactions to the Watts Riot. *Social Problems, 16*, 312–324.

Karan, O.C., & Knight, C.B. (1986). Developing support networks for individuals who fail to achieve competitive employment. In F.R. Rusch (Ed.), *Competitive employment issues and strategies* (pp. 241–255). Baltimore: Paul H. Brookes Publishing Co.

Lakin, K.C., Burwell, B.O., Hayden, M.F., & Jackson, M.E. (1992). *An independent assessment of Minnesota's Medicaid Home and Community Based Services Waiver Program*. Minneapolis: University of Minnesota, Center for Residential Services and Community Living.

Levy, J.M., Jessop, D.J., Rimmerman, A., & Levy, P.H. (1992). Attitudes of *Fortune 500* corporate executives toward the employability of persons with severe disabilities: A national study. *Mental Retardation, 30*(2), 67–75.

Lutfiyya, Z., & Reidy, D. (1991, November). *Personal relationships and social networks: Facilitating the inclusion of people with disabilities*. Presentation at the annual meeting of The Association for Persons with Severe Handicaps, Washington, DC.

Lynch, J.J. (1977). *The broken heart: The medical consequences of loneliness*. New York: Basic Books.

McKnight, J. (1987). *Regenerating community*. Paper prepared with support of District 1, Massachusetts Department of Mental Health.

Mount, B., & Zwernik, K. (1989). *It's never too early, it's never too late: A booklet about personal futures planning*. St. Paul: Metropolitan Council.

Newton, J.S. (1989). *Social support manual*. Eugene: University of Oregon, Neighborhood Living Project.

O'Brien, J., & O'Brien, C.L. (1992). *Remembering the soul of our work*. Madison, WI: Options in Community Living.

O'Connell, B. (1983). *America's voluntary spirit.* New York: Foundation Center.

O'Connell, M. (1988). *The gift of hospitality: Opening the doors of community life to people with disabilities.* Evanston, IL: Northwestern University, The Community Life Project.

O'Connell, M. (1990). *Community building in Logan Square: How a community grew stronger with the contributions of people with disabilities.* Evanston, IL: Northwestern University, The Community Life Project.

O'Connor, G. (1976). *Home is a good place: A national perspective of community residential facilities for developmentally disabled persons.* Washington, DC: American Association on Mental Deficiency.

People First of Washington. (1985). What we want from residential programs. In J. O'Brien & C.L. O'Brien (Eds.), *Framework for accomplishment,* Version 2.4, 1991 (pp. 29–36). Lithonia, GA: Responsive Systems Associates.

Perske, R. (1988). *Circles of friends: People with disabilities and their friends enrich the lives of one another.* Nashville: Abingdon Press.

G. Allan Roeher Institute. (1990). *Making friends: Developing relationships between people with a disability and other members of the community.* Downsview, Ontario, Canada: York University.

Spierman, G. (1991). *Everyone welcome: Powell River's Community Life Project.* Powell River, British Columbia: The Powell River Association for Community Living.

Steinbeck, J. (1937). *Of mice and men.* New York: Modern Library.

Taylor, S.J., & Bogdan, R. (1989). On accepting relationships between people with mental retardation and non-disabled people: Toward an understanding of acceptance. *Disability, Handicap, & Society, 4*(1), 21–36.

Tyne, A. (1988). *Ties and connections: An ordinary community life for people with learning difficulties.* London: King's Fund Centre.

Vandercook, T., York, J., & Forest, M. (1989). The McGill Action Planning System (MAPS): A strategy for building the vision. *Journal of The Association for Persons with Severe Handicaps, 4*(2), 205–215.

Vanier, J. (1971). *Eruption to hope.* Toronto, Ontario, Canada: Griffin House.

Wade, P. (1991, November). *Community inclusion for adults with profound and multiple disabilities.* Presentation at the annual conference of The Association for Persons with Severe Handicaps, Washington, DC.

Wolfensberger, W. (1976). The origin and nature of our institutional models. In R.B. Kugel & A. Shearer (Eds.), *Changing patterns in residential services for the mentally retarded* (pp. 35–82, rev. ed.). Washington, DC: U.S. Government Printing Office.

Wolfensberger, W. (1988). Common assets of mentally retarded people that are commonly not acknowledged. *Mental Retardation, 26*(2), 63–70.

17

Steps for Supporting Community Connections

Angela Novak Amado

Man is a knot, a web, a mesh into which relationships are tied.

Saint Exupéry

Many different approaches have been used over the years to support relationships between persons with disabilities and community members. Many of these efforts started outside the human services system with citizen advocacy, community leisure-recreation programs, self-advocacy groups, and community-based bridge-builders. As the importance of typical relationships and friendships has received greater recognition, more human services agencies have taken on the role of connecting people to the community. In fact, many human services programs are now required to do so by federal and state regulations and the standards of professional organizations such as the National Accreditation Council.

The information in this chapter presents a planned, intentional approach to connecting persons with disabilities to community life. The information is written for human services agencies that have taken on or wish to take on this role, and in a manner that would support the efforts of agency staff. However, other individuals, families, groups, or organizations can certainly apply the information to

Information contained in this chapter pertaining to the Friends Project is in the public domain.

The development of some of the information in this chapter was funded through Grant No. 17673 to the Human Services Research and Development Center from the Minnesota Governor's Planning Council on Developmental Disabilities under provisions of the Developmental Disabilities Act of 1987 (PL 100-146). This content does not necessarily reflect the position or policy of the Minnesota Governor's Planning Council on Developmental Disabilities or the Minnesota State Planning Agency.

their situations and can find it useful for supporting people to be more connected to their communities and to have more friends.

DIMENSIONS THAT SHAPE
COMMUNITY-CONNECTING EFFORTS

As a poet once said, "A man is what he does with his attention." Where we are putting our attention defines who we are as well as the results that are produced.

As described in the previous chapter, many different strategies in a variety of arenas have been used to promote community connections. In assisting human services agencies to change their focus toward more support of friendship with community members, several overriding dimensions have been discovered that shape and frame those community-building efforts. A number of overall issues, which are discussed below, will affect both the efforts and the resulting degree of success.

1. An Alteration in the
Larger Context of the Job Is Necessary

Most services for persons with disabilities are designed around the deficits of those individuals. After all, persons only receive services because they are by definition in need of support; that support is funded and based on what's "wrong" with a person. Virtually all government entities require an assessment and determination of "need" to use public dollars for services to an individual. The vast majority of assessment processes that are currently utilized direct the assessor to and result in a focus on physical care and skill training. If relationships are considered at all, they are usually entered under the domain of "social skills" or "leisure-recreation," or they appear as issues in programs to control or alter inappropriate social behavior, such as hitting or spitting. Although there is also much more focus now on community integration in many services, most of this "integration" activity consists of *doing* things in the community, such as shopping or going to the movies, rather than participating with other community members in shared activities. In one study of the most physically integrated services in one state (Lakin, Burwell, Hayden, & Jackson, 1992), only 5% of the individuals regularly participated in community activities with friends who did not have disabilities.

Working on friendships and relationships first requires a deep recognition of their importance. Relating to others is at the very heart of existence for all people, whether they have disabilities or not. Even though many individuals with disabilities are surrounded by people (usually staff and other persons with disabilities) all day, many are often starved for attention and recognition. They want to be known as unique individuals and to be liked and known as themselves, not just somebody's "job." Working on friendships requires an alteration in the definition of staff roles, from caregiver or skill trainer to community connector. It also requires replanning and rescheduling staff priorities and activities.

The focus in the design of many individualized program plans (IPPs) and in professional preparation and education for the field has been teaching increased independence and improvement of skills. Increased independence may lead to greater productivity, but also to isolation and loneliness. For example, some group home residents become "independent" enough to move to an apartment; after they do so, staff sometimes become aware of their social isolation. Some agencies have responded to this loneliness by ensuring people get together with old friends from the group home, supporting them in attending special recreational activities (i.e., segregated), or even moving them back to a group setting. However, a different solution is also possible: supporting relationships with community members. Support for community relationships requires a different kind of work than the experience or training of human services professionals has provided. Rather than a focus on an individual's degree of *independence*, success in building relationships requires a focus on building *interdependence* and mutual contribution between people with and without disabilities.

2. Not Doing "More," But "Different"

Human services staff are already overburdened with too much to do. When the importance of community connections and friendships is realized, sometimes "helping people have friends" gets added as one more item on an already too-long list of "things to do." If support of relationships is recognized as critical, staff time must be allotted for it. If staff efforts are devoted to working on community connections, something else will probably need to be eliminated or reduced.

Another avenue not to do "more," but to do things "differently," is to change or shift the focus of what is being done. For instance, time already set aside for "community integration" can be changed from shopping or recreating with little opportunity for real interactions to thoughtfully planning where individuals can go to connect meaningfully with community members. Agencies may have to undertake an entirely new way of operating. An administrator of one agency in the Friends Project (Amado, Conklin, & Wells, 1990), for example, said, "I used to think that 'community integration' meant doing activities in the community; now I know it means helping people have friends."

When people are asked or the unspoken communications in their behavior are "heard," it is often found that relationships with community members are very important—they want and prefer other people in their lives who want to be with them and who like them. (This issue is discussed in A.N. Amado, chap. 16, this volume, as one of the main reasons to work on friendships.) A person also likes to be with people whom they see as valuable or important. Many individuals who receive services are explicit about their preference for people other than staff and other people with disabilities. One friend of this author is insistent that friends be "not a client," and refuses to go to community club events with a staff person. Another man who volunteers at a local library is adamant about never introducing the library staff to his residential services staff; he wants to keep his two "worlds" separate.

Stepping beyond the illusion that we can do *everything* for people, decisions can be made about specific areas on which to concentrate our efforts. What are the most important things to work on? What are the areas that will affect other areas and create the most change for the person? In Chapters 4 and 16 of this volume, examples were given of how people changed in several areas of their lives once they made friends who were community members or after they were given a chance to contribute meaningfully to their community. It is possible that in using a "different" approach (concentrated work on community relationships), many of the other items on the "to-do" list that is too long will also disappear.

3.   Meeting Many People May
Be Necessary To Develop Real Friendships

The work of supporting friendships does not necessarily mean focusing on finding *one* friend for each individual served. When any two people meet, they do not necessarily or immediately "click" as friends. Sometimes it takes a long time before any two people become friends, before the right "chemistry" is apparent. If the entire social context is opened up, each person served will have the opportunity to get to know many different kinds of people and be more fully included in community life. A variety of different types of relationships can be supported, for example: companions, acquaintances, fellow club members, partners, family members, co-workers, neighbors. Rather than just focusing on one relationship or connection, the point is to support individuals in getting to know and be known by many different people, expanding the social network and maximizing the variety of relationships. In addition to ensuring a wide network of relationships for an individual, the chances will also then be increased to make at least one friend. The more people one meets, the more opportunity there is for two people to "click" as friends.

4.   Supporting Relationships Means the Work Is Never Done

Once the work of supporting relationships and friendships is started, it is an illusion to think it will end. There may be many failures before there is any success. Having a friend is not a goal or objective that can be reached with 100% effectiveness. The friendships of persons with disabilities are like those of anyone—they have ups and downs and they may last a short while or a long time. While some friendships are continuing, others may start and some may end. Friends of 2 years ago may be gone now and replaced with others in yet another 2 years. All relationships change and fluctuate throughout people's lives.

In terms of these kinds of changes over time, one cannot expect that relationships for persons with disabilities will be or should be any different. Significant effort may be put into establishing one community relationship for one individual, only to have the community member move out of the state in a year. Even after connections are established, support may continue to be needed to overcome the sadness when people leave, to meet new people, to resolve the ups and downs of existing relationships, and to continue to expand both the breadth and depth of the social network.

5.   The Problem Is Often Not
Community Members, but Staff and Agencies

Working with six residential services agencies in the Friends Project, Amado et al. (1990) found that staff often felt before starting connecting efforts that community members or community attitudes were their largest barrier. Some staff held the view that community members might not be interested or would need a lot of convincing; other staff were reluctant to speak to community members. However, when concrete and specific efforts were actually implemented, it was found that the real barrier was staff attitudes rather than community members. Building bridges to community is not an activity in which human services staff have been trained or with which they have much experience. Once community members were finally asked, staff were often very surprised to find them overwhelmingly open and interested in getting to know individuals with disabilities. It might be necessary for staff to catch themselves in their own generalizations and professional habituation about both individuals with disabilities and community members. Often underneath reluctant attitudes toward community members are unconscious opinions on the part of staff that the individual with disabilities is not as valuable a person to know as other community members, that others would not want to spend time with him or her, or there is a lack of appreciation and belief in the importance of these relationships for both community members and individuals with disabilities.

The success of this work will depend on staff perspectives toward three things: the individuals with disabilities, community members, and the importance of this work. Community members can be seen as: dead, rejecting, dangerous, incompetent, the enemy, or the "client," or as:

—having the potential for welcome, appreciation, tolerance, sharing, assistance, and love;
—lacking connections to people;
—deprived—by human services policies and practices—of the opportunities and resources to get to know individuals who have been labelled. (O'Brien & O'Brien, 1989)

Besides staff attitudes, agency structures and practices often interfere with establishing community relationships and increase the amount of distance between a service recipient and a community citizen. Goals and objectives for greater independence, staff–client ratios, "active treatment," and subcontract production deadlines all often leave insufficient time and energy for the work involved in connecting individuals to community members. Other program practices directly increase distance with community members. Sometimes people get moved from one residence to another with no thought for where their current friends live and how hard it will be to get together in the new residence. Traveling in the community with small groups of people, imposing residential agency rules on community members, and scheduling with minimum flexibility or thoughtfulness regarding friendship are all examples of potential interference with a natural flow in a relationship. For example, a friend of this author attends a day treatment program in the morning and comes home at noon. Her residential support staff arrives at 2:00 P.M. and stays until 6:00 P.M. Because of the medications she is currently taking, this 33-year-old woman usually goes to bed a little after 6:00 P.M. She has no time on weekends because of her staff schedule. The only time she sees that she has to get together with friends is from noon to 2:00 P.M. during the week. In addition, her staff devote no time in their busy schedules to helping her get together with her friends, and this woman prefers to keep her "staff" time and her "friend" time separate. The schedule and the ingrained perception of "services" prevent more opportunities for companionship and certainly interfere with her getting to know others.

Supporting people's relationships can also include rekindling old relationships. In the Friends Project (Amado et al., 1990), it was found that the attitudes of some staff can also interfere with these efforts. For example, for certain individuals it is reported that their family is not interested or gave up on the person long ago. However, when other staff were unsure about "the story" about the family, and did some investigative work to find out what was really the truth, they were often surprised (see Shapiro, chap. 11, this volume, for an example). Sometimes it takes some work to reconnect people to old relationships. One mother insisted that no one in the family and none of her other children were interested in her son with mental retardation; however, when the staff persisted and contacted some of the adult siblings, the sisters reported they were indeed very interested in spending time with their brother. The sisters offered that they had different attitudes than their mother.

In the late 1980s and early 1990s, this author conducted workshops in several different states about supporting all types of friendships and relationships, including rekindling lost ones. Since then, some staff have been trying to find family members who have not seen their siblings with disabilities in 5, 30, 40, or, in one case, 60 years. After staff do the work of locating families, some of the parents and siblings are very willing to be reconnected. It is difficult to say what the reasons are for this willingness; perhaps it is due to the increased public knowledge of disability, different attitudes from the time when families were originally separated, other children's discomfort with parental actions long ago to place their siblings out-of-home, a continuing interest in contact even though in prior years family members had felt discouraged by professionals from contacting their sister or brother, or some other reason. Whatever the cause, these siblings are willing to contact, write, and see their brother or sister again, even across hundreds of miles, different states, and in their advanced years.

Successful work in supporting relationships will take shifting staff and agency attitudes from "building community happens after everything else—if we have time" to "building community is central to everyone's job" (Jacob, 1991). Staff time must be freed up for this work; staff must also be allowed time for gathering together to reflect and celebrate triumphs, failures, and the day-to-day hard work.

6. A Friend Is Not a Volunteer

Volunteers are extremely valuable and make necessary and worthwhile contributions; however, to ask someone to volunteer is very different from asking him or her to be someone's friend. When someone volunteers for another person, there is often an imbalance and lack of reciprocity in the relationship—it is someone doing something *for* someone else. Volunteer relationships are also often formalized and time-limited. Of course, some volunteer relationships lead to genuine and long-lasting friendships; however, asking someone to enter into a relationship with an individual with disabilities as a volunteer can perpetuate the notions of dependence, caretaking, and neediness.

Some formal regulations regarding volunteers also distance the individual being assisted from the community member who might be volunteering. Requirements might include a certain number of training hours, criminal background checks, reporting of volunteer hours, and other paperwork that formalizes a relationship. Often a volunteer is attached and serves the program or agency rather than being there for the individual with disabilities. Often, it is also a "functional" rather than a "personal" relationship (see A.N. Amado, chap. 16, this volume).

In contrast, a friend is there for someone because he or she likes the person and wants to be with him or her. Both people contribute and are contributed to in the relationship. In Powell River, British Columbia, one of the families who became involved with an individual with disabilities had this to say:

> When people see us together, I don't want them to think it's because we're part of a program. . . . We get a lot out of having (Bob) in our family life and like most of our friends we expect he'll be part of our life for a long time. So even though our relationship started through the Community Life Project, I don't want anyone to think that the time we spend together now is a volunteer activity. It's not. It's just a friendship. (Spierman, 1991, p. 12)

7.   "Community" Is an Experience, Not a Place

Sometimes the idea of assisting individuals to be more a part of their community seems difficult; the picture or definition of what that would look like or what is really involved might be vague or confusing. One element that often contributes to the perceived difficulty and confusion is the erroneous concept of "the community" as a defined geographical space.

For a human services program, "community" can mean anything outside of the facility. In many agencies, persons served have goals and objectives in their individualized service, habilitation, or program plans regarding community integration or community activities. Such goals are required for federally funded programs, in the standards of the National Accreditation Council, and in the regulations of many states. People have "community outings;" they work on their "community goal" one to five times a week, and they "go out to the community." Typically these opportunities mean going anyplace else in town outside the program building, such as visiting a shopping mall, store, museum, zoo, or bowling alley. Yet, when staff members in their own day-to-day lives go shopping or visit the museum or zoo, they do not say they are going to "the community." Rather, they say, "I'm going to run an errand," "I'm going to do the grocery shopping," "Let's go to the museum (or zoo) today," or "I'm going down to the club." The relationship of staff persons to their community is different, even in their language, than that of program participants to their community (even when that "community" is the same geographical place). For persons in human services settings, "the community" is often like a foreign country; people with disabilities take tours with their staff as tour guides.

If this notion of physical space is examined more closely, it continues to be clear that a "community" is not defined by geography. One person may belong to many different communities—the communities of golfers, single mothers, or *Star Trek* fans; these communities can crisscross wide physical spaces and many different groups of people. One person living on a particular street may not know anyone else on that street; yet, someone else on the same street may know almost everyone living there. The first person attributes no importance for social companionship to the block on which he or she lives, but for the second person, the block may be one of the most important components of his or her total social network.

One geographical area that appears to be a "community" may not even be such in terms of people's actual experience in that place. Even in small rural towns, there can be great divisiveness among different "communities" within the town—the people who live on the hill, the ones across the tracks, the more conservative and the less conservative Lutherans, the city council crowd, the serious softball players, and the folks who are promoting tourism and those opposed or indifferent to it. In one small Minnesota town, one of the frequent conversations among town citizens is who "belongs" and who does not "belong" to that town. Staff from one of the residential agencies in the town felt that one of the community attitudes was that none of their residents "belonged." However, when the staff started investigating the public conversation, they found that probably a majority of *all* of the people in town felt they did not "belong." Someone whose grandfather was one of the founders of the town still felt she did not "belong." Someone else who had lived there only 5 years felt that she *did* "belong." Instead of meeting some set of criteria, "belonging" was definitely a person's experience.

Rather than relating to any characteristic of a place, perhaps the best way to think about community is as the set of "ties and connections" that a person has with others. Tyne (1988) has explained this concept of community as "the ways that ordinary people live their lives. Community is the set of connections or ties a person has with others, whether or not it is based in a place on the map" (p. 2). It is the experience of being known by others, being liked, being seen as a unique person, and belonging with others. Based on a survey of more than 40,000 people, Davis (1985) characterized qualities of friendship as including enjoyment, acceptance, understanding, and spontaneity (feeling free to be ourselves)—all familiar elements in the relationships of true community.

In terms of this confusion with geography, staff have sometimes argued that they do not know their own neighbors or that they are not necessarily well-connected in their own communities (especially in larger cities, suburbs, or bedroom communities). The work of community-connecting often starts with looking to the immediate geographical space around the program, in the neighborhood, town, or city; if staff are not from that immediate area, they often experience difficulty initiating efforts. They may argue against understanding or knowing "community."

However, when community is viewed as "ties and connections" rather than geographical space, it can be seen that these staff do have their own communities. Their social networks may not include their neighbors or people from the immediate vicinity of their own town or city; however, staff members do have relationships in which they are at ease, known, comfortable, and liked for themselves. They have people they hang out with, complain to, do things with, and care about. They have ties and connections *somewhere*—even if those relationships are not in one geographical area or are in other towns or states.

Building community, therefore, is a matter of assisting persons in being related to others, no matter where those others may live. It is a matter of building social networks, establishing ties and connections, and crossing wide arenas of sources for relationships. Primarily, it is a matter of bringing people together to have them experience each other and supporting individuals with disabilities to be known, liked, and appreciated by others, as well as to contribute, be contributed to, and be with people they value and who value knowing them.

BASIC STRATEGIES

Several projects and agencies have developed useful and successful methods for assisting people with disabilities to meet community citizens, be more fully included in their communities, and have friendships with typical community members. Some of these projects include:

The Friends Project in Minnesota, 1989–1990 (Amado et al., 1990)

Options for Individuals, Inc., in Louisville, Kentucky (see Bartholomew-Lorimer, chap. 10, this volume)

The Community Life Project in Logan Square, Chicago (O'Connell, 1988, 1990)

The Community Life Project in Powell River, British Columbia (Spierman, 1991)

The work of Deborah Reidy and others in Massachusetts to assist persons to join community organizations and groups (see Reidy, chap. 19, this volume)

Description of Different Projects

The methods used in these efforts and described here are based on the work of several different thinkers committed to reshaping the experience of community life. These authors include: John McKnight (1987) who has written extensively about the power and strength of communities to include the gifts of all citizens; Beth Mount, the developer of Personal Futures Planning, which helps people understand and see an individual as gifts and capacities rather than as deficits (Mount & Zwernik, 1988); and John O'Brien and Connie Lyle O'Brien (1989) who have articulated a "basic strategy" to assist human services agencies develop specific opportunities and build concrete connections to community life for the people they serve. The ideas of these individuals have provided the foundation for the work in the following efforts.

The Friends Project   Many of the techniques and processes described below were tried out with six residential services agencies in Minnesota in the Friends project (funded by the Minnesota Governor's Planning Council on Developmental Disabilities). This project worked with staff in both rural and urban agencies in 1989 and 1990. It focused on 23 individuals with developmental disabilities who ranged in age from 11 years to 72 years, in living settings from their own apartment to a 15-bed group home, and in degree of independence from fairly independent persons who worked competitively to persons who could not walk or speak.

The purpose of the project was three-fold:

1. To assist individuals to have more friendships with persons without disabilities and to be more fully included in their communities
2. To develop the role of staff as "community connectors"
3. To assist agencies in determining internal structures that support more relationship-building and community connectedness for the people served

A "focus group" was formed around each of the 23 focus individuals in the Friends project. This group went through a planning process utilizing some of the components of Personal Futures Planning and then met approximately once a month to develop and try out different strategies. The groups ranged in size from two to seven people and always included residential services staff; some groups also included family members, case managers, day program or school staff, and other community friends. More detail about the exact processes used in the Project is contained in *Friends: A Manual for Connecting Persons with Disabilities and Community Members* (Amado et al., 1990).

Options for Individuals, Inc., Louisville   Options provides adult day services to support 25 people in a variety of ways. Staff start by getting to know people and identifying each person's unique capacities and interests. Then, places are sought out where people can contribute and become a part of the everyday life of the community. (See Bartholomew-Lorimer, chap. 10, this volume, for more description and examples.)

Community Life Project, Chicago   A project sponsored by the Center for Urban Affairs and Policy Research at Northwestern University worked in one neighborhood of Chicago called Logan Square to strengthen the community with the contributions of persons with disabilities. The project was hosted by the Logan Square Neighborhood Association. Project staff identified resources and became familiar with associational life in the neighborhood, interviewed community members, and introduced approximately 30 people with disabilities on a one-to-one basis to individuals and groups (O'Connell, 1990).

Community Life Project, Powell River   The Community Life Project in Powell River was sponsored by the British Columbia Association for Community Living and built upon the work in Logan Square, Chicago. It particularly used the idea of asking interested community citizens to act as "hosts" for persons with disabilities to guide isolated people into groups of community citizens (Spierman, 1991).

Western Massachusetts   In various towns and communities in

Massachusetts, conscious efforts are applied to assisting persons with disabilities become members of community groups and associations. This work is explained in detail in Chapter 19, this volume.

These are, of course, not the only community-building efforts that have occurred. Many other projects and efforts have been initiated, and numerous useful materials are available (Arsenault, 1990; Curtis, Dezelsky, & Coffey, 1990; Newton, 1989; Tyne, 1988). Parts of the strategies and methods used by these different groups are similar in nature and overlap; some groups use a variety of approaches. These different strategies are summarized into the sequential process described below.

BASIC PRINCIPLES

The methods used in the Friends Project and the other four projects and initiatives described above have been successfully used by residential services staff, day program and employment agencies, individual families, and other groups such as advocacy organizations, developmental disabilities councils, and community organizations. There are at least three basic principles shaping the work of these projects, including: 1) act as if almost anything can happen, 2) start small—one to one, and 3) plan and implement based on a capacity-based view of the person.

1. *Act as If Almost Anything Can Happen* When people from Connecticut who implemented the Personal Futures Planning process for several years were asked why they were having such extraordinary results, they responded that one of their operating guidelines was to: "act as if almost anything can happen" (Mount, Ducharme, & Beeman, 1991). They strongly believed in the purpose and vision of their work and trusted both people with disabilities and community members. It takes real confidence and belief in the work of community-building for it to be successful, especially through the high and low points.

2. *Start Small— One-to-One* It would be a mistake to start out with the premise that "I have to find friends for everyone on my caseload" (Jacob, 1991). Because this work is often new and different from the current operating practices of most agencies, it takes learning over time. It makes sense for a staff person or other community connector to start with one person rather than everybody. It also helps if the person the staff starts with is someone they like and about whom they can speak easily to others (this is a more important factor than any particular characteristics the individual might have).

It is very difficult to implement the processes described here if one staff member is attempting to take three people with disabilities out into "the community" at a time. It is even very difficult if it is one staff with two individuals. Each person is unique, with different interests. It is harder for community members to see and relate to two or three people than it is for them to relate to one person.

3. Plan and Implement Based on a Capacity-Based View of the Person   Whereas the services system encourages us to see people as their deficits and to focus on what is missing, many authors have encouraged more positive views of people (Mount & Zwernik, 1988; Taylor & Bogdan, 1989). Specific processes, such as Personal Futures Planning, help people see an individual as their gifts and capacities and to see what he or she has to offer and contribute to others. Such processes also help individuals to be appreciated just as they are, with nothing needing to be "fixed." The whole scope of community-building efforts, including planning, implementing, and working through issues, requires a view of individuals as their gifts and capacities, a belief in their right to belong fully and be included, and a deep and rich appreciation of their humanity.

Although different approaches can be utilized to access and develop this view of an individual, one method that has been very useful for the planning process is to draw on the basic tenets and components of Personal Futures Planning (Mount & Zwernik, 1988). This form of planning is a possibility-based, interactive approach to understanding a person and to envisioning a future for him or her. A group of persons who care about an individual and his or her future gather together, usually in more informal and comfortable settings than typical meetings. Rather than stacks of files and records, the process uses large sheets of paper taped up to walls; colorful markers are used to create drawings and images that keep a group focused on the individual. As opposed to more traditional forms of planning that are typically focused on a person's deficits, it is a process that allows a person to be seen as his or her gifts and capacities. The different charts that can be completed include:

The person's past life experiences
A relationships map of current relationships, importance of various
    relationships, and his or her role in any given relationship
The places where the person goes, including frequency and type
What works and does not work for the person (preferences and upset-
    ting situations)
The person's interests, gifts, and contributions to others
What assistance the person needs in meeting and getting to know
    others (These charts are described in Mount and Zwernik, 1988,
    1990.)

The process supports a group in seeing and understanding an individual as a complex human being, with needs and wishes and dreams similar to those that all people have. Even when a group member has known an individual for years or thinks he or she knows the person well, the process often allows very surprising insights and understanding; individuals are often seen in new ways and with a fuller appreciation of their lives and current situations.

In Personal Futures Planning, dreams and images for the person's future are agreed upon by the group and people are inspired to move into action for that individual. Then the group continues to meet and to work on having the dream become a reality. In the Friends Project, the Futures Planning process was not used to address all aspects of the person's future, but rather was focused on his or her friendships and relationships. Other projects have also been based on a capacity-based view of the person, and project staff have taken steps to get to know individuals as their interests, gifts, and possible contributions.

THE STEPS OF THE PROCESS

Friendship is like sex: we always suspect there's some secret technique we don't know about.

Pogrebin (1987, p. 5)

Supporting friendship is not a linear process that means following steps A-B-C. Each person is unique, every relationship is different, and every situation needs to be thought through carefully. If efforts are made and are unsuccessful, then the actions regarding the individual with disabilities, the community person or group, and staff practices need to be re-examined. Many methods and models may need to be tried.

As noted by other authors in this volume, these methods should not be taken as "written in stone." One way will certainly not work with everyone. A variety of different methods and strategies should be drawn upon, for each has its own strengths and weaknesses. Four steps that can be used are: 1) identify interests, gifts, and possible contributions; 2) explore and identify possible connections; 3) make introductions; and 4) continue to support the relationship.

1. Identify Interests, Gifts, and Contributions

No one should have to wait to gain more social skills or to have his or her behavior "fixed" before having more relationships. A focus on what is wrong with or missing from someone will leave that person waiting for a long time. Rather, the work can start with accepting people the way they are. A capacity-based approach looks at the person now and asks: What does this person have to offer? How and where can he or she be included, just the way he or she is?

Sociological and psychological research indicates that people become friends with individuals with whom they share mutual interests (Santrock, 1989). Therefore, identifying interests that might be shared with others is a critical component of the planning process, as is clarifying gifts that the person has to offer to others. Physical proximity is also a key factor in whether or not two people become friends —people must be in the same place to get acquainted and to get to know each other (Santrock, 1989). Once interests are identified, then the places to meet others, get acquainted, and share interests with community members can be explored.

Interests are those things that express the meaning in a person's life (O'Brien & O'Brien, 1989), or that seem to express a person's "calling." A person's gifts are those qualities or characteristics that are appreciated by others. Sometimes gifts can be very obvious, such as a good sense of humor or being a hard worker; sometimes they are more subtle, such as a great smile or an ability to inspire others to care. Wolfensberger (1988) has eloquently written of the many gifts that persons with disabilities bring to the world. Many human services workers also report that they are in this field because of the enjoyment they experience in working with people with disabilities— there is something they really appreciate about the people with whom they work.

Listening carefully to many people who know the individual well or have spent many years with the individual helps to flush out the list of interests and gifts. Usually, direct care staff or someone who spends more day-to-day time with the person is more helpful. Seeking information from many different sources also helps, such as the residence, day program, family, or any community members the person knows. Sometimes residential staff and day program staff have very different information about a person. Being very specific about interests is also important; for instance, what kinds of food, television shows, cars, or movies does the person like? Does he or she like all sports or just some; watching, playing, or helping out; women's sports as well as men's; or watching on television or sitting in noisy arenas?

For some individuals, it is difficult to identify interests. Perhaps years of deprivation in institutions, restricted life experiences, lack of conscious encouragement and stimulation, perpetuation of a self-fulfilling prophecy that the person is not interested in anything, or other reasons may make some individuals appear to have few interests. For these people, it is important to spend time exploring. The question to ask and to spend time answering is: What could the person explore to clarify and develop his or her interests? Although interests may not be easy to define, they can be developed and expressed in action, that is, by trying out things. For this exploration, it also takes knowing someone well enough and spending enough time with him or her to be able to "read" or interpret their reactions. For instance, Reidy (chap. 19, this volume) tells the story of a woman with severe disabilities with whom the community builder spent a long time before discovering (almost accidentally) her interest in walking. This discovery led to her joining a walking club.

Sometimes it takes just strolling down the street and noticing very subtle things, such as when the person turns his or her head or opens his or her eyes wider. One staff mentioned that a man with very profound disabilities preferred to eat at Perkin's rather than McDonald's because he responded to the ceiling fans at Perkin's. It can take long periods of "walking with" or sharing life with people and deep sensitivity to really understand their interests.

It is important to clarify interests because they are the sources for identifying what can be shared with community members and what can be contributed to others. They also help identify potential memberships and associations to which the person might belong.

2. Explore and Identify Possible Connections

When the person is deeply understood and appreciated, and some of his or her interests and gifts are identified, the next step is to plan possible connections. There are at least five different approaches that can be utilized to explore and develop possible connections. One or a combination of more than one of the following approaches can be used.

A. Where Are All the Places This Interest Can Be Expressed? After a group has selected and focused on just one of the identified interests, the members can generate a list of all the places where this interest is expressed and all the types of places where people engage in anything related to this interest. For example, one man was very enthusiastic about cars. His group came up with the following list of places where cars were worked on or talked about and where this interest could be expressed or shared with others:

Auto repair body shops
Auto parts dealers

Service departments
Used car lots
Auto inspection centers
Car washes
Auto rentals
Performance racing tracks
Auto stereo stores
Race tracks
Mechanics' garages and schools
Gas stations
Parking lots and/or garages
Tire stores
Auto magazine publishers (Mount, 1991)

Once a list of places or areas is generated, the group members can ask: For each of these places, whom do we know there? Whom can we ask to be involved at any of these places? If we don't know anyone, who knows somebody they can ask who might know someone at one of these places?

Another way to generate ideas is to identify one interest or gift and determine where the person could contribute that gift and where his or her gifts would be appreciated. Where are people or places where this individual could bring this interest and fit in? Often community members are better at seeing how and where someone can use his or her gifts than staff people.

An individual may do something that is perceived by staff as a barrier to community members' interest or as an insurmountable problem, such as being very loud, banging his or her head, or wearing a helmet. Staff might use the behavior as a reason not to begin any community-connecting efforts or might wait and try to "fix" the behavior first. However, at least two different approaches can be used in these instances in order to support community connecting: first, ideas can be generated for places where that particular behavior would not be a problem. For instance, where do other people hang out who are loud? Loading docks and rock concerts are two examples. Where are places where "normal" people bang their heads? Two places are wrestling matches and boxing clubs. Where are other people who wear helmets? Football and hockey teams are examples. For almost any behavior considered odd or undesirable in a human services program, that same behavior is also exhibited by ordinary people in specific types of settings. Those settings might provide excellent opportunities for an individual to be included. A second way to generate ideas is to ask: Where could we find places where this individual could be included and the other people there would not mind this person doing what he or she does? One individual who was echolalic and made sounds that were often irritating to others was able to work in a family-run business owned by a Chinese family who did not speak English very well; they simply thought the individual spoke that way because he was "from New York" (Mount, 1991). Bartholomew-Lorimer (chap. 10, this volume) gives an example of selecting a neighborhood food service as a community site for a person because it was big and open with people hanging around the trucks. It was a place where a person could yell and it would not bother anyone.

B. Identify Opportunities for Community Relationships   Unfortunately, most efforts called "community integration" for persons in the services system are focused on *doing something*—a community activity. Many of these community activities present no opportunity to meet others or form relationships. Outings such as shopping, going to the park, eating at restaurants, or visiting museums or fairs present very little opportunity for a unique individual to be known and appreciated by others.

One of the most significant changes that a program could make, which would substantially alter the likelihood of developing relationships for the persons served, is to shift the focus of community integration from *activities* to *opportunities for relationships*. There are two critical factors to consider in exploring community places as having potential for opportunities for relationships:

1. *Seeing the same people over time is important.*   To become familiar and be known as an individual, it is necessary to see the same people over and over. For all people, friendships have developed as a result of seeing the same people repeatedly and over time. It makes a difference to become a "regular" (Bartholomew-Lorimer, chap. 10, this volume) or "member" (Reidy, chap. 19, this volume).

2. *Some basis for exchange is needed.*   Places that hold opportunities for relationships are those in which there is some basis for people giving back and forth and for participating with each other. Shopping or 8-week community education classes are often insufficient. Opportunities such as recreating together on the same team, being in the same club, or being volunteers together at the museum all provide some basis for exchange and for an individual becoming known for what they have to offer.

These two dimensions define, at a minimum, places where opportunities for relationships could be present or could be developed. In addition, that the community members in a particular place are or could be interested and welcoming will also affect whether real connections develop.

C. Look for Potential Welcoming Places The approach for community-building used in Louisville (Bartholomew, 1985; Bartholomew-Lorimer, chap. 10, this volume) was to identify what were called "interest sites." Staff explored the local areas and neighborhoods around people's homes and identified places that they thought held the potential for individuals with disabilities to be included. Ultimately, they found that the places with which they had the most success were local places, such as small, family-owned businesses or neighborhood groups and clubs (e.g., small prayer groups or coffee clubs). They explored places where someone could contribute in some way and become known over time. In investigating different sites, staff would go into the cafe or store, talk to club members, and determine if the owners or members would be open and interested in welcoming a particular individual with disabilities. They were careful and discriminating about people and places, looking for the "right" community members and the best potential matches.

They also applied the "one person, one environment" rule and never introduced more than one person with disabilities into any setting. In each environment, they also explored and sorted out what the individual with disabilities could contribute in that particular setting, even small things such as washing the dishes or sweeping the floor in a cafe, greeting people in a pet store, or helping out with children in a daycare program.

D. Explore the Local Community: Local History, Leaders, and Associational Life Sometimes research must be done to find out what is available, what kind of formal and informal associations exist, and who local leaders are and whether they would be willing to be allied with community-building efforts. In the Logan Square neighborhood of Chicago, for instance, one of the first steps of the Community Life Project was to interview business owners and leaders of the neighborhood association to discover what they knew about people with disabilities in their area and to find out the neighborhood resources (O'Connell, 1990).

A day program agency in Buckley County, Ohio, wanted to develop specific opportunities for individuals to be involved in regular community life (Wade, 1991). At first it was difficult because, as in many places, a large majority of the citizens worked during the day. If the persons who attended the day program were not in supported or competitive employment, it was difficult for the agency to identify specific community opportunities during the Monday–Friday daytime schedule. In order to fully explore their options, staff began researching their own community. Starting with the assumption that not everyone worked, they explored what the community members who were not working did during the day. They discovered six categories of places and activities in which typical community members participated:

1. *Personal business:* banking, laundry, many kinds of shopping, going to the beauty shop or post office, other errands
2. *Leisure and/or recreation:* restaurants and cafes, parks, library, cinema, theatre, music, tours and trips, other recreation
3. *Hobbies:* art, fishing, crafts, collecting, pets
4. *Continuing education and/or personal development:* many different kinds of classes and physical fitness activities
5. *Club and/or organization activities:* groups that met during the day, such as seniors, sororities and fraternities; churches, political, social and/or service organizations
6. *Volunteerism:* hospitals, universities, libraries, public administration and elected officials' offices, parks, animal shelters, free stores, churches

The agency then assisted individuals in becoming established in environments where they could contribute and be with the same people regularly and over time. Other resources list various ideas for how to "get involved" and find out about what is going on in the community. The Community Life Project in Logan Square (O'Connell, 1988) identified three main sources for finding out about neighborhood groups: 1) using printed sources, such as phone books and directories; 2) contacting local institutions, such as churches and libraries; and 3) completing surveys of individuals. Arsenault (1990) calls the exploration of community resources "going on a treasure hunt."

E.   Look for Interested People   The last way to explore possible connections is to look directly for people who might be interested in getting to know an individual with disabilities. When looking for such people, questions to ask among staff and others include: Do you know somebody who might be interested in becoming (John's) friend? Whom do you know who might like (John)? Where could we find somebody who might like to be (Linda's) friend? It helps to have a sense of what kind of community member would be preferred or what characteristics that person should have. It does not necessarily have to be someone who has considered it before or who knows anything about disabilities.

Sometimes staff have very extensive social networks. In some small towns, the social networks of just the agency staff include virtually everyone in town. However, staff have to be willing to cross the usual boundaries. They might have to be willing to examine their own networks of relationships and be willing to ask their own friends or relatives to become interested in a particular individual.

Another avenue to pursue is staff joining clubs or groups, meeting more people, and finding out more about their own community. Some staff members have joined a group with an individual with disabilities, become acquainted with the members, made sure the individual was included, and enjoyed the associational life themselves.

3. Make Introductions

Once possible connections are identified, the next step is to introduce people. Two broad categories of introduction are one-to-one and to a group.

A. One-to-One Introductions How introductions are made is probably one of the most critical factors affecting the success of community-building work. Many times, efforts at community-connecting have been what human services agencies call "educating the community" and have consisted of speeches or talks to churches, Kiwanis, or other groups on what people with disabilities are like and why group members should "get involved." Or, efforts to build connections have consisted of a staff person saying to a community member, "I work at the Village Group Home and the people there really need friends. Would you be interested in becoming somebody's friend?" Although both of these types of efforts have, from time to time, miraculously unearthed someone willing to become involved in an individual's life, they are far less productive than a more personal, one-to-one approach.

The person who is functioning as the community connector should know the individual with disabilities well enough to be able to speak personally about him or her and his or her interests and gifts. Then, a particular community member should be identified and asked about getting to know that individual. It helps if the community connector also knows the community member well enough to know why he or she might be interested in getting to know the individual with disabilities. As opposed to the broad general methods described in the previous paragraph, it is an entirely different approach to say, "Joan, I think you would be interested in meeting Robin. She really likes sports. Robin, this is Joan who is really into baseball." The relationship gets initiated not on the basis that people feel they *should* get involved or because the person with disabilities *needs help*. Rather, it is an opportunity for two people to get to know each other on the basis of *enjoying the relationship* (Spierman, 1991).

It also makes a difference to let the community member know, either directly or indirectly, that this individual is someone worth knowing, someone important. Staff may need to start with their own values and attitudes on this issue and let go of ideas that they have to "apologize for" or "explain" the person, or introduce the person as "one of my clients" or "someone I work with." Rather, staff need to start with their own view that others would really appreciate getting to know this individual because he or she is worth knowing as a person and because he or she is a wonderful individual who really has something to offer.

It helps to work through what to say and how to best surround the individual with messages that he or she is important and worth knowing. For instance, consideration should be given to *where* the initial introduction should take place. It might not be the best idea to have the community member come to the group home or the workshop. Attention should be paid to how the individual is dressed, who the person is making the introductions, the number of nondisabled people accompanying the individual (i.e., do many people find him or her worth knowing), if the individual with disabilities is one of a group of others with disabilities or if he or she stands out as a unique person, and if the community connector is respected by the group to whom the person is being introduced.

What is said about the individual in the initial introductions will affect the future concepts and attitudes of community members. Because individuals with disabilities have ways in which they are different (as all people do), it takes thinking and planning to decide how much to tell the community person about the individual before the introduction, such as what they are like, what they may or may not do, or how they might act. It is also important to consider how best to express this information. Similar to setting up a blind date for two friends, it should be an individualized process based on both the person with disabilities and the community member. Some people may be more comfortable knowing as much as possible before the introduction and others may not care. Technical and program jargon never works as well as simple, straightforward communication, such as "Sometimes John gets anxious when he meets new people, but after he has a chance to know you he will relax." Also, individuals who receive services will often act differently with a community member or away from human services settings; the person conducting the introductions will have to be wary of his or her own predetermined concepts of how the individual and the community member will act or respond.

At times, the question of "confidentiality" in introducing people has been raised. Confidentiality will not be an issue if there is a commitment to, permission for, and support for particular community-building efforts by the person and his or her guardian.

Enough support should be provided in the introductory process to the individual with disabilities and the community member so that they are both comfortable. It might be that a staff person will have to accompany the person with disabilities, to "translate" his or her communications, to assist with physical care, for sufficient support for the individual or community member, or for other reasons. The staff should be sensitive, however, to letting community members and individuals with disabilities meet and connect with each other on their own terms.

B.   Introductions of Individuals to Groups   Individuals with disabilities also have the opportunity to become connected and meet many more potential friends by joining large or small groups or clubs and formal or informal associations. Reidy (chap. 19, this volume) provides excellent advice for these types of introductions. Spierman (1991) describes the process and methods used to support people joining the associational life of the community in Powell River, British Columbia. The person who was doing the community-building work in this city became familiar with a group and identified at least one person in the group who would act as a "host" or "sponsor" for the individual with disabilities; that host or sponsor would act as a guide for the person, introducing them to other group members and assisting group members to include that person.

Either type of introduction, one-to-one or to groups, should be done by a community connector who has confidence in his or her understanding of the person with disabilities, trust in community members, and high expectations. The community connector should also be someone who can trust people to work out problems on their own, but at the same time be sensitive to and gently assist when there are problems or difficulties.

4.   Continue To Support the Relationship

Probably the most difficult aspect of this work is supporting an acquaintance relationship to become a real friendship. Sometimes this process happens on its own, sometimes support helps it happen, and sometimes it just does not happen no matter how much assistance is provided. Understanding what support is needed to help it happen and when to allow it to happen on its own requires a delicate appreciation of people and situations.

Once connections are made, some relationships will continue to need support. The staff or community connector can check from time to time; informally ask people in the setting about how things are going; and verify that the individual with disabilities is really being included, especially if he or she is in a group or club. Sometimes the staff person who is supporting the community connection will need to continue to accompany the person with disabilities, perhaps even for a long time. The connector should assist the community member or members in becoming more comfortable with and knowledgeable about the individual with disabilities and realize that every situation is different. When an individual with disabilities and a community member can be left "on their own" will vary with each situation. An individual may be without staff support for a while and then need additional assistance again, depending on the person's life situation or changes in the community group (see Bartholomew-Lorimer, chap. 10, this volume, for an example). Community connectors also need to be sensitive to letting individuals with disabilities and other community members resolve their own difficulties in their relationships and know when it is time to "let go" after they have guided someone into the community (O'Connell, 1988).

The Roeher Institute (1990) has pointed out several concerns about the movement from acquaintance to real friendship. For instance, if people join associations, they might simply be going to meetings rather than having the door opened to real friendship. People may expect too much of formal recreation programs or membership in community associations, which sometimes never leads to friendship. Supports need to be built in to ensure that relationships develop. Again, what seems to help is that no more than one individual with disabilities be included in a particular environment or group; interdependence is supported; sufficient communication is provided; and mutual contribution, even in small things, is assisted.

There may be problems or difficulties in many relationships over time. It seems almost impossible in human life for a person to have *any* relationship in which there are not some occasional problems. All relationships go up and down over time. Sometimes community members and people with disabilities should be allowed the room and space to work out their own problems; sometimes they will need assistance. As opposed to many of the problems people spend their time worrying about in human services, the problems related to supporting real friendships and caring relationships are problems worth having.

CONCLUSION

The failure of society and its institutions derives more from their failure to face the right problems than from their failure to solve the problems they face.

Russell Ackoff

The dimensions, basic strategies, and steps presented in this chapter are intended to be useful to those engaging in their own efforts at supporting friendships and building community. They are starting places and also represent lessons already learned over time. If certain efforts are not working, these ideas can be re-examined to discover what might be potentially missing in attitudes or in the strategies that are attempted, and to help deepen connections and relationships that are established.

There are three over-arching contexts to remember as the determinants of success. The first, and perhaps most important, is the community connector's values toward and personal appreciation of the individual with disabilities. As one direct care staff person expressed, "I can't ask somebody else to do what I'm not willing to." The staff or persons who are acting as community connectors must care deeply about, fully appreciate, and be willing to spend time themselves with the individual whom they are supporting in relationships. If the connector is not willing to have a personal relationship with a person, it is unlikely that he or she will be successful in asking a community member to be in a relationship with that individual. The key factor here is not that the connectors *must* develop their own friendship with each individual with disabilities, but rather that they would have the types of feelings, caring, and liking that they would be *willing* to do so. That willingness translates into having no hesitation in calling on and requesting others' willingness.

The second key context is faith and trust in community members' openness to know and befriend individuals who may be different. Staff must be willing to cross the usual boundaries separating their own networks of relationships from the people with whom they work; that is, they must be willing to ask people they know both to befriend their "clients" and for help in linking them to others. The openness and willingness of community members, when asked and when properly introduced, to be in relationships with persons with disabilities are often in striking contrast to the preconceived perceptions of reluctant staff members. Professional attitudes and actions need to catch up to the current knowledge and values of community members, who have frequently been deprived of opportunities to know and befriend particular individuals with disabilities simply because they have not been asked or directly introduced.

Perhaps professional attitudes may still lag behind in assumptions or generalizations about community attitudes because of some negative incidents or failed attempts at connecting and introducing. However, negative attitudes on the part of some community members do not mean *all* persons in the same community share the same attitude, nor do some failures in supporting community connections mean that more learning and other strategies should not be tried. Rather than being stopped by assumptions about community attitudes or particular incidents, staff can actively take on community-building for both the profession and the community. They can make bold requests and develop partnerships with those community members who are willing to be friends and, thus, leaders toward fully inclusive communities.

The last key context is the belief in the importance of the work of community-building for individuals with disabilities, for other community members, and for society as a whole. That belief can sustain committed persons through the failures and mistakes that will occur.

Inside of these three contexts, the strategies and steps to take will follow. Inside of these three contexts, anything is possible.

REFERENCES

Amado, A.N., Conklin, F., & Wells, J. (1990). *Friends: A manual for connecting persons with disabilities and community members.* St. Paul: Human Services Research and Development Center.

Arsenault, C.C. (1990). *Let's get together: A handbook in support of building relationships between individuals with developmental disabilities and their community.* Boulder, CO: Developmental Disabilities Center.

Bartholomew, K. (1985, November). Options for Individuals. *Institutions, Etc.* Alexandria, VA: National Center on Institutions and Alternatives.

Curtis, E., Dezelsky, M., & Coffey, C. (1990). *Using natural supports in community integration.* Salt Lake City, UT: New Hats, Inc.

Davis, K.E. (1985, February). Near and dear: Friendship and love compared. *Psychology Today,* 22–29.

Jacob, G. (1991, July). *Person-centered organizational change.* Presentation at "Quality lives: Person-centered services" conference sponsored by Human Services Research and Development Center, Minneapolis.

Lakin, K.C., Burwell, B.O., Hayden, M.F., & Jackson, M.E. (1992). *An independent assessment of Minnesota's Medicaid Home and Community Based Services Waiver Program.* Minneapolis: University of Minnesota, Center for Residential Services and Community Living.

McKnight, J. (1987). *Regenerating community.* Paper prepared with support of District 1, Massachusetts Department of Mental Health.

Mount, B. (1991). *Personal futures planning.* Paper presented at "Quality

Lives: Person-Centered Services" conference sponsored by the Human Services Research and Development Center, Minneapolis.

Mount, B., Ducharme, G., & Beeman, P. (1991). *Person-centered development: A journey in learning to listen to people with disabilities.* Manchester, CT: Communitas, Inc.

Mount, B., & Zwernik, K. (1988). *It's never too early, it's never too late: A booklet about Personal Futures Planning.* St. Paul: Metropolitan Council.

Mount, B., & Zwernik, K. (1990). *Making futures happen: A manual for facilitators of Personal Futures Planning.* St. Paul: Metropolitan Council.

Newton, J.S. (1989). *Social support manual.* Eugene: University of Oregon, Neighborhood Living Project.

O'Brien, J., & O'Brien, C.L. (1989). *Framework for accomplishment: A workshop for people developing better services.* Lithonia, GA: Responsive Systems Associates.

O'Connell, M. (1988). *The gift of hospitality: Opening the doors of community life to people with disabilities.* Evanston, IL: Northwestern University, The Community Life Project.

O'Connell, M. (1990). *Community building in Logan Square: How a community grew stronger with the contributions of people with disabilities.* Evanston, IL: Northwestern University, The Community Life Project.

Pogrebin, L.C. (1987). *Among friends: Who we like, why we like them, and what we do about them.* New York: McGraw Hill.

G. Allan Roeher Institute. (1990). *Making friends: Developing relationships between people with a disability and other members of the community.* Downsview, Ontario, Canada: York University.

Santrock, J.W. (1989). *Life-span development.* Dubuque, IA: Wm. C. Brown Publishers.

Spierman, G. (1991). *Everyone welcome: Powell River's Community Life Project.* Powell River, British Columbia, Canada: The Powell River Association for Community Living.

Taylor, S.J., & Bogdan, R. (1989). On accepting relationships between people with mental retardation and non-disabled people: Towards an understanding of acceptance. *Disability, Handicap, & Society, 4*(1), 21–36.

Tyne, A. (1988). *Ties and connections: An ordinary community life for people with learning difficulties.* London: King's Fund Centre.

Wade, P. (1991). *Community inclusion for adults with profound and multiple disabilities.* Paper presented at the annual meeting of The Association for Persons with Severe Handicaps, Washington, DC.

Wolfensberger, W. (1988). Common assets of mentally retarded people that are commonly not acknowledged. *Mental Retardation, 26*(2), 63–70.

18

Partnerships at Work and in the Community

*Sheila Conway Wilson and
Marian Cecelia Coverdale*

In Antoine de Saint-Exupéry's *The Little Prince* (1943), the prince encounters a fox who states he cannot play with the little prince until the fox has been "tamed."

> "It is an act too often neglected," said the fox. "It means to establish ties."
>
> "To establish ties?"
>
> "Just that," said the fox. "To me, you are still nothing more than a little boy who is just like a hundred thousand other little boys. And I have no need of you. And you, on your part, have no need of me. To you, I am nothing more than a fox like a hundred thousand other foxes. But if you tame me, then we shall need each other. To me, you will be unique in all the world. To you, I shall be unique in all the world . . . if you tame me, it will be as if the sun came to shine on my life. I shall know the sound of a step that will be different from all the others. Other steps send me hurrying back underneath the ground. Yours will call me, like music, out of my burrow. . . ."
>
> "One only understands the things that one tames," said the fox. "Men have no more time to understand anything. They buy things all ready made at the shops. But there is no shop anywhere where one can buy friendship. . . . If you want a friend, tame me . . ." (pp. 80–84)

WHO NEEDS COMMUNITY?

"Tamed" may, at first, be an awkward and objectionable word to use to refer to intimate friendships, but its application in the broader and literary context addresses the very heart of this chapter and this book—to be connected, to be "a part," not "apart"; and to have others care for us. The idea that individuals with severe disabilities may have the same desires and aspirations for relationships as everyone does is only now gaining wider consideration and attention. The five individuals highlighted in this chapter traditionally had goals and objectives for their life plans that addressed laundry tasks, first-aid skills, pedestrian skills, identification of the four basic food groups, time orientation, and so forth. Yet, nowhere was there any mention in their plans of the fostering of a relationship with *anyone*, let alone with a community member. A person labeled by society has historically been denied access, excluded, and generally considered uninterested in what the rest of society expects and desires in the natural course of daily living. As a featured speaker at the 15th Annual TASH Conference in Washington, D.C., in 1989, Patrick Worth movingly addressed the effect of these noninteractions when he declared:

> Being labeled retarded denies us of that love. If we are not seen as people we will be denied the human right to be loved. And that is the biggest kind of mistake that people in this society could ever make, is denying us the common right to be loved. We are people who are poor, but I'm not talking about money, when I mean poor. Of course we don't have very much money. But poor in the fact that we are people who are unloved, by our neighborhoods, by a society who made decisions to institutionalize us and segregate and congregate our lives. (p. 2)

Barriers by service systems—human services agencies, residential programs, schools, and workshops—have effectively cut labeled individuals off from the rest of society (Lutfiyya, 1991). Consequently, there exists a society parallel to mainstream society with cursory to minimal informal interaction between the two. The individuals in the parallel society have been consigned to special education, special bowling and swimming, Special Olympics, separate schools, segregated group homes—the list is endless. This parallel society developed from well-intentioned, although misdirected, attempts to assist; assumptions or misinterpretations about what was needed; or viewing the process of inclusion as being too troublesome and challenging (King's Fund Centre, 1988).

However, whatever the rationales, mainstream society is diminished by this separation. Society "fails to thrive" by the lack of participation of all its members. Society withers when all lives are never fully developed or fully realized. Mary O'Connell eloquently writes:

> The community, meanwhile, loses something when it exiles people into the social service system. It loses the gift of each individ-

ual: Those who are exiled, like the rest of us, have their own beauty and their own potential . . . When the community cuts itself off from people who are disabled, it also denies part of what it is to be human. A community that has no place for those who cannot speak, or walk, or do higher mathematics is finally impoverishing itself. It becomes intolerant of differences, thus narrowing the path we all must travel. And it makes itself an impotent place, a place that doesn't help each of us live through disappointment, and failure, and sickness, and sorrow, and death—experiences that cannot be isolated because they come to everyone. (1988, p. 4)

All people must be guaranteed inclusion and participation into every aspect of society.

WHAT DOES FRIENDSHIP
HAVE TO DO WITH EMPLOYMENT?

In the past 2 decades, supported employment initiatives through such efforts as "state systems change" grants, individual agency efforts, transitional school programs, state developmental disabilities councils, and university projects have effectively challenged the very premise of "separateness" by eliminating the concept of sheltered workshops and/or prevocational or in-house training as a necessity before placement at a community job site. Evidence has mounted that the most efficient and commonsense approach to learning a job is to be at the job site itself. Throughout the country, individuals perceived as having even severe intellectual disabilities are now working side by side with fellow co-workers in regular community job sites. Though such initiatives represent actions toward community participation, it must be remembered these job placements are only the first of many steps on the journey. Working alongside typical community members is an initial entry into the outside world, but it also opens the door to a wealth of other roles to experience. Besides the role of co-worker, both the person with a disability and the typical community member now also have the opportunity to experience the roles of friend, chum, buddy, mentor, neighbor, and companion.

Nisbet and Hagner (1988) found that when persons with severe disabilities are placed at typical job sites, co-worker support happens naturally and is typical in those workplaces. Job satisfaction and job tenure can be enhanced by the informal interactions that constitute the "culture" of that business. Mutually beneficial interdependence is a common by-product. Sharing common work experiences reinforces the concept of "playing for the same team." In a survey of persons with disabilities employed in community jobs conducted by

Shafer, Rice, Metzler, and Haring (1989), although much attention was focused on work performance by job coaches, often little attention was paid to social interactions. Shafer et al. concluded that not only is there an absolute need to address this area of social interactions during all aspects of the workday, but also to extend beyond the "9 to 5" schedule. This observation was echoed during a Georgia Mental Retardation/Mental Handicaps (MR/MH) planning retreat (O'Brien, 1990) and stressed as an emerging issue by John Kregel (1989) in his summary of national issues in the field of supported employment. In society, people gain a sense of self-worth, value, connectedness, and identity from their job and accompanying outside activities. Individuals perceived as having an intellectual disability should have the same opportunities for this growth and development.

Whereas existing literature has suggested the need to explore a possible relationship between job site networks and job retention, there is much anecdotal material and many case studies that unquestionably support the importance of connections (Mount, 1990) and friendship (Forest & Lusthaus, 1989; Perske, 1980; Perske, 1988; Snow, 1989). Grenot-Scheyer, Coots, and Falvey (1989) wrote, "The challenge to professionals is to create the optimal environment that encourages individuals with and without handicaps to want to be friends with one another" (p. 354).

However, there has been much debate surrounding that idea. Charges have been leveled that endeavors to facilitate connections at work sites are "unnatural" and "artificial." These criticisms overlook the concerted efforts all people exhibit in pursuing and fostering relationships. Maintaining a friendship, or even a passing acquaintance, demands attention and work. Whereas rapport can be instantaneous, sustaining that connection requires planning for anybody and even more work and support for persons with disabilities. The concept that friendships between persons with and without disabilities should be "spontaneous" is a red herring. Research to document the spontaneity of connections at work sites or the amount or type of work necessary to sustain these connections should not be the pivotal factors for addressing this area. The emptiness and disconnectedness endemic to segregation mandate more immediate action.

PATHWAYS TO PARTNERSHIPS: THE TASH FRIENDSHIP PROJECT

In October 1989, the national professional organization The Association for Persons with Severe Handicaps (TASH) received funding for 3 years from the federal Rehabilitation Services Administration

(RSA) to address the social network needs of three possible groups of individuals with severe disabilities: 1) those in supported employment; 2) those who, in time, would have work as an outcome; and/or 3) students exiting the school system into supported employment. The purpose of the grant was to go beyond only supporting connections with fellow co-workers at supported employment sites and to extend into the whole social network of community life. The intents of the TASH Friendship Project, as outlined in the grant proposal, included: 1) the development of connections for individuals perceived as having severe disabilities, 2) forming organized volunteer groups at the chosen project sites with social network expertise who will continue to facilitate and advocate for the networks once federal funding ends, 3) infusing the service delivery system with those values and attitudes that facilitate the creation of these networks, and 4) examining the effects of the social networks on all participants.

Adding six new state sites in October 1991 to the four started in the first 2 fiscal years (1989 and 1990), the project was brought up to 10 state efforts nationwide. In its first 2 years, the participating areas were California (Los Angeles and San Diego), Delaware (statewide), New York (White Plains), and Indiana (Indianapolis). Florida (Tallahassee) was a site the first year, but became inactive due to circumstances that are addressed later in this chapter. The most recent sites were Montana (Billings), Washington (Des Moines/Seattle), West Virginia (Clarksburg), North Carolina (Charlotte), Louisiana (Baton Rouge), and Maryland (Rockville/Silver Spring). At each of the 10 sites, the applicants proposed and implemented an individualized approach that met their local needs and the requirements of the project. Each site is unique, as is the nature of friendships and relationships. Some of the sites focus on connections through an individual's current supported employment position, whereas others address the more communitywide connections of a person's life. The focus is determined by the targeted individual's own wishes and desires.

In each area, there are two identified lead facilitators; these are individuals who are employed by a local agency, school system, or project. At the Delaware, California, and New York sites, the lead facilitators have to coordinate project commitments with their ongoing job responsibilities. These project facilitators do not have the freedom to focus exclusively on fostering work or job connections for individuals with severe disabilities. The job duties of the project facilitators at the newest six state sites are to concentrate on the development, facilitation, and maintenance of community and work relationships and friendships. This attention will allow full focus on the social aspect of an individual's life. The Indianapolis site (highlighted later in this chapter) illustrates how beneficial this intense concentration is in the facilitation of social networks.

The project has provided the facilitators a variety of consultants (i.e., acknowledged leaders concerning the issues of friendship and/or supported employment) and a wealth of resource materials to reiterate and stress the project's philosophy that no single "model" should be or will be constructed or formulated by grant end. The facilitators are familiar with the various tools, strategies, and processes proffered by the leaders in order to individualize each person's network.

The essence of the project is in the lives that are changing—not just those of the "targeted" individuals, but of all the participants. Although there are beginnings to all the stories, there are no endings. With each problematic situation brought to some resolution, another emerges in response to the changed circumstances, reflecting the first law of thermodynamics that "for every action, there is an equal and opposite reaction."

To illustrate some of the lessons learned and problems encountered in project attempts to support friendship in supported employment, the Indianapolis site is described below.

NOBLE CENTERS, INC., INDIANAPOLIS, INDIANA

Noble Centers, Inc., a nonprofit organization in Indianapolis, Indiana, provides services to children and adults labeled with developmental disabilities. Since 1953, the agency has grown to include residential programming, sheltered employment, and supported employment options to adults. The mission of Noble Centers, Inc., is to facilitate the inclusion of individuals perceived as having severe disabilities in the community through work, education, and recreation, and create systemic and social occasions that empower those persons to make choices concerning their lives.

Noble Centers, Inc., responding with a deep commitment to the Marion County individuals perceived as having severe disabilities, has been a leader in developing strategies to support those individuals to participate and live more fully in community life. However, it was discovered that there were several individuals remaining at home without services, either due to lapses in supported employment opportunities or labels of severely challenging behaviors. To be more responsive to their needs, some key staff members decided that a total community-based emphasis was needed, not an adherence to traditional settings. Motivation for this shift in thinking was the realization that even individuals who received a substantial amount of programming and effort continued to remain on the "fringes" of their communities with almost no friendships or relationships. It was determined that there was only *one* way to begin: "You Just Do It!" A proposal from Noble Centers, Inc., accepted by the Indiana Department of Mental Health coincided with the TASH Friendship Project's call for project sites. Consequently, Noble Centers, Inc., started on a course to include persons who had been institutionalized for most of their lives into the community before, during, and after jobs were secured.

Administrative Leadership and Staff

This new project at Noble Centers, Inc., was placed under their division called Noble R & D (Research & Development), Inc., in an effort to continue to define and answer the unmet needs of persons labeled with developmental disabilities and their families. Programs under the R & D umbrella are established to initiate research and to pilot new ventures at the agency. This proposal accepted by the Indiana Department of Mental Health was designed to provide support to the individuals who are at home with no services.

All "training" was to occur in natural environments in the community while personal networks of support were developed and established. The program offered a 3:1 staff ratio and 30 hours of support in community settings per person per week. Initially, the vocational emphasis was excluded due to restrictions mandated by the funding source. However, midway through the first year, staff at the Indiana Department of Mental Health agreed that work was critical to an individual's development and they supported work experiences, even on a part-time basis, with local Indianapolis employers. The total cost for the first fiscal year was approximately $140,000, which covered the hiring of 5 facilitators and service to 15 individuals. Only individuals who recently exited large intermediate care facilities for persons with mental retardation (ICFs/MR) or nursing homes were deemed eligible for this project as stipulated by the Department of Mental Health. (This mandated requirement is addressed in Jon's story later in this chapter.)

Although initially apprehensive due to the newness of their efforts, staff of the community-based project had faith in themselves, the individuals, and the Indianapolis community, and held an unshakeable belief in the moral rightness of inclusion. Personal characteristics sought in the hiring and selection of the facilitators included creativity, flexibility, resourcefulness, connectedness to the community, and outgoing natures.

Although freed of behavior plans, bureaucratic rules, and clinical theories, the staff still found the lack of standard guidelines and benchmarks rather disconcerting at first. With these traditional foundations ignored, they felt compelled to continue to seek reassurances that the course they were pursuing was correct. These community-based specialists, having been steeped in the traditional service delivery ways, continue to struggle with the absence of a formal design or plan; they openly admit that "it has been our hardest year in this field."

Most importantly, these staff have seen friendships blossom, witnessed tremendous gains in individuals' feelings of self-worth and self-esteem, and have been involved in the orchestration of organizational and systemic change. Their ongoing concerns do not signify a lack of commitment to the paths that are being taken, but are testimony to how difficult it can be not to have the kneejerk reaction to problems of responding with a "systems" solution. Noble Centers, Inc., administration has consistently reiterated that: 1) there are no right or wrong answers; 2) "mistakes/failures" will be made, but they should be considered as "redirections" (Siegel, 1986); 3) barriers and obstacles are to be viewed as challenges and opportunities; 4) others should be treated the way you would like to be treated; and 5) the individuals are the guiding light—they control, they are *not* controlled.

When Others Do Not Understand

This Indianapolis effort is guided by the principle that all persons correlate happiness with the degree of control over their own lives, their connectedness to others, and the presence of an array of meaningful activities and challenges in their life. The validity and value of these community efforts have been questioned from the beginning by fellow colleagues. Comments have ranged from "This program discriminates against people with disabilities by excluding them from segregation" to "What does the community have to do with supported employment anyway?" to "This seems like an eternal community field trip!" These remarks have only strenghthened and emboldened the community-based staff in their resolve and commitment to the individuals.

Stories

One can talk theory, philosophy, and programming endlessly, but power and essence come with the personal stories of the Indianapolis individuals. Some of these stories are about what happened at people's places of employment, some are about what happened with other community connections, and some are about both.

Jenny[1]   Jenny, 64 years old in 1991, resided with her mother until her mother's death in 1964 when Jenny was 37 years old. From 1964 to

---

[1]This name is a pseudonym.

1989, she lived in three different state hospitals, one nursing home, and one large intermediate care facility for persons with mental retardation (ICF/MR). She has been labeled with diagnoses of mental retardation and chronic schizophrenia. After group home placement in 1989, she sat for more than a year, doing nothing because she chose not to go to a sheltered workshop and "the system"believed she was too old to work. However, Jenny wanted a job, so Noble Centers pressed Rehabilitation Services to effect supported employment for her.

Jenny's first job was working in the floral department of a greeting card manufacturer. Jenny loved the work and was described as an "excellent worker" by her supervisor. He has also commented on how much she brought to the lives of the other employees. Jenny continued to work for this corporation for a period of time and voiced concern relating to the wages. Due to cutbacks in the retail industry, it was impossible to see the potential for career mobility. Jenny made the decision to seek employment where she could command a higher salary with benefits and greater opportunity to enhance her skills. Jenny's current job is that of clerical assistant in a marketing distribution center. Jenny secured the job based on the recommendations and awards received from her previous employer.

Jenny has been instrumental in bringing about positive changes in the lives of her co-workers while working to enrich her own. Through the development of personal relationships at the work place, Jenny has succeeded in changing negative perceptions that were held by co-workers regarding persons with disabilities just by allowing them the opportunity to know her and experience her enthusiasm for life. She has recommended holding small gatherings to celebrate co workers' birthdays, and encouraged management to install coat racks and purchase lab coats to safeguard clothing. The manager of the department describes her as a "valued member of the team" and further reports that "Jenny is forever coming up with new ways to improve the work environment." To launch the birthday celebrations, Jenny planned and organized the first event. Jenny has not only made friends in her own department, but extended her "circle" to include people working in the nearby warehouse, including a woman named Kathy. Jenny shares a common interest with Kathy, sports. Kathy stressed that she "feels better about the company as a whole since working with Jenny. She is part of the family. I would be very upset if she would decide to leave. She has met my new baby and we talk a lot about our family and sports. Other people made fun of her at first. They feel bad about that now. I think we have all learned something" (personal communication with Kathy, August 1991).

Another impetus for Jenny's community connections has been her after-hours activities. During her leisure time, she participates in a group known as OASIS (Older Adult Services and Information Systems) in which the members volunteer to organize and sponsor various events. Activities for the senior citizens consist of classes for enrichment, book reviews, attendance at the opera, lectures on travel adventures, beginning drawing, museum tours, lectures on health-related issues, learning to garden, and many other subjects. Jenny has become so entrenched in this group that she volunteers her time greeting other members as they enter before the start of a session.

OASIS's Senior Movie Club is sponsored by the East Washington Branch of the Indianapolis Public Library. Since attending the movies every Wednesday, Jenny has become friendly with another woman named Muriell. The two ladies chat on the phone during the week and socialize each week before the movie begins. Muriell became concerned when Jenny missed two consecutive weeks of movies. She was unable to contact Jenny because up until that time, Jenny had not given her number to Muriell. Jenny had not realized that people share their phone numbers with their friends and acquaintances.

The facilitator, Laura, realized early on that because she is only 25 years old her presence could be intrusive in any of the senior activities. She attended a few gatherings, became assured that Jenny was making connections, and knew it was time for Jenny to "sail solo."

When asked what she appreciates about her life, Jenny replies, "I enjoy being nice to other people and trying to be happy. I try to make friends with other people and I like them all very much."

Dennis[2]   Dennis is a very outgoing and talkative young man in his twenties. At their first meeting, the community-based staff learned that Dennis had been "discharged" from several workshops and had lost three supported employment positions. His father felt Dennis's firings were due to lack of continued support at the job sites. His father, a strong advocate, expressed his belief that with support and a well-matched job, Dennis's employment would last. During this meeting, Dennis informed the community-based staff that he was accustomed "to reinforcers for good behaviors at intervals every day" and asked that he be allowed "to review his new behavior plan." He was quickly told that there would be no major plan and that he was responsible for his own behavior.

Dennis was very interested in finding a new job; therefore, with the facilitator, Kim, he spent countless hours exploring various job opportunities. He utilized the library and its resources in conducting his career search and to research information. He, along with two other individuals from the program, were offered the opportunity to work

---

[2]This name is a pseudonym.

part-time for a local Indianapolis lawn company; outside yardwork was a preference all three had voiced. Over the spring and summer, they learned to plant flowers, prune trees, and landscape. Future responsibilities included raking leaves, thatching in the fall, and snow removal during the winter months. By summer's end, Dennis had so impressed the employer with his attention to his assigned duties and thoroughness that he was offered the job full-time.

A good working relationship and camaraderie developed between Dennis and his co-workers at the lawn company. Because Dennis has a tendency to be rather garrulous, his fellow workers will tell him when he needs to listen more so that they can have a chance to talk! Obviously, he is learning about the give and take in relationships.

Dennis has led a rather eventful life involving some cross-country adventures. Given her appreciation for Dennis's personality, Kim is proceeding slowly and working to strengthen the evolving ties at the work site. Because Kim had the opportunity to spend countless hours getting to know Dennis in a variety of settings and to review the information detailing the jobs, relationships, and activities in which he had participated in the past, she was determined and confident that Dennis would succeed if given the necessary supports. Over the summer, Kim came to realize how much Dennis valued his position at the lawn company and how meaningful the job responsibilities were to him. According to Noble Center's organizational structure, when Dennis was offered the full-time position he would have been transferred to the responsibility of an employment training specialist in the supported employment division of Noble Centers, Inc. Upon Dennis's full-time hire, the community-based staff advocated to the administration that Dennis needed the continuity and support of Kim, someone he knew and trusted. Fortunately, the administration recognized that Kim had come to know Dennis as a *person*, not a client, during their exploration of job opportunities and subsequent work at the lawn company. Therefore, Kim was tapped to provide the ongoing assistance to Dennis. She completed an agency-sponsored 2-week orientation to supported employment strategies and techniques. This readjustment and acknowledgment of personal connections signified a shift in organizational philosophy. After a year of project implementation, the community-based and supported employment programs at Noble Centers, Inc., merged to combine staff talents and to support both *co-worker* and *community* connections.

Margaret Mary[3]   Margaret Mary is a 43-year-old woman who, before 1990, resided in a large ICF/MR on the north side of Indianapolis.

---

[3]This name is a pseudonym.

At one time, she lived with her family while attending a large sheltered workshop. Unfortunately, due to what the workshop reported as "behavioral difficulties," her workshop slot was terminated and her family placed her in an ICF/MR. However, the power of Margaret Mary was not to be denied. One day, she entered the office of the director of the residential facility and offered this pact: "I will improve my behavior and lose weight if you will move me out of here." A deal was struck and Mary Margaret was moved into a smaller residential setting—a group home.

When Margaret Mary first met with the Noble Centers, Inc., community-based staff, she listed the highlights of her life as: 1) going to the group home from the ICF/MR; 2) losing weight; 3) the Special Olympics; and 4) meeting people through Noble Centers, Inc. When she was asked about her friends, everyone she named was a staff member of one agency or another.

During a recent surgery, Margaret Mary received an abundance of cards, flowers, and balloons from her co-workers at a major research and medical diagnostics corporation where she works part-time. It was the first time she ever received attention and recognition from people other than her family or staff.

Before her participation in the community-based program, Margaret Mary had few leisure pursuits. After 6 months of exploring and experiencing different community activities, she discovered a love for the symphony and choir. She loves and is stirred by the sound a baritone produces while singing various songs. Margaret Mary is also interested in travel destinations and will readily discuss the pleasures of visiting new places. She talks about her new life experiences with enthusiasm, "I like meeting new people. I have a job and friends at work. I have learned much about the city and have done things I've never done and never thought of. I found things I enjoy."

Gus   Gus is a 26-year-old gentleman with a passion for music and art. He was considered so "unsuccessful" in past attempts at sheltered employment through three different agencies that he was never given a chance at supported employment. Case notes state that he did not do well in "high stimulus environments or large crowds." Gus himself openly admitted to a fear of crowds. However, his community-based facilitator helped him to learn how to ride the city bus. This past spring they attended the NCAA Final Four together along with 40,000 other spectators. When asked how he tolerated the crowd, Gus just gave the "thumbs up" sign. At a recent workshop, the community-based facilitator was asked what "therapeutic method" was employed in order to achieve that wonderful result. She stumbled, knowing she could not think of the clinical term, and finally replied that through mutual support, taking it slowly, and going step by step, Gus was able to face the crowds. However, her audience only seemed satisfied with the outcome when another participant defined her explanation as "systematic desensitization." Their comfort level was restored with the label!

Gus's love of art manifests itself in very detailed, free-hand depictions of various aircrafts. To further and share that interest, he joined a hobby club whose members build model airplane replicas, which requires absolute precision plus creativity. In a recent club competition, he was awarded third place for his model. When asked to explain his experiences over this past year, Gus responded, "It's neat. I get to meet new friends. I still don't like to take the bus. I learned to value money."

Jon Jon is a 28-year-old man with mental retardation, cerebral palsy, and left eye blindness. Jon was the first participant in Noble Centers, Inc.'s, new community-based venture. He had been a long-time recipient of segregated services. He "followed procedures" and worked his way through the service continuum of adult day activities, work adjustment, sheltered employment, and finally arrived at an assembly job at a construction company. By that time, he was living with eight other individuals and complained about the lack of privacy and constant noise. With company cutbacks, his job was eliminated. He sat at the group home for more than a year waiting for his "turn" at another job placement. Jon, like so many others, spent much of his life waiting for others to fill out a form, make a decision, or send in a voucher.

Initially, funding for Jon's entry into the community-based project was denied due to the previously mentioned Department of Mental Health stipulations regarding program eligibility. He had received services in the past, but had not recently moved from a nursing home or ICF/MR and was, therefore, ineligible under the regulations. Advocacy by many individuals immediately began to move for an exception in Jon's case. Jon himself wrote letters to the commissioner of the Indiana Department of Mental Health requesting attention to the problem. Soon after, a department head called to announce that either the funding would be arranged or she would "personally fund Jon." However, Jon's was not an isolated case. This funding struggle highlighted a whole area that needed changing, not just making Jon's case a single exception to the rule. Changes were made so that others who followed Jon in the community-based venture also received the necessary dollars.

His last psychological evaluation reported that Jon was "unable to describe in any detail a usual day for himself, and he provided only the crudest and grossest behavioral description. If we are to take at face value the things he says, he appears to be without friendships, without ADL skills, without basic school skills, without community involvements, without church attendance, without pastimes and hobbies, and the like." However, despite these observations of a rather empty existence, the evaluation team chose not to address these sorely lacking areas at all. One *important* recommendation they made, however, was for Jon to learn the four basic food groups.

When Jon started in the project, attention was focused on his capacities, talents, and interests. He commented that he enjoyed shopping, bowling, watching television, listening to the radio, playing video games, and the Indiana Pacers basketball team; things he disliked included, "having my teeth pulled; hospitals; crazy bus drivers; cleaning my room; cold water; the yelling, fighting, and lack of privacy in the group home." He had infrequent contact with his family and he had a few people he considered friends from a local church he had stopped attending. When asked what he would do if he could do anything, he responded, "The best thing would be to have my own place, a good job, and money to go shopping. I would like to go to an apartment of my own, so nobody can scream and yell at me."

Jon and his facilitator, Sally, began to establish a relationship built on mutual respect and trust through the undertaking of a multitude of shared community experiences. Initially, they spent an extraordinary amount of time talking on the phone at night, exploring what community activities Indianapolis had to offer during the day. Jon became involved in a neighborhood garden plot that was started by volunteer community members to grow food for homeless people in the Indianapolis area. Because a great deal of time is required to nurture a garden, Jon became recognized by the neighborhood's residents. It was at the garden that Jon met Leah, a well-known fabric artist and teacher. Leah began inviting Jon and Sally to lunch in her patio garden. Given this budding friendship, Sally encouraged Jon to call Leah in the evenings and make the trips to the garden a regular occurrence. One day, while a neighbor had stopped by his garden area to chat, Jon mentioned what a great time he had attending a practice of the Indiana symphony. When the neighbor stated she loved the symphony, arrangements were made for the neighbor, Leah, and Jon to attend an evening performance.

Jon's zucchini, grown in this communal garden plot, won a prize at the Marion County State Fair. However, the true prize was the growing relationship between Jon and Leah. When cold weather moved in, efforts turned to sharpening Jon's telephone skills and learning new bus routes and the trolley system in order to visit Leah on the weekends.

One day while he was downtown, Jon noticed a bicycle repair shop. He discovered it housed a nonprofit organization that trades bicycle ownership in return for 24 hours of work. Deciding to participate, he soon learned how to patch tires and straighten frames. He also had the pleasure of meeting the French racing team that was in town for a race at the Veledrome.

Also during this time, Jon moved from the group home to an apartment with two other men. Although it is not totally his own place, he is pleased to have more peace and quiet. The rules and regulations that so annoyed him at the group home do not intrude in this new setting. Following up his voiced interest in returning to church and becoming active again, he met with a local minister, Jim, who invited him to join in their services. Now, he attends both services and Bible readings on a weekly basis.

However, Jon's greatest worries were those concerning employment. His initial meeting with Jill, the supported employment specialist, did not begin smoothly. Jon did everything to antagonize her in an effort to avoid this change in his life. After so many false starts and losses in his life, Jon was afraid to believe that the current changes and upcoming ones were "for real," that the people now in his life would stand by him. However, Jill saw through his hassling and gave him the reassurance he needed. While Jill explored job possibilities, Jon continued to work part-time at two job sites in addition to his volunteer time at the Salvation Army and the bike shop.

After a few months, Jill approached Jon about a job polishing silverware at a university hotel and conference center. He observed the job, expressed an interest, was interviewed, and was offered the position. Although excited, he immediately began to express concerns. Chief among them was the thought that he would lose all his newfound friends. When assured that would not happen, he became visibly relieved and stated with surprise, "You mean I can have a job and friends, too?" Attention at this new job site was given to the bus stop and bathroom locations, places to buy snacks and sodas, where to eat lunch, and what would happen and what he would do if he missed his bus stop. Jon needed to run through every aspect to reassure himself, not just take the word of Sally or Jill.

Since starting his job at the university hotel and conference center, he has become acquainted with several co-workers with whom he eats dinner in the evenings. Now that he is earning money, he is saving for a waterbed, a CB radio, and a vacation. Jon also started seeing a new girlfriend who attends Noble Centers, Inc. He plans on celebrating his birthday with a party and will start inviting friends and acquaintances to his home for dinner.

Selection of Individuals

The people served in the Noble Centers, Inc., community-based project are labeled with the "dual diagnoses" of both mental retardation and mental illness (MR/MI). These are the persons about whom the respective state programs constantly attribute "ownership" to the other, with the result being minimal to nonexistent support or attention to these individuals. They are the people no one wanted to touch because of their perceived difficulties; they do not *cleanly categorize*! However, at Noble Centers, Inc., the decision was made for the community-based venture to focus on these individuals whom others had given up on, the people who always got the proverbial "short end of the stick."

The other TASH Friendship Project state sites have primarily selected individuals who are more typical supported employment recipients, those labeled as "mentally handicapped." At the root of all efforts at all project sites, however, is the critical need for relationship building for all concerned.

The Facilitators' Experience

The facilitators at Noble Centers, Inc., began to see their role as that of the catalyst "to assist individuals to find themselves and help them bring about positive changes in their lives." Their own friendship with an individual was based on genuine mutuality and reciprocity, unlike their past client and/or staff relationships fostered by "the system." However, the facilitators sometimes struggle with being on both sides of the coin—friend and paid staff. For most people, there are many people paid to be in one's life—minister, teacher, counselor—and these "paid staff" probably make a tremendous impact on one's behavior, thinking, and quality of life. These people may be responsible for steering someone in a new direction or giving them the self-confidence to try again.

The Noble Centers facilitators are witnessing the emergence of persons too long denied. Sally poignantly notes, "People used to think of themselves as things, things that other people control. Individuals would often make up stories about their lives. Once their own lives began to unfold, this was no longer necessary." When one is party to these major life changes, there is no turning back. The traditional frames of reference—continuums, readiness—are no longer acceptable or palatable. Kim was recently offered a better paying job opportunity that required a return to segregated services. She rejected it with, "I found it too confining. I could never again work in strictly segregated settings. I know I have had a change in values."

CAUTION: THE FRANCHISING OF FRIENDSHIPS

In the Irish legend of the leprechaun, he must give a pot of gold to the person who catches him. A story that has been passed on through generations tells of a man who was able to induce a leprechaun to take him to the very bush where gold was buried. Immediately, the man tied a red handkerchief to the bush in order to recognize the spot upon returning with a shovel. Though gone just a few short moments, he returned to find a red handkerchief tied to every bush in the field. Although the leprechaun's intent was to confound and disguise, the field of mental retardation often does the same thing: overindulgence in an unabating tendency to replicate what "works." Although the field is adept at defining "best practices" in such areas as job training, skill acquisition, or behavior modification, it then tries to replicate those best practices *everywhere.* However, the very personal and intimate nature of relationships, friendships, and connections prevents a similar approach. Each person is unique and distinctive, therefore the process to facilitate connections must mirror those same characteristics. Personal Futures Planning, circles of support, McGill Action Planning System (MAPS), lifestyle planning, and so forth, are all, for instance, excellent tools and strategies to use to understand and appreciate each person more uniquely; they are not inflexible processes that should be "standard operating procedure." In addition, they must never be mandatory, such as the individualized habilitation plan (IHP) or the individualized education program (IEP). The process of building friendships and connections should remain fluid and open to draw on many ideas and approaches.

We shall not cease from exploration
And the end of all our exploring
Will be to arrive where we started
And know the place for the first time.
Through the unknown, remembered gate
When the last of earth left to discover
Is that which was the beginning; . . .

Eliot (1943, p. 59)

It is this very lack of systematization and having to start anew with each person that has led some supported employment programs to shy away from the difficult, although absolutely essential and exhilirating, area of relationships and friendships.

STRATEGIES

There are no surefire methods that guarantee development of an acquaintance or relationship at the jobsite or in the community. Notwithstanding the cautions in the above section, some factors and strategies have been found to be effective in "setting the tone" in the fostering of ties and connections. Some are not new revelations and have been mentioned in other resources. However, these issues were found to affect success in Indianapolis and the TASH Friendship Project and they bear repeating because of their absolute importance.

1. Appearance is extremely important, as is appropriate dress for the occasion, weather, and person's age. Atypical hair or clothing style (or lack of) spotlights the already existing gulf with society.

2. Individuals often need assistance in learning how to be a friend or acquaintance. Help can be provided by showing and/or explaining how to work an answering machine (their own or leaving a message on another's), the value in sending greeting cards, planning a small dinner party, explaining the importance of initiating and maintaining periodic contact with co-workers and community members, discovering the art of "hanging out" and just being in someone's company, or listening to another person's point of view without interrupting. All these elements make up the "dance" of interaction.

3. Responsibility and control need to be transferred to the individual, where they rightfully belong. Behavioral difficulties subside greatly when people are treated as equals and peers, "masters of their own fate." The rigid behavior management plans that did not work were discarded in favor of the "real world" methods of dignity and respect.

4. Facilitators must understand the value of community connections and be well connected themselves. This point has been stated by others who have been involved in the facilitation of relationships for labeled individuals, but it needs to be trumpeted. Busy, socially aware people have proven to be the most interested and willing to invest their time and energies. These same characteristics have proven valid and essential in the hiring of facilitators. Ideally, a community facilitator should not be an individual new to an area who has little knowledge of the

community and no connections. If the person is new, that facilitator must be allowed *ample* time to develop community knowledge and personal networks, although it will most likely delay any facilitation for the individuals in the program. It would be best not to have that situation occur in the first place.

5. Being exclusively in the community and at real jobsites exposed the individuals to everyday role models. The learning process was stimulated because of this daily focus. These individuals were seeing and experiencing for themselves what people did at work, play, and in community activities, and what was acceptable and unacceptable.

6. Social errors made while in the community also subsided when the facilitators took the time to explain to the individual why certain behaviors were considered unacceptable in the community. When an inappropriate behavior occurred, the subsequent learning atmosphere was not punitive, controlling, or threatening, nor were negative consequences enforced. "Faux pas" were accepted and quickly forgiven. When offered real choices, interested role models, and meaningful activities, problems diminished. Inappropriate responses were replaced with newly learned ways of interacting with others.

7. People need as much time as necessary to begin thinking of themselves as a singular and separate person rather than only having the member identity of the larger group. Segregation and exclusion have typically limited a given individual's exploration of interests. It was discovered that one Indianapolis participant, labeled with an IQ of 15 and reported to have had communication difficulties for years, can read and spell. The extended and concentrated sharing of time by the facilitator and individual in varied settings brought these unknown skills to light.

8. The value of acquaintances, not just friends, should not be underestimated. Attention was directed to facilitating the development of these less intense, although no less vital, community and job connections. Acquaintanceships added variety to daily situations and became a lead to other potential resources.

9. Facilitators must be available for evening and weekend activities. Flexibility *must* be given to allow staff to structure their work week to best suit the individual, not what best suits the agency.

10. Sensitivity to age differences is critical. The long-term presence of a 25-year-old facilitator is inappropriate and intrusive in a seniors' group. If group (or member) support for the individual has not yet become established, then the younger facilitator could

be present, but in a less visible manner—preparing lunches in the kitchen, and so forth. Also, close attention needs to be paid to the subtle rituals or nuances of cultural groups. The best situation would be to have a facilitator who shares in that particular culture or who personally knows someone who does. An acceptable alternative is to research and learn as much as possible about the group before contact, especially directly from its members or close affiliates. Other bits of information that may need to be known are whether or not dues are paid, work is shared, members bring baked goods regularly, and so forth.

11. The wonderful diversity of community members and co-workers should be utilized. What a staff person in the system may see as a barrier and obstacle, a community member or co-worker sees as a surmountable challenge and opportunity.

12. A detailed, factual history on the involved individuals should be completed before beginning efforts to connect them to their community. Although past reports will probably be quite negative and deficit-oriented, they may contain information that will assist a facilitator to understand a possible recurring response. Past physical abuse, a stated fear of crowds, or an aversion to noise may explain why an individual is withdrawn or hesitant to participate. Persons with medical needs may require ongoing assistance from their new friends once the facilitator has faded. Information regarding seizures or different communication methods may be warranted. Information-sharing with community members can be accomplished respectfully and without the use of language steeped in professional jargon. Assurance that needed supports are in place is necessary before leaving an individual with a group. Organizations burned by agencies that have "dumped" individuals are leery and skeptical to opening their doors again. Above all, every attempt needs to be made to ensure that the individual will be safe from harm and that emergency contact numbers are readily available or known.

13. Human services organizations must be responsive to the needs of the served individuals and be willing to reallocate necessary resources to explore new options. As new ideas and processes to support people in establishing and developing relationships are learned, new focus and direction must be evidenced in the current programs and services.

14. The powerful influence of family relations needs to be understood and supported. Many of the Indianapolis participants suffered the heartache of long separations from their family, or

became completely disconnected. For some, their family's whereabouts were completely unknown. The facilitators worked hard to find and reunite family members. Sometimes, when ties were reestablished, there were struggles over control and guardianship. In these situations, the facilitators were available to help the individual and their family in examining and probing these core issues.

15. The focus of friendship cannot be exclusive to one setting. While one of the intents of the TASH Friendship Project was to facilitate job connections for individuals in supported employment, it was quickly discovered that some individuals were more interested in developing *community* connections or that a particular worksite culture was not conducive to fostering relationships. Efforts needed to be extended based on the person's interests and need for relationships, rather than a specified job setting.

OBSERVATIONS AND IMPLICATIONS

Besides the steps listed above that are specific strategies, there are other observations and implications that will affect the success of efforts to build connections.

1. The facilitators found it anxiety-provoking to balance the support of individuals as they made their own choices with being alert to any potential exploitation. Protection and a conflict-free environment were the traditionally sought standards. Dependency occurs because it is fostered and encouraged. However, risk must be allowed to flourish in people's lives. Being an adult means living with your decisions and the accompanying consequences. Who does not ascribe to the adage, "You learn from your mistakes"? Is it not one's poorest choices that typically produce the greatest growth toward maturation?

2. Some discussion has diminished the idea of working on relationships because it is currently "fashionable." Although there is a great deal of attention currently being focused on this area, that attention should not diminish the value and importance of this issue. Being an active community participant and having varied relationships are rights to be enjoyed and experienced by all. The accusation of trendiness insults those involved in this journey.

3. Working in the community exposes one to many experiences and opportunities. However, in the past, most supported employment programs attended to the vocational aspects of the job with little, if any, consideration to the social and humanistic ele-

ments. Compartmentalization of a person into different skill areas or to different agency divisions often engenders more work and frustration for all involved. A complete person is placed in a job, not just the skills of that person. At the Indianapolis site, efforts are underway to staff according to the person's needs rather than agency needs. However, until the complete conversion is made, the supported employment specialists and community-based facilitators will work side by side to generate co-worker supports and desired relationships and activities both on and off the job.

4. In Indianapolis, the Noble Centers, Inc., community-based facilitators are able to focus solely on connections, both in the community and at jobs. Because they have had the "luxury" of this intensive focus, greater and more numerous strides have occurred than at the California, New York, and Delaware sites. The newly added six state sites utilize processes that will more closely mirror the approaches used in Indianapolis. While the other three state sites learned important strategies and contributed critical information, it is clear that the degree of effectiveness is correlated with the amount of total attention provided. The project facilitators at the other three state sites have been able to coordinate their other agency job responsibilities with those of the project, but there have been difficulties with time constraints. This time difficulty caused the Florida site to become "inactive" and motivated one of the original California facilitators to drop out. Common sense dictates that daily contact and focus facilitates swifter changes than infrequent and variable contact.

5. The Indianapolis site discovered the worthlessness of classifications, labels, and descriptions of people such as "behaviorally challenging" or "unable to sustain community placements." The past restrictive and controlled environments to which the Indianapolis individuals were subjected shaped their responses in those settings. When people work together jointly with mutual regard and treat each other with dignity and respect, adult expectations are sensed, observed, experienced, and practiced. This is the flip side to labels: favored ones can have a positive effect. There is great value and worth imbued in the label of employee, friend, co-worker, and confidante. Favorable images are triggered from those societal roles.

6. The very nature of community and its lack of concreteness makes it an easy target for systems naysayers. Such naysayers point to the absence of "measurable objectives" and "predictors of outcomes." Whereas information gathered in projects oriented

toward objectives and outcomes may translate into spectacular graphs and charts, such information does little to tell of the essence of an individual. A person cannot be factored down to his or her common denominators. At the Indianapolis site, outside agencies that initially were skeptical of the community-based effort, now value what is occurring because they have seen the wonderful changes for the individuals.

CONCLUSION

All the persons involved in the TASH Friendship Project are moving beyond theory and conceptual ideas, the thinking and passive aspect, and into the "real"—the happening and doing aspect. Mary Ellen Sousa (1991) of San Diego's Interwork Institute and a California Project facilitator wrote, "It is ironic that traveling life's 'hills and valleys' with people is exactly what the institutional movement sought to avoid by making life so uneventful as to seem surreal" (p. 3). When the expressions of a person's life are controlled and monitored, their existence lacks the mystery, lacks the suspense, and lacks the very heart of life. What ensues and emerges through connections and relationships can be exciting, messy, fulfilling, frustrating, but at the root is being open and expectant to the spectacular vitality of life. There are no guarantees with this exploration, no neat syllogisms, "if p, then q." It is the neverending adventure!

---

dive for dreams
or a slogan may topple you
(trees are their roots
and wind is wind)

trust your heart
if the seas catch fire
(and live by love
though the stars walk backward)

e. e. cummings

REFERENCES

Cummings, E.E. (1958). "60." In *Complete poems, 1904–1962* (p. 732). New York: Liveright Publishing Corporation.

Eliot, T.S. (1943). Little gidding. *Four quartets* (p. 59). New York: Harcourt Brace Jovanovich.

Forest, M., & Lusthaus, E. (1989). Promoting educational quality for all students. In S. Stainback, W. Stainback, & M. Forest (Eds.), *Educating all students in the mainstream of regular education* (pp. 43–57). Baltimore: Paul H. Brookes Publishing Co.

Grenot-Scheyer, M., Coots, J., & Falvey, M.A. (1989). Developing and fostering friendships. In M.A. Falvey, *Community-based curriculum: Instructional strategies for students with severe handicaps* (2nd ed.). Baltimore: Paul H. Brookes Publishing Co.

King's Fund Centre. (1988). *Ties and connections: An ordinary life for people with learning difficulties.* London: King's Fund Centre.

Kregel, J. (1989). Opportunities and challenges: Recommendations for the future of the national supported employment initiative. In P. Wehman, J. Kregel & M. Shafer (Eds.), *Emerging trends in the national supported employment initiative: A preliminary analysis of 27 states.* Richmond: Virginia Commonwealth University.

Lutfiyya, Z. (1991). *Personal relationships and social networks: Facilitating the participation of individuals with disabilities in community life.* Syracuse, NY: Center on Human Policy, Syracuse University.

McKnight, J. (1987, Winter). Regenerating community. *Social Policy*, 54–58.

McKnight, J. (1989, January/February). Why servanthood is bad. *The Other Side*, 38–41.

McKnight, J. (1989, Summer). Do no harm: A policymaker's guide to evaluating human services and their alternatives. *Social Policy*, 1–16.

Mount, B. (1990). *Imperfect change: Embracing the tensions of person-centered work.* Manchester, CT: Communitas, Inc.

Nisbet, J., & Hagner D. (1988). Natural supports in the workplace: A reexamination of supported employment. *Journal of The Association for Persons with Severe Handicaps, 13,* 260–267.

O'Brien, J. (1990). *Working on . . . A survey of emerging issues in supported employment for persons with severe disabilities.* Syracuse, NY: Center on Human Policy, Syracuse University.

O'Connell, M. (1988). *The gift of hospitality: Opening the doors of community life to people with disabilities* (p. 4). Evanston, IL: Center for Urban Affairs and Policy Research.

Perske, R. (1980). *New life in the neighborhood.* Nashville: Abingdon Press.

Perske, R. (1988). *Circles of friends.* Nashville: Abingdon Press.

de Saint-Exupéry, A. (1943). *The little prince* (pp. 80–84). New York: Harcourt Brace Jovanovich.

Shafer, M., Rice, L.R., Metzler, H., & Haring, M. (1989). A survey of nondisabled employees' attitudes toward supported employees with mental retardation. *Journal of The Association for Persons with Severe Handicaps, 14,* 137–146.

Siegel, B.S. (1986). *Love, medicine, and miracles.* New York: Harper & Row.

Snow, J.A. (1989). Systems of support: A new vision. In S. Stainback, W. Stainback, & M. Forest (Eds.), *Educating all students in the mainstream of regular education* (pp. 221–231). Baltimore: Paul H. Brookes Publishing Co.

Sousa, M.E. (1991, December). Report to the TASH Friendship Project director.

Worth, P. (1989, May). The importance of speaking for yourself. *TASH Newsletter*, p. 2

19

Friendships and Community Associations

Deborah Reidy

In his classic book, *Democracy in America* (1835), Alexis de Tocqueville characterized Americans as a nation of joiners. He wrote:

> Americans of all ages, all stations in life, and all types of disposition are forever forming associations. There are not only commercial and industrial associations in which all take part, but others of a thousand different types —religious, moral, serious, futile, very general and very limited, immensely large and very minute. Americans combine to give fetes, found seminaries, build churches, distribute books, and send missionaries to the antipodes. Hospitals, prisons, and schools take shape in that way. Finally, if they want to proclaim a truth or propagate some feeling by the encouragement of a great example, they form an association. (p. 485)

This tendency is as true today as it was in 1835 when de Tocqueville was writing. Indeed, in one city of 35,000 people in the Northeast United States, a cursory survey of voluntary associations numbered 200. These include groups such as the Christian Motorcycle Association, the Gufus Magic Club, and the Society of the 17th Century, as well as more commonly known groups, such as the Knights of Columbus, the Rotary, and Kiwanis. A group seems to exist for every conceivable interest!

This particular community is not unique in its rich assortment of clubs and organizations. The *Encyclopedia of Associations* (Burek, 1992) lists 23,000 nonprofit membership associations currently active in the United States. Why do so many of these groups exist?

Anyone who has ever been a member of an association or group knows the benefits first hand. A community's associational life is where its "real business" is conducted. People find one another jobs, recommend hairdressers and mechanics, make and carry out *de facto* public policy, swap recipes, give advice, explore and challenge their values, form relationships, and exercise leadership. In addition to the practical benefits of association membership, the mere fact of *belonging* to a group with common interests can provide a powerful sense of personal fulfillment (Berger & Neuhaus, 1977; Milofsky, 1988).

John McKnight of the Center for Urban Affairs and Policy Research at Northwestern University in Evanston, Illinois, writes and speaks extensively about the potential for voluntary associations to play a role in helping people with disabilities gain entry into community life. He writes, "The primary problem of most people who are labelled is that they are excluded from the power and protection of community life" (1989, p. 10).

This chapter describes why community organizations, such as the Knights of Columbus, stamp collecting clubs, and others, have great potential to foster relationships and a sense of inclusion for people with disabilities. It provides real-life examples and offers principles and strategies for assisting people with disabilities to become members of organizations.

George: One of the Guys

Several times each week, George Gagnon, a man in his mid-forties, spends his evenings at the Knights of Columbus hall near his home. Weekly, he helps with the bingo games. He likes to work in the kitchen preparing the meal they serve on bingo nights. Sometimes, George and his girlfriend share a meal with fellow Knights. Other times, George attends by himself and visits with the other members. He has rarely missed a meeting. He also marches in the annual Saint Patrick's Day Parade, and participates actively in all fund-raising activities sponsored by the organization.

George has been a Knight since 1988. He is a Third Degree Knight, a very respectable position to hold within the organization as Fourth Degree is the highest level. He recently sponsored another man to join the organization.

His involvement with members is not limited to his time at the Knights of Columbus Hall. Other members have invited George to their homes, and he has reciprocated. In 1990, when it came time for him to move to a new apartment, several of his friends from the Knights came over to give him a hand.

George's contribution to the organization is significant. The Grand Knight commented on his helpfulness: "George is always willing to help out with any project." In fact, he was commended in a recent issue of their newsletter for selling a large number of raffle tickets. He works tirelessly at bingo games, helping to prepare and serve meals, and he recently worked 12 hours straight at their summer picnic.

Up until a few years ago, George, diagnosed with mental retardation, spent most of his life living in a state institution. He then lived in a community residence for several years before moving into a staffed apartment with a roommate. During the day, he attends a sheltered workshop.

Before joining the Knights, most of his free time was either spent watching television or riding his three-wheel bicycle up and down the street near his house. He had few interests and fewer friends outside his program.

Although George is not a talkative man, "before" and "after" photographs, along with testimonies from staff and friends, highlight the change in his personality. One photo, taken the night of his initiation into the Knights, shows George with a serious, almost fearful, expression on his face. A recent photo, taken at the "K of C" Hall, shows him relaxed, smiling, with a warm twinkle in his blue eyes. Another photograph shows George proudly wearing his Knights of Columbus pin on his lapel.

Other members describe George as being very shy when he first joined. They say he is much more outgoing now and participates in the joking and bantering that is part of the atmosphere.

When George is asked what he enjoys about being a member, he says, "I like that they ask me to help." He also likes the teasing that goes on: "I like joking around with them; we joke about my cat."

For George, his initiation into the Knights of Columbus has also been a true initiation into community life.

Emily: Expanded Horizons

Most girls who join the Girl Scouts look forward to learning new skills and making friends. For Emily Griffin,[1] membership in the Girl Scouts also means a chance to expand her horizons beyond the special education class she attends at the local high school.

Emily is a 16-year-old girl with mental retardation. She is vivacious and enjoys socializing tremendously. In June 1990, she joined a Girl Scout troop that meets near her home. Before attending her first troop meeting, she had already read the entire handbook and identified the badges she wanted to earn. Within 2 months, she earned two badges: pet care and toddler tending.

During the first few months of participation, Emily's enthusiastic

---

[1]This name is a pseudonym.

and sometimes unpredictable behavior disconcerted some of the other members, but the troop leader tactfully explained about Emily's disability. The other members were relieved to learn that there was a reason for her behavior and became very accepting of Emily from that point on. In fact, Emily made a friend in the troop with whom she spent some time outside of meetings until the girl moved away.

After 8 months of membership, Emily started spending time with other members outside of troop activities. Her mother was thrilled at the way her horizons expanded. Emily became involved with writing letters to the troops during the Persian Gulf War, selling Girl Scout cookies, and attending a sleepover with other Scouts at the Boston Science Museum. She researched the countries of France and Greece, and made a presentation to her troop on each country. The other girls also enjoyed the Greek cookies Emily baked to supplement her talk.

In addition to these activities, Emily was recommended by her troop leader for a new program called Wider Opportunities, in which Girl Scouts age 14 years and older have the chance to travel and learn new things. Emily is interested in traveling to Little Rock, Arkansas, to participate in a 2-week course on sign language. To be nominated for this program is a real honor. Each nominee must fill out an application and deliver a presentation explaining why she should be chosen. Whether she is chosen or not, Emily will continue expanding her horizons through her membership in the Girl Scouts.

This year, she was assisted to become a volunteer at a local hospital. She works one afternoon a week. Her current placement is in the marketing department where she stuffs envelopes. She also has the opportunity to bring beverages to patients in the hospital.

Sharon, Emily's mother, considers this volunteer position to be an excellent stepping stone into paid employment for Emily. She says, "This is very maturing for her. She has to get there on time and remember her badge. She comes right home from school and gets ready. She doesn't even ask for a snack on the day she goes to the hospital." These days, Emily's life looks very much like that of a typical teenager.

Dee: Walking for Fun and Fitness

Dee is an active, energetic woman who lives in a two-person residence run by a community agency. At times, her staff describe her as having "behavior problems": she can be stubborn if she does not want to do something. She is a woman in her thirties who has spent the majority of her life living in an institution for people with mental retardation. She has a very limited vocabulary and uses a few signs to communicate.

Until the fall of 1988, Dee's activities were limited to what was happening in her program. She had few outside relationships or activities. Through the efforts of a "community guide," Karlene Shea, Dee was assisted to join a walking club that meets once a week.

Photographs of the Holyoke Evening Walking Club show a determined group of women striding purposefully along a path by a lake. The women appear to range in age from 20 years to 60 years. There is nothing about Dee that makes her stand out in the group of eight women; her pace is perfectly matched to the other walkers.

Despite Dee's limited communication abilities and sometimes stubborn personality, her presence is fully accepted by the other members of the club. She is a strong walker, which is the most important requirement for membership in this group.

It was almost an accident that Karlene helped Dee to join the walking group. She spent several weeks trying to identify possible interests of Dee's to find a group for her to join. Karlene had taken Dee to the high school to see if she might be interested in learning how to play volleyball. That was immediately eliminated as an option because before they even got into the gym to watch the players, Dee sat down on the floor and refused to budge. Karlene then took Dee to a festival to see if there might be something promising there, but nothing revealed itself.

Between these trips, Dee and Karlene would walk from Dee's house to get ice cream. These outings started because Dee refused to get out of Karlene's car on several occasions after returning from their trips. Instead, she would bang on the windshield and window until her staff convinced her to get out of the car and go into the house. Karlene was afraid Dee might hurt herself with her banging, so she proposed the walking trips. After several trips to the ice cream store, Karlene noted that Dee seemed to enjoy walking as much as she enjoyed ice cream. She had no trouble keeping pace with Karlene, no matter how fast or far they walked. Thus, the idea for the walking club.

Because Karlene is an occasional member of the club, she had no difficulty arranging for Dee to join them. What took time, however, was helping the other members feel comfortable enough with Dee's presence so that Karlene did not need to attend. Now, after several years, other members sometimes pick Dee up and drive her to their meeting spot. She also attends parties at the homes of members. In addition, the women are trying to teach her new words as they walk.

Dee's staff report that she has lost weight and is having fewer difficulties with her behavior. In fact, Dee is gaining the same benefits that anyone might gain from an exercise program: fun, fitness, and a chance to make new friends.

FORTUNATE ACCIDENT OR CAREFULLY CRAFTED OPPORTUNITY?

Years of exclusion cannot be reversed overnight. How, then, have George, Emily, Dee, and others with disabilities become active and contributing members of community organizations? Across the country, a growing number of people and groups are beginning to explore innovative ways to assist people with disabilities to become integrated within their communities by involving ordinary citizens in their lives. Sometimes called bridge-building, circles of friends, or associational integration, these activities emphasize the ways individuals, rather than programs, can facilitate the integration. McKnight (1989) describes common features of people who fill these roles, whom he terms "community guides":

They focus on the gifts and capacities of excluded people.
They are well connected in associational life.
The paths they walk into community life are based on relationships of trust rather than the authority of systems.
They believe strongly that the community is filled with hospitality for strangers.
They learn to leave the person they guide so that the community can surround them and become responsible for their lives.

These efforts have emphasized integration into recreational and leisure activities, religious congregations, and the development of personal relationships between persons with and without disabilities. People with disabilities have become members of community organizations and religious congregations (Osburn, 1988; Reidy, 1989; Shea, 1987–1990); they have developed and been assisted to develop circles of support (Forest & Snow, 1987; Mount, Beeman, & Ducharme, 1988; O'Connell, 1988; Perske, 1988); and they have become regular visitors at libraries, bakeries, coffee shops, and other public places (O'Connell, 1988).

Such approaches represent various possibilities for assisting people with disabilities to become more connected within their communities. Although they do not offer rigid blueprints for action, they are intentional, rather than accidental efforts. As such, they suggest principles, guidelines, and strategies that can be used to develop similar approaches.

In the next section, approaches that have been successful in assisting George, Emily, Dee, and others to become members of their respective organizations are described. It does not matter if it is a person's job to be a community guide or if a friend, family member, or agency staff person is simply interested in the idea. These approaches can work if the person is committed to assisting an individual with a disability join a group.

APPROACHES THAT WORK

There is a great deal that can be said about designing successful programs with the explicit purpose of facilitating community integration. That is not the purpose of this chapter. Most people do not have the luxury to work in an environment that is especially set up to assist in the process of integration. Instead, most people are residential staff, parents, or people with a personal interest in the well-being of an individual with a disability. They are often concerned with day-to-day living (e.g., a place to live, adequate money, health and safety), as well as assisting in the integration process. To be truly successful in helping a person to join a group, the focus must be on the essential ingredients: What will make this effort work?

Four guidelines appear to be vital to the success of any effort to help someone join a community organization.

1. Know the Person

Knowing the person seems self-evident until it is considered how superficially most individuals know people with disabilities. Too often, contacts are influenced by the person's status as a client, service recipient, or person with disabilities. Professionals are trained to see people through the dual lenses of neediness and impairment, making it difficult to clearly view a person's gifts and talents, interests, and motivations.

This difficulty is compounded by the fact that a large majority of people with disabilities lack opportunities to develop their interests and talents. Although Dee was in her thirties, it took Karlene weeks of spending time with her to discover her enjoyment of walking. Up to that point, Dee's potential interests had not been considered important factors affecting how she spent her time.

It may take some time and experimentation to really know a person, even if that person has been an acquaintance for years. With some people, it may mean trying a range of activities to see what the person seems to enjoy. With others, asking them, "What would you like to do?" can assist in determining their interests.

It is not unusual for young people to try out a number of activities before settling on something that suits them. Emily was assisted to join a gymnastics class before she became a Girl Scout. She had expressed an interest in gymnastics for some time before joining and was initially very enthusiastic. After a couple of weeks, her interest waned. At the end of a month, she stopped going to class. Emily's mother and Susan Sawyer, the person assisting Emily, were discouraged until they realized that it is natural for young people to try many different activities. This may also be true with adults whose interests have not been developed.

2. Know and Respect the Group

People who work in human services are often disconnected from their local communities. It is rare that a human services worker is a member of various groups or even knows what groups exist in a community.

Family members may not have the time to become familiar with the possibilities of community participation because of their time-consuming roles of caregivers and advocates for their son or daughter. Whatever the reason for not being familiar with a community's associational life, it is important to thoroughly explore what is available when assisting someone to join a group. If the person already has a clearly defined interest, such as gardening, the task is much simpler. Then the task is only to research gardening groups. This includes: When and how often does the group meet? Who are the members? (Perhaps the staff person knows someone?) Are there dues? Are there membership requirements? What are the members like? Do certain types of people join? Why do most people join? What kinds of skills do members need to possess?

The more that is known about a prospective group, the better the chances of a good match between the person being introduced and the activities and culture of the group. This match is crucial: experience has shown that a good match between the person and the group is the most important factor in determining the success of a person's experience. In fact, the type and degree of a person's disability is not nearly as important.

For example, someone who wants to join the Junior League, a prestigious women's organization that teaches and involves women in volunteer activities in the local community, would have to meet certain requirements. She would need to be capable of and interested in attending lengthy and sometimes abstract meetings, carrying out community service, and otherwise filling the qualifications for membership and participation.

Ruth Sienkiewicz-Mercer is a woman who fits that description. She is a dynamic and charming woman who has written a book about her life, published by a major publishing company. In addition, she and her husband regularly deliver presentations about the situation of people with disabilities and serve as advisors and advocates to disability groups and others interested in integration.

Ruth has severe cerebral palsy, limiting any movements to her head and, to some extent, her arms. She usually communicates with the help of a communication board, a series of eye movements, and another person who points to words. This process is slow and arduous, but it enables her to communicate clearly. Ruth recently began using a new computerized device. She relies totally on others for all of her physical care. Prior to moving into an apartment with her husband, she spent a number of years living in an institution for people with mental retardation.

Although Ruth's identity and personality fit well with the Junior League in many respects, her membership has not lacked controversy. Some members were unprepared for the severity of Ruth's disability and found her method of communication difficult to accommodate. Other members questioned Ruth's contribution to the League and to the local community. They felt that the charter of the Junior League is to train young women to become community leaders, volunteers, board members, and public speakers and were not sure how Ruth's involvement fit that mandate.

Ruth herself has been frustrated by the limited role she is allowed to play within the organization. She, too, finds it hard to communicate with other members because they have not learned to use her system. At the same time, she is proud that her membership can serve as a model for other people with disabilities and as a way of educating League members about the contributions that can be made by people with disabilities.

In spite of the controversy, Ruth's membership in the Junior League has continued for years. Accommodations have been made to enable Ruth to attend meetings; most meetings were held in members' homes that were not wheelchair accessible. One member tried to initiate a learning program on how to use Ruth's communication boards so the women could communicate with her directly rather than through a personal care attendant. The group's president, after describing several of the challenges associated with Ruth's membership, went on to say, "I found Ruth's presence to be very motivational and educational."

If there had not been a good match between Ruth and the Junior League, it is almost certain that her membership could not have withstood these challenges. Most groups, and the Junior League is no exception, are understandably committed to maintaining their basic membership requirements and carrying on with their regular activities. Once these conditions are met, however, members can be quite flexible about accommodating other differences.

Many groups have aspects that are not to the liking of some people—they may be too liberal or too conservative, others may have restrictive membership requirements, still others may have paternalistic qualities. However, the primary goal is membership for people with disabilities, *not* changing the group. Some aspects, especially those related to inclusion of people with disabilities, may change given sufficient time. Other group traditions were established long before our interest in introducing people with disabilities into groups and deserve to be respected.

An assistant to a person with a disability may have his or her tolerance for difference challenged. If, for example, the person being assisted is eager to join a rod and gun club and the assistant is an animal rights activist, the assistant needs to be aware of his or her biases and be prepared to deal with them.

3. Know Yourself

An assistant needs to know his or her own gifts and talents and be able to enlist the help of others to compensate for any limitations.

Many limitations can be compensated for. If the assistant is new to a community, he or she can get help from others to find out what groups exist and who's who in town. If the assistant does not own a car, he or she can enlist the help of a group member to drive the person to and from meetings. In fact, sometimes it is better to have a substantial array of limitations because, that way, there is more for other people to do. One of the main points of this endeavor is to bring a person with a disability into contact with people who might become friends and associates.

There is one quality, however, that is absolutely essential: an assistant needs to be a "people person." He or she needs to have an enduring confidence in the capacity of people to do what is right, knowing they will not always live up to his or her ideals. He or she needs to have a continually replenished capacity to forgive others (including him- or herself) for mistakes, at the same time remembering that people with disabilities cannot afford to have more mistakes made in their lives. Flexibility, maturity, and a willingness to laugh when things go wrong are also necessary. The most exciting and infuriating aspect of this work is that it is about people and their interactions.

4. Remember What Is at Stake

Earlier in this chapter there was reference to the exclusion of people with disabilities from the "power and protection of community life." This exclusion has a long history and many consequences. One consequence, of course, is that most people with disabilities lack friends and other social relationships.

For instance, a study of the "social supports" of 11 people with mental retardation served by community programs in Western Massachusetts found that none of the clients had a "best friend" and that people had few or no close friends and few enduring relationships. Instead, relationships were almost exclusively with staff and care providers (Specht & Nagy, 1986).

McKnight (1989) described his meeting with five men with developmental disabilities living in their own New England homes:

> When the opportunity came to talk to each of the men, I inquired as to their lives, experiences and relationships in the town. To my surprise, the response of each man made clear that they had almost no social relationships with their neighbors or the other citizens of the town. . . . and none were involved in any kind of organization, association or club. (p. 1)

In addition to the long history of exclusion and isolation, people with disabilities are commonly stereotyped in negative ways. Such stereotypes include "child," "nonhuman," "needing to belong with their own kind," "menace," "incompetent," and so forth. These negative stereotypes commonly lead people to expect individuals with disabilities to act in certain ways. Because people tend to live up to (or down to) the expectations held about them, a "self-fulfilling prophecy" may be created. People interested in breaking the cycle of negative stereotypes and expectations must be particularly sensitive to helping people with disabilities be seen in the best possible light.

Remembering what is at stake means taking seriously this history of exclusion, negative stereotypes, and low expectations. Some potential implications follow.

Recognize that People with Disabilities Lack Experience Participating in Community Life   It must be understood that introducing a person with a disability into a community organization needs to be done carefully and thoughtfully, with the full realization that the "little things" make a difference. It is important to ensure that a person's dues are paid, that a ride to and from the group meeting has been arranged, that they are dressed appropriately for the group's activities, and that they are able to carry out membership responsibilities (even if it means having someone else assist them). An assistant may need to stay involved with the group for a while. It may be a long time before a person's membership fully "takes hold."

Pay Special Attention to the Process of Introducing a Person with a Disability   Because of the history of exclusion, some diplomacy may be required when introducing people with disabilities to group members. Someone may need to smooth the way, dispel misunderstandings, and serve as an ambassador in uniting people from essentially different cultures.

Brief the Person with a Disability on the Special Rituals and Routines of a Group   Because people with disabilities often lack experiences of the typical world, such as going to a fancy restaurant, taking a taxi, or hosting a party, some extra coaching may be required. Take care to explain in advance what is expected, and, if appropriate, model the behavior.

One woman who had just begun to attend an Episcopal church did not realize that Communion is not the time to strike up a conversation with the priest. After an explanation by her sponsor, she chose another time to chat.

Introduce Only One Person with a Disability to an Organization   Because one of the common negative stereotypes plaguing people with any kind of disability is that they "belong with their own kind" or "are happier with their own kind," special attention must be paid to introducing only one person with a disability to a given organization. People need the chance to be known as their own person, not as "one of the disabled members."

It can be tempting to overlook this consideration, especially if a group is very welcoming of people with disabilities or if there are several people who could benefit from group membership. In addition, sometimes an individual with a disability enjoys his or her membership so much that he or she wants to invite a friend to join. Although it would be inappropriate to make a hard and fast rule that there can *never* be more than one member with a disability, a useful point to remember is that there are often chapters of a certain group in other towns or neighborhoods. For example, the Knights of Columbus in Chicopee was especially welcoming to George. Rather than introduce other men with disabilities into that chapter, the Knights of Columbus in Holyoke, an adjacent city, was identified as a different prospect for membership of another individual. Even within the same organization, there are sometimes subgroups and varied activities that can be tapped for different individuals. For instance, a church may have numerous Bible study groups, committees, and so forth.

Help the Person with a Disability Become a Valuable, Contributing Member Not only should a person with a disability be able to join a group, but he or she should also be valued as a member. This is much more difficult to accomplish than simply helping a person gain membership, but it will pay off in the long run. People who are seen as valued, important group members will find it much easier to make friends and will have their membership more secure over time.

In addition, the satisfaction of knowing that one is not a token or a mascot is a boost to the person's self esteem. George likes being a member of the Knights because he likes to have a chance to help. Ruth's major criticism of her role in the Junior League is that she is not allowed to use her full potential in the organization.

Not all groups have a range of ways in which a person can be seen as a valued member. The walking club in which Dee is a member has basically one role: walker. Yet, even within that type of group it is possible to "carve out" a special and important role. For instance, one of the members is a new grandmother who sometimes brings her baby granddaughter on walks. Dee greatly enjoys pushing the stroller and other members noticed a positive difference in her once the baby started coming on the outings: Dee began to talk more. Her assistance also gives the grandmother a break from pushing the baby.

HOW TO START?

There is no recipe for assisting someone with a disability to join a group. There are, however, certain steps that will greatly add to the chances for a successful experience. These steps flow in a logical sequence, the same sequence that anyone who seeks to join a group might follow.

Before the Introduction

1. Get To Know the Person It is important to find out a person's needs and expectations, as well as what kind of group the person is looking for. Does he or she want a small and close-knit group, a large and dynamic group, or a physically active group? Is the person looking for a hobby, a chance to practice a skill, or is he or she primarily interested in forming relationships? Although it is sometimes difficult to identify a person's interests, everybody has special qualities that can be enhanced.

The person's gender needs to be considered also. Some groups are male only or female only. In other groups, it is traditional to find mostly one gender and members may not welcome people of the opposite sex.

Age is also a factor. Certain groups, either intentionally or accidentally, attract certain age groups. A person who falls outside the expectable range might not fit in as a member.

2. Find Out About Local Groups   In some communities, the chamber of commerce keeps a listing of groups and organizations. This list is usually not exhaustive, however. There is also the *Encyclopedia of Associations*, Volume 1 (Burek, 1992), which lists 23,000 national and international nonprofit membership associations. There is also a five-volume companion to the encyclopedia that lists 53,000 regional, state, and local organizations. The *Encyclopedia* can be found in most public libraries. Most newspapers also list special events and meetings of local groups. However, the most effective way to find out about what groups exist in a community is to talk to people. Once an interest area has been identified, people in the community may know of groups with that focus. Retail stores that are frequented by persons with a particular interest or hobby (e.g., a camera shop, fabric store) are a good source of information.

Once one or more possible groups are identified, information about each group can be researched. What are a group's expectations of its members? Do they earn badges, participate in fund-raisers, carry out work projects, door-to-door solicitations, or public speaking activities? Is there a very formal organizational structure with long meetings? The activities of some organizations are actually quite dull, but people participate to advance their business or civic interests. Such groups may not appeal to someone who is looking for fun or friendship.

Certain questions about the membership should also be answered. What is the age range, gender, and typical socioeconomic or ethnic background? These factors can influence a person's enjoyment. For example, a young woman who wanted to join a prayer group attended several meetings of a group that met near her home. Although the group met at a convenient time and location and was very welcoming of her, she decided not to continue her involvement. She said, "The other women in the group are much older than me. They have different interests like their children and getting along with their husbands. I'm not even married."

The location of group meetings is an important consideration. How easily can the person with a disability get to and from the meeting? Initially, transportation might be the responsibility of staff or family, rather than other group members. In time, it is possible for other members to assist with rides, but people will usually not go very far out of their way to give someone else a ride. Transportation is a big consideration in a person's long-term participation; therefore, it is important to make travel as convenient as possible.

Another possibility is to look for a group that accommodates transportation. For example, some groups of older persons assume that a fairly large percentage of their membership does not drive; therefore, carpooling is a common occurrence. Other groups are neighborhood-based, which makes it possible to walk to and from group activities.

3. Contact Current Members of the Group   It helps to know someone in the group as plans are being made. He or she can provide information about people in the group and what *really* goes on. They can also introduce the assistant and the person with disabilities to other members, including people in leadership roles. Once the person with disabilities becomes a member, the contact person can be the "eyes and ears" in the group to ensure that everything is going smoothly.

A little investigation will result in meeting someone who knows a group member. Introducing the person who has a disability to a current member can make that person's initial contact with the group a more enjoyable and successful experience. Some organizations, such as the Knights of Columbus and the Junior League, have official sponsors and advisors for new members. In other groups, inviting a current member to serve in an informal capacity can be very beneficial. While this groundwork takes time, it can play a crucial role in the long-term success of a person's involvement in a group.

4. Put the Best Foot Forward   People who assist individuals with disabilities to join groups are often confronted with a delicate situation: what to tell group members about the person. The nature or extent of a person's disability should not be minimized, yet, the person should be presented as positively as possible. There is no magic rule for this dilemma. One guideline is to describe the person in very human terms, such as, "Joan has some difficulties communicating with words, but she is very capable of making herself understood," as opposed to human services jargon, such as "Joan has mild M.R., is nonverbal, and uses total communication to get her needs across."

Another guideline is to emphasize the person's capabilities and potential rather than his or her limitations and deficiencies. After all, a person joining a group is not likely to say, "Well, I'm divorced, a very messy housekeeper, I'm always late for appointments, and I commonly break my promises!"

Another guideline, a very important one, is to ask the person how he or she wants to be described before talking to group members about particulars. Confidentiality, as well as basic etiquette, is a consideration here. This is the time to obtain the person's permission (or a guardian's) to provide a description to group members. At the same time, the assistant and the person with disabilities (or guardian) can discuss how to describe the person.

At the Time of the Introduction

Several steps should be followed at the time of introduction:

1. The prospective member should formally meet group leaders and possibly some other members. It is best to have a sponsor arrange the introduction.
2. If a sponsor has not been identified in advance of the person's initial contact with the group, one or more willing group members should be paired with the person to ensure full inclusion in group affairs. This aspect is crucial. Once a person with a disability has joined a group, it is easy for him or her to be overlooked as the group continues with their regular activities. It can take a special effort of hospitality for someone to be fully included.
3. Group leaders should be asked to discreetly inform other members that the new member might need more time to become acclimated to group activities. Coach group leaders on respectful ways to interact with a member who has a disability, such as speaking directly to the person rather than talking to an aide who might be present. It is important not to feel awkward about being this direct. People who have little contact with individuals with disabilities welcome information about how to interact with the person. In Emily's Girl Scout troop, the other members were relieved to learn some facts about Emily's disability because it helped to explain why she acted in certain ways. The information freed them to fully welcome her as a peer.
4. Group leaders should be assured that an assistant will attend a few meetings with the person, if necessary. The assistant's behavior can serve as the example for other group members to follow regarding their interactions with the person who has a disability.
5. Group leaders should explain the group's expectations and history to the new member.
6. If there is an initiation ceremony, the new member should be encouraged to participate. These rituals can mean a great deal to the person. The day after George was formally initiated as a member of the Knights of Columbus, he called a friend and proclaimed, "I'm a card-carrying Knight!"

After the Introduction

Several steps should be followed after the introduction:

1. Assistants should stay informed about the person's participation in the group. Sometimes that means attending the meeting; other times a sponsor, group leader, or the person with a disability can update the assistant. Particular attention should be paid to whether the person is being included in group activities and interactions, whether other group members feel comfortable, and so forth.
2. If it seems appropriate, a follow-up meeting can be scheduled between the assistant and other group members. This can be an informal, brief discussion about how things are going. It can also be helpful to talk to nongroup members who are aware of the group's activities to learn of any "scuttlebutt" associated with the person's membership. Sometimes group members are reluctant to talk about problems and concerns.
3. Problems should be anticipated and viewed as a natural part of the process, not a sign of failure. They should be heard receptively and nondefensively. The goal is to ensure the success of a person's participation if possible. Sometimes that requires hearing and responding to criticisms that may seem unfair. These criticisms may come from anyone, including the person, their family, other group members, or service providers. It is important to listen, consider, and address the obstacles to that person's full participation.
4. Assistants should continue to seek ways for the person's talents to grow and be recognized. As mentioned earlier, finding positive roles for the person to play within the group has many benefits, but it does not always happen spontaneously. Sometimes, a nudge in the right direction is necessary. For example, "Wouldn't Myra really enjoy hosting a meeting at her house next month?" might be planted as a suggestion.
5. The extent of the assistant's ongoing involvement should be carefully considered. This is another delicate balancing act. On the one hand, a desirable goal is to ensure that the person is well accepted within the group and outside assistance is not required. On the other hand, there may be reason to stay involved in supporting the person on an ongoing basis—helping the person remember to pay dues, for example, or assisting them to carry out some other membership requirement. If such involvement is

ongoing, it is helpful to strive for a behind-the-scenes role, unless one becomes so interested in the group that one joins it, too!

FROM MEMBERSHIPS TO FRIENDSHIPS

Helping a person to become a *member* of a group is a relatively straightforward process. Although there can be obstacles and pitfalls, most can be overcome with persistence. Translating a membership into friendships is much more elusive. Friendship is the undefinable spark between two people that cannot be fabricated with any amount of effort.

However, it is possible to create the *conditions* that encourage a friendship to flourish. Group membership can provide several important elements for these conditions to occur.

First, people need to be together. In the past, friendships between people with and without disabilities were unusual because there were not many opportunities for contact. Membership in a group can provide the context for people to come together.

Second, people need to be peers. Even though there is greater contact today between persons with and without disabilities, there is still a great deal of inequality in the roles they play. Quite often, individuals with disabilities are perceived as dependent or needy persons, without the recognition that they also have something to contribute to a relationship. This inequality of status makes it difficult to form peer relationships. Group membership emphasizing the contributions made by the person with a disability is an excellent way to enhance status, and thereby shift the relationship to more equal footing.

Third, having shared interests and experiences helps to encourage friendship. Most friendships are formed through common experiences or common interests. These shared experiences offer the basis for a relationship in which the presence or absence of a disability is irrelevant. Group membership certainly provides shared experiences and a chance to pursue shared interests.

A final element is reciprocity. Reciprocity is the bridge between group membership and friendship. It is not an automatic result of group membership; it takes extra effort. Reciprocity means giving as well as receiving, contributing as well as being contributed to. It can mean taking the initiative to invite someone to dinner; having them over to one's home after enjoying dinner at theirs, sending a thank you note if someone has done a favor, or offering to carpool instead of depending on someone else to provide a regular ride. Reciprocity implies equality—a peer relationship. Instead of continuing to function in the role of recipient, reciprocal relationships challenge people with disabilities to "pull their own weight." Only when this shift is accomplished can people with disabilities participate in true friendships with other people.

People with disabilities must often rely on staff or family members to help them learn and carry out gestures of reciprocity. They may not have experience with such relationships and with the "giving" end of friendship. In addition, they may not have the means to follow through on the action. While the effort required to help a person act reciprocally may entail inconvenience, it is such attention to the little details that can make the difference between merely being a member and having friends. One couple who has a son with disabilities makes a point to invite the neighborhood children over after school for snacks and play. They know their initiative is one important way to ensure that their son will be invited over to neighbors' houses. Extra effort is needed, but the payoff is knowing that their son has friends in his neighborhood.

Helping to foster reciprocal relationships also means paying attention to the unique qualities brought by each individual to a relationship. A person who is "nonverbal" may be a wonderful friend to someone who needs to share her secrets. A man who relies on a fellow church member to provide a ride each week may offer his driver companionship and someone to sit next to during the service. If the analogy of a symphony orchestra is used, it is possible to appreciate the uniqueness of each person's contribution to a relationship. All the instruments in an orchestra have their own sound, their own part to play. No one would claim that the trumpets make a greater contribution than the flutes or the drums. Each instrument plays an essential and singular part in producing a symphony. So it is in relationships, whether one person has a disability or not. Sometimes people need to remind one another of this truth, especially when a person's contribution does not appear comparable to that of another.

If assistants become discouraged by the time and effort needed to assist individuals with disabilities to develop friendships, they should keep in mind the comments made by Karlene Shea, who has reflected upon her experiences as a "community guide":

> We have learned much in these past three years, not the least of which is why having friends in the community is especially important for people with disabilities. What better safeguard could be built into their lives? Friends look out for each other, friends help each other and friends don't let you get put away in an institution no matter how pretty a picture is painted by someone who says it's for your own good. Friends know better. Friends can speak up for

you if you are too shy or nervous to do it, and friends can give you the confidence you need to do it yourself.

They say that it's good to have friends in high places; we say it's good to have friends, period. (1987–1990, p. 2)

CONCLUSION

Developing friendships and promoting membership in associations can be satisfying work. It offers chances to make contributions that are real and meaningful, as well as the potential to learn more about oneself and one's community. Susan Sawyer, who assisted Emily and other young people to become involved in integrated activities, describes the benefits to herself: "On a personal level, it helps me to better understand my own kids, the changes they go through in what they like and don't like . . . how to take it in stride. Also, talking to a parent who has had real success with their child, watching them blossom and grow, you feel like you're doing something worthwhile."

No matter what a person is paid to do, he or she can sponsor a person with a disability and help that person gain access to all the benefits of community membership. The principles and strategies suggested in this chapter are just a beginning—many more are waiting to be discovered.

REFERENCES

Berger, P., & Neuhaus, R. (1977). *To empower people: The role of mediating structures in public policy.* Washington, DC: American Enterprise Institute for Public Policy Research.

Burek, D.M. (Ed.). (1992). *1993 Encyclopedia of associations* (2nd ed.) (vol. 1). Detroit: Gale Research, Inc.

Forest, M., & Snow, J. (1987). *The Joshua Committee: An advocacy model.* In D.B. Schwartz, J. McKnight, & M. Kendrick (Eds.), *A story I heard: A compendium of stories, essays and poetry about people with disabilities and American life* (pp. 48–54). Harrisburg, Pennsylvania: Developmental Disabilities Planning Council.

McKnight, J. (1989). *Beyond community services.* Center for Urban Affairs Paper. Evanston, IL: Northwestern University.

Milofsky, C. (1988). Scarcity and community: A resource allocation theory of community and mass society organizations. In C. Milofsky (Ed.), *Community organizations: Studies in resource mobilization and exchange* (pp. 16–41). New York: Oxford University Press.

Mount, G., Beeman, P., & Ducharme, G. (1988). *What are we learning about circles of support? A collection of tools, ideas, and reflections on building and facilitating circles of support.* Manchester, CT: Communitas, Inc.

O'Connell, M. (1988). *The gift of hospitality: Opening the doors of community life to people with disabilities.* Evanston, IL: Center for Urban Affairs and Policy Research, Northwestern University & Department of Rehabilitation Services.

Osburn, J. (1988). *Welcome to the club: Report of an external evaluation of the Association Integration Project conducted for Education for Community Initiatives*. Unpublished manuscript.

Perske, R. (1988). *Circles of friends*. Nashville: Abingdon Press.

Reidy, D. (1989). *Integrating people with disabilities into voluntary associations: The possibilities and limitations*. Unpublished manuscript, Education for Community Initiatives, Holyoke, MA.

Shea, K. (1987–1990). *"Dear friend" letters: Quarterly reports of the progress of the Association Integration Project*. (Unpublished letters of limited circulation between 1987 and 1990 available from Education for Community Initiatives, 187 High Street, Suite 302, Holyoke, MA 01040.)

Specht, D.I., & Nagy, M. (1986). *Social supports research project: Report of findings*. Holyoke: Western Massachusetts Training Consortium.

de Tocqueville, A. (1966). *Democracy in America*. In J.P. Mayer & M. Lerner (Eds.). (G. Lawrence, Trans.). New York: Harper & Row (Original work published 1835).

20

Afterword

Angela Novak Amado

Currently, society is crying out for more caring, friendship, and community for all people. At the same time, the human services field is in a process, a transition, and a gradual unfolding of better understanding of the lives of individuals with disabilities and of what is possible in real community. There have been some useful and successful ways discovered to support friendship and community. And of course, some of the progress that looks wonderful now will later be understood as damaging mistakes. As people learn from these mistakes, yet more effective approaches will be discovered.

Also unfolding in this process is different understanding of the roles of professional services and of community members. On one hand are those who say human services staff can never do real community-building, that it can only happen when the community is empowered to take it on themselves. On the other hand are those who are committed to the quest for human services that are more responsive and effective at understanding people and supporting them in really being part of their communities. They are working to make the services that they do provide more sensitive to the needs of individuals with disabilities so that these individuals might have a life as free from services and as "real" as possible.

Supporting friendships can be fragile, delicate, magical, and sensitive work. It is not work that easily fits into formalized systems and agency patterns. Often, a tremendous amount of failure must be tolerated before any success is experienced. As more human services agencies and staff see the importance of supporting community friendships and struggle to be more effective in that work, a dilemma often arises. Whereas formal program plans, regulated priorities, and agency accountabilities push one way, the informalities and heart and soul of supporting relationships pushes the other way. Some agencies initially try to support community-building by keeping it fun, special, and informal. However, as more individuals are supported by such efforts and as more staff take on the responsibility, it often seems necessary to make community-connecting more formalized. With the demands of service plans, licensing rules, and reporting requirements, to carve out any time at all for supporting friendships seems to necessitate setting aside the time in formal programs. Sometimes it seems that the only way to ensure that time is spent on connecting is to ensure that it is written into formal goals and objectives, staff schedules, and program plans. Given that intentional efforts are needed for supporting community connections, it seems that intentional structures must be in place.

Although guaranteeing time and structures for community connecting may be necessary, other dangers then loom as a result. Human services often formalize and systematize to the point of making everything just another "service" used to strengthen formal bureaucracies and to separate and diminish people's lives. Given the sensitive nature of supporting friendships, connecting isolated individuals to community members is not as easy or straightforward as writing a program with specific measurable performance objectives. Friendship cannot be "programmed." This dilemma in human services' support for community building reflects the current era of questioning and confronting the balancing act required when systematized structures are applied to real people and when formal ways seem to make no sense for real lives.

The current era can be seen as one phase in the long-term movement of building more accepting and diverse communities for all people. Working on friendship for persons with disabilities can translate into a greater understanding of building community throughout society. As part of the current evolution, people working for more accepting communities may need to become more aware of their own attitudes and habits that divide rather than bring together. True architects for inclusion promote all people belonging. An all-inclusive community makes no divisions between "persons served" and "community members," between "professionals" and "community citizens," or between "members" and "nonmembers." In true community, there are no "good guys" (those believing in and working for community) and "bad guys" (administrators opposed to full inclusion or state licensers imposing rules that result in segregation). Any such divisions of any people are, after all, just another form of exclusion. Today's path must include the capacity to recognize any expression of "us" and "them," even in ourselves, and then bringing the spirit of belonging everywhere.

All human services staff are also community members—they belong to softball teams, service clubs, and churches. Some staff are also family members of individuals with disabilities. Some staff include the people they serve in their own family and community life. Many community members are also family members of individuals who receive services and many have disabilities themselves. Perhaps the divisive lines need to become even more blurred.

It is possible that this era is only serving to strengthen agencies and professional services by allowing them to "take over" the additional territory of community building. Yet, perhaps communities are being strengthened by developing stronger partnerships and relationships with both individuals with disabilities and those who provide services to them; perhaps all parties are coming closer together.

This era will only be understood, if at all, in retrospect. In the meantime, the isolation and loneliness of many individuals who receive services must be faced. Action and efforts need to start immediately. For many individuals with disabilities, their current service providers are the only source for these efforts; for thousands of individuals, if agencies do not provide support for friendships, such relationships simply will not happen at all. Through these efforts, the best and most immediate ways that people can be supported to have friends can continue to be explored and developed.

Right now, there is also cause for celebration for the people who have been and continue to be brought together—the greater number of individuals who for now have even one more friend or one more community place in which they are included, and the increased number of community members who come to appreciate and see even one individual not as a "retarded person" or "one of them," but as Joe or Mary or Linda. One by one, relationship by relationship, the people who are brought together will affect others.

In a real sense all life is inter-related. All men are caught in an inescapable network of mutuality, tied in a single garment of destiny. Whatever affects one directly affects all indirectly . . . I can never be what I ought to be until you are what you ought to be, and you can never be what you ought to be until I am what I ought to be. This is the inter-related structure of reality.

Martin Luther King, Jr.

Index

Page numbers followed by "f" indicate figures;
those followed by "t" indicate tables.